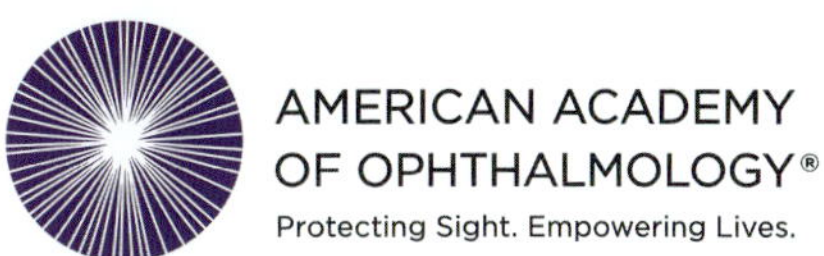

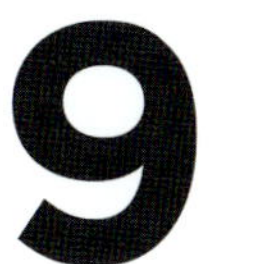

Uveitis and Ocular Inflammation

Major Revision Edition

2023–2024

BCSC

Basic and Clinical Science Course™

Published after collaborative review with the European Board of Ophthalmology subcommittee

The American Academy of Ophthalmology is accredited by the Accreditation Council for Continuing Medical Education (ACCME) to provide continuing medical education for physicians.

The American Academy of Ophthalmology designates this enduring material for a maximum of 10 *AMA PRA Category 1 Credits*™. Physicians should claim only the credit commensurate with the extent of their participation in the activity.

CME expiration date: June 1, 2026. *AMA PRA Category 1 Credits*™ may be claimed only once between June 1, 2023, and the expiration date.

BCSC® volumes are designed to increase the physician's ophthalmic knowledge through study and review. Users of this activity are encouraged to read the text and then answer the study questions provided at the back of the book.

To claim *AMA PRA Category 1 Credits*™ upon completion of this activity, learners must demonstrate appropriate knowledge and participation in the activity by taking the posttest for Section 9 and achieving a score of 80% or higher. For further details, please see the instructions for requesting CME credit at the back of the book.

Cover image: Figure 10-2B in BCSC Section 9, *Uveitis and Ocular Inflammation*. Image courtesy of Sam S. Dahr, MD, MS.

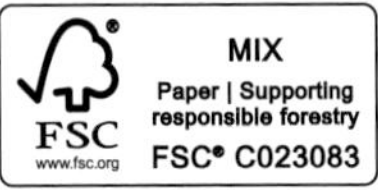

Printed in South Korea.

Basic and Clinical Science Course

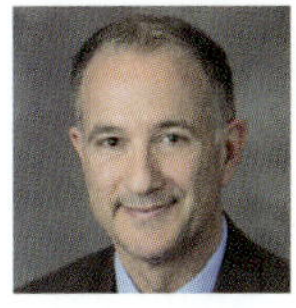

Christopher J. Rapuano, MD, Philadelphia, Pennsylvania
Senior Secretary for Clinical Education

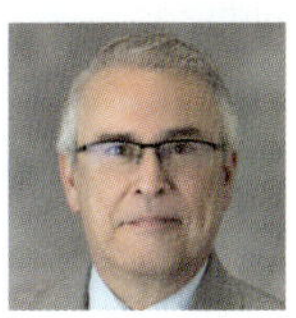

J. Timothy Stout, MD, PhD, MBA, Houston, Texas
Secretary for Lifelong Learning and Assessment

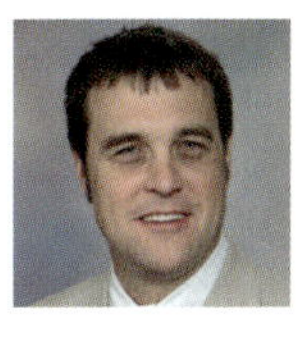

Colin A. McCannel, MD, Los Angeles, California
BCSC Course Chair

Section 9

Faculty for the Major Revision

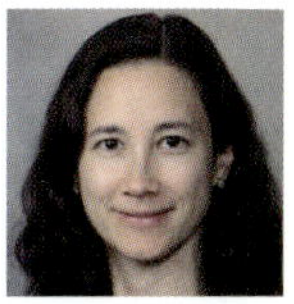

Wendy M. Smith, MD
Chair
Rochester, Minnesota

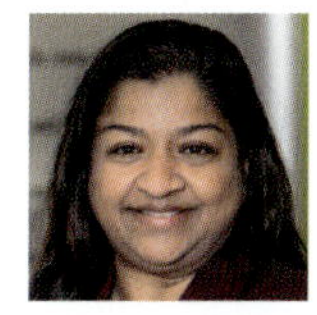

Sapna Gangaputra, MD, MPH
Nashville, Tennessee

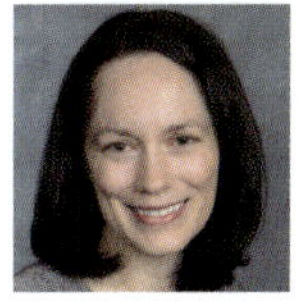

Karen R. Armbrust, MD, PhD
Minneapolis, Minnesota

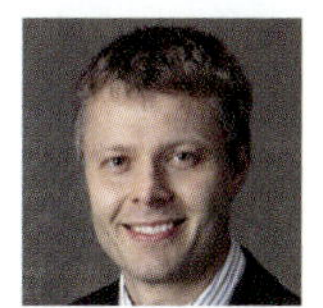

Jared E. Knickelbein, MD, PhD
Pittsburgh, Pennsylvania

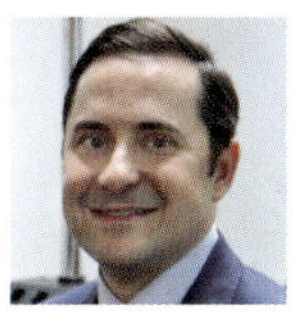

Sam S. Dahr, MD, MS
Houston, Texas

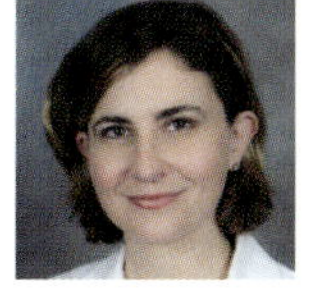

Thellea K. Leveque, MD, MPH
Seattle, Washington

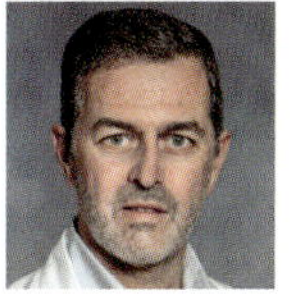

Emilio M. Dodds, MD
Buenos Aires, Argentina

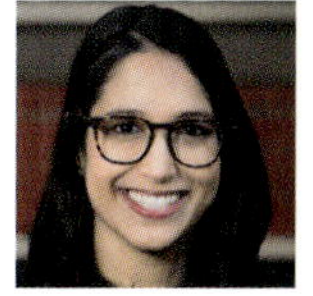

Jessica G. Shantha, MD, MSc
San Francisco, California

The Academy acknowledges the following committees for review of this edition:

Committee on Aging: Rosa Kim, MD, Houston, Texas

Vision Rehabilitation Committee: Marie A. Di Nome, MD, Scottsdale, Arizona

BCSC Resident/Fellow Reviewers: Sharon L. Jick, MD, *Chair,* St Louis, Missouri; Maria Paula Fernandez, MD; Hong-Uyen Hua, MD; Danny Mammo, MD; Margaret McDougal Runner, MD

Practicing Ophthalmologists Advisory Committee for Education: Gaurav K. Shah, MD, *Primary Reviewer,* San Francisco, California; Bradley D. Fouraker, MD, *Chair,* Tampa, Florida; George S. Ellis Jr, MD, New Orleans, Louisiana; Kevin E. Lai, MD, Carmel, Indiana; Philip R. Rizzuto, MD, Providence, Rhode Island; J. James Rowsey, MD, Largo, Florida; Scott X. Stevens, MD, Bend, Oregon; Troy M. Tanji, MD, Waipahu, Hawaii

The Academy also acknowledges the following committee for assistance in developing Study Questions and Answers for this BCSC Section:

Resident Self-Assessment Committee: Evan L. Waxman, MD, PhD, *Chair,* Pittsburgh, Pennsylvania; Zachary Koretz, MD, MPH, San Diego, California

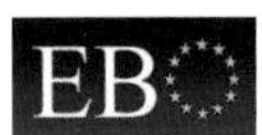

European Board of Ophthalmology: Anna P. Maino, MBBS, PGCert, *Liaison,* Manchester, England; Laura R. Steeples, MBChB, *Chair,* Manchester, England; Chiara Giuffrè, MD, Manchester, England; Ines Leal, MD, Lisbon, Portugal; Sasa Pockar, MD, Manchester, England; Joanne Wong, MD, Manchester, England

Recent Past Faculty

Thomas A. Albini, MD
Bryn M. Burkholder, MD
H. Nida Sen, MD, MHSc
Daniel V. Vasconcelos-Santos, MD, PhD

In addition, the Academy gratefully acknowledges the contributions of numerous past faculty and advisory committee members who have played an important role in the development of previous editions of the Basic and Clinical Science Course.

American Academy of Ophthalmology Staff

Dale E. Fajardo, EdD, MBA, *Vice President, Education*
Beth Wilson, *Director, Continuing Professional Development*
Denise Evenson, *Director, Brand & Creative*
Susan Malloy, *Acquisitions and Development Manager*
Stephanie Tanaka, *Publications Manager*
Jasmine Chen, *Manager, E-Learning*
Sarah Page, *Online Education and Licensing Manager*
Rayna Ungersma, *Manager, Curriculum Development*

Lana Ip, *Senior Designer*
Amanda Fernandez, *Publications Editor*
Beth Collins, *Medical Editor*
Kenny Guay, *Publications Specialist*
Debra Marchi, *Online Education Specialist*

Financial Disclosures

Academy staff members who contributed to the development of this product state that within the 24 months prior to their contributions to this CME activity and for the duration of development, they have had no financial interest in or other relationship with any entity that produces, markets, resells, or distributes health care goods or services consumed by or used in patients.

The authors and reviewers state that within the 24 months prior to their contributions to this CME activity and for the duration of development, they have had the following financial relationships:*

Dr Fouraker: Addition Technology (C, L), AJL Ophthalmic SA (C, L), Alcon Laboratories (C, L), OASIS Medical, Inc (C, L)

Dr Gangaputra: MERIT CRO, Inc (C)

Dr Knickelbein: Alexion Pharmaceuticals, Inc (S), Apellis Pharmaceuticals, Inc (S), EyePoint Pharmaceuticals, Inc (S), Gilead Sciences, Inc (S), Novartis Pharmaceuticals Corporation (S), Outlook Therapeutics, Inc (S), Regeneron Pharmaceuticals, Inc (S), Santen, Inc (S)

Dr Lai: Twenty/Twenty Therapeutics LLC (C)

Dr Leal: AbbVie, Inc (C, L), Alimera Sciences, Inc (L), Merck & Co, Inc (S), Novartis Pharmaceuticals Corporation (C)

Dr Rowsey: HEO3 (P)

Dr Shah: Allergan (C, L, S), DORC International (S), Focus Vision Supplements (O, S), Regeneron Pharmaceuticals, Inc (C, L, S)

All relevant financial relationships have been mitigated.

The other authors and reviewers state that within the 24 months prior to their contributions to this CME activity and for the duration of development, they have had no financial interest in or other relationship with any entity that produces, markets, resells, or distributes health care goods or services consumed by or used in patients.

* C = consultant fee, paid advisory boards, or fees for attending a meeting; E = employed by or received a W2 from a commercial company; L = lecture fees or honoraria, travel fees or reimbursements when speaking at the invitation of a commercial company; O = equity ownership/stock options in publicly or privately traded firms, excluding mutual funds; P = patents and/or royalties for intellectual property; S = grant support or other financial support to the investigator from all sources, including research support from government agencies, foundations, device manufacturers, and/or pharmaceutical companies

American Academy of Ophthalmology
655 Beach Street
Box 7424
San Francisco, CA 94120-7424

Contents

Introduction to the BCSC

The Basic and Clinical Science Course (BCSC) is designed to meet the needs of residents and practitioners for a comprehensive yet concise curriculum of the field of ophthalmology. The BCSC has developed from its original brief outline format, which relied heavily on outside readings, to a more convenient and educationally useful self-contained text. The Academy updates and revises the course annually, with the goals of integrating the basic science and clinical practice of ophthalmology and of keeping ophthalmologists current with new developments in the various subspecialties.

The BCSC incorporates the effort and expertise of more than 100 ophthalmologists, organized into 13 Section faculties, working with Academy editorial staff. In addition, the course continues to benefit from many lasting contributions made by the faculties of previous editions. Members of the Academy Practicing Ophthalmologists Advisory Committee for Education, Committee on Aging, and Vision Rehabilitation Committee review every volume before major revisions, as does a group of select residents and fellows. Members of the European Board of Ophthalmology, organized into Section faculties, also review volumes before major revisions, focusing primarily on differences between American and European ophthalmology practice.

Organization of the Course

The Basic and Clinical Science Course comprises 13 volumes, incorporating fundamental ophthalmic knowledge, subspecialty areas, and special topics:

1 Update on General Medicine
2 Fundamentals and Principles of Ophthalmology
3 Clinical Optics and Vision Rehabilitation
4 Ophthalmic Pathology and Intraocular Tumors
5 Neuro-Ophthalmology
6 Pediatric Ophthalmology and Strabismus
7 Oculofacial Plastic and Orbital Surgery
8 External Disease and Cornea
9 Uveitis and Ocular Inflammation
10 Glaucoma
11 Lens and Cataract
12 Retina and Vitreous
13 Refractive Surgery

References

Readers who wish to explore specific topics in greater detail may consult the references cited within each chapter and listed in the Additional Materials and Resources section at the back of the book. These references are intended to be selective rather than exhaustive, chosen by the BCSC faculty as being important, current, and readily available to residents and practitioners.

Multimedia

This edition of Section 9, *Uveitis and Ocular Inflammation,* includes videos related to topics covered in the book and interactive content, an "activity," developed by members of the BCSC faculty. The videos and the activity are available to readers of the print and electronic versions of Section 9 (www.aao.org/bcscvideo_section09) and (www.aao.org/bcscactivity_section09). Mobile-device users can scan the QR codes below (a QR-code reader may need to be installed on the device) to access the videos and activity.

Videos

Activity

Self-Assessment and CME Credit

Each volume of the BCSC is designed as an independent study activity for ophthalmology residents and practitioners. The learning objectives for this volume are given on page 1. The text, illustrations, and references provide the information necessary to achieve the objectives; the study questions allow readers to test their understanding of the material and their mastery of the objectives. Physicians who wish to claim CME credit for this educational activity may do so by following the instructions given at the end of the book.*

Conclusion

The Basic and Clinical Science Course has expanded greatly over the years, with the addition of much new text, numerous illustrations, and video content. Recent editions have sought to place greater emphasis on clinical applicability while maintaining a solid foundation in basic science. As with any educational program, it reflects the experience of its authors. As its faculties change and medicine progresses, new viewpoints emerge on controversial subjects and techniques. Not all alternate approaches can be included in this series; as with any educational endeavor, the learner should seek additional sources, including Academy Preferred Practice Pattern Guidelines.

The BCSC faculty and staff continually strive to improve the educational usefulness of the course; you, the reader, can contribute to this ongoing process. If you have any suggestions or questions about the series, please do not hesitate to contact the faculty or the editors.

The authors, editors, and reviewers hope that your study of the BCSC will be of lasting value and that each Section will serve as a practical resource for quality patient care.

* There is no formal American Board of Ophthalmology (ABO) approval process for self-assessment activities. Any CME activity that qualifies for ABO Continuing Certification credit may also be counted as "self-assessment" as long as it provides a mechanism for individual learners to review their own performance, knowledge base, or skill set in a defined area of practice. For instance, grand rounds, medical conferences, or journal activities for CME credit that involve a form of individualized self-assessment may count as a self-assessment activity.

Objectives

Upon completion of BCSC Section 9, *Uveitis and Ocular Inflammation,* the reader should be able to

- describe the immunologic and infectious mechanisms involved in the development of and complications from uveitis and related conditions, including AIDS
- identify general and specific pathophysiologic processes in acute and chronic ocular inflammation that affect the structure and function of the uvea, lens, vitreous, retina, and other adjacent tissues
- distinguish infectious from noninfectious uveitic entities
- state appropriate differential diagnoses for ocular inflammatory disorders and identify systemic associations or implications
- based on the differential diagnosis, select examination techniques and appropriate ancillary studies to distinguish infectious from noninfectious causes
- describe the principles of medical and surgical management of infectious and noninfectious uveitis and related ocular inflammation, including indications for and adverse effects of immunosuppressive drugs and monitoring of patients who use them
- describe the main principles for distinguishing masquerade syndromes from uveitis and increasing clinical suspicion for these conditions
- describe the structural complications of uveitis, their prevention, and their treatment

CHAPTER 1

Basic Concepts in Immunology: Effector Cells and the Innate Immune Response

Highlights

- An immune response is the process for eliminating an offending stimulus. The clinical evidence of an immune response is inflammation.
- The immune system is composed of tissues, cells, and molecules that mediate response to infection or foreign material.
- Immune responses are broadly defined as innate or adaptive with close interaction between the two.
- Innate (natural) immunity provides immediate protection and requires no prior contact with the foreign substance or organism.
- Adaptive (acquired) immunity develops more slowly than innate immunity but provides more specific defense against infections.

Definitions

An immune response is a sequence of molecular and cellular events intended to rid the host of a threat: offending pathogenic organisms, toxic substances, cellular debris, or neoplastic cells. There are 2 broad categories of immune responses, *innate* and *adaptive*.

Innate immune responses, or *natural immunity*, require no prior contact with or "education" about the stimulus against which they are directed. Adaptive (or *acquired*) responses are higher-order, more specific responses directed against unique antigens. The term *antigen* refers to any substance (eg, toxin, foreign protein, bacterium) that can induce an immune response. Chapter 2 discusses adaptive responses in detail. This chapter introduces the crucial cells of the immune system and their functions in innate immunity.

Abbas AK, Lichtman AH, Pillai S. *Basic Immunology: Functions and Disorders of the Immune System*. 5th ed. Elsevier/Saunders; 2016.

Abbas AK, Lichtman AH, Pillai S. *Cellular and Molecular Immunology.* 9th ed. Elsevier/Saunders; 2018.

Murphy KM. *Janeway's Immunobiology.* 8th ed. Garland Science; 2012.

Cellular Components of the Immune System

White blood cells, or *leukocytes,* include several kinds of nucleated cells that can be distinguished by the shape of their nuclei and the presence or absence of cytoplasmic granules, as well as by their uptake of various histologic stains (Fig 1-1). They can be broadly divided into 2 subsets:

- myeloid (neutrophils, eosinophils, basophils and mast cells, monocytes and macrophages, and dendritic cells and Langerhans cells)
- lymphoid (T lymphocytes, B lymphocytes, and natural killer cells)

See BCSC Section 4, *Ophthalmic Pathology and Intraocular Tumors,* for additional discussion of leukocytes and findings on histologic examinations.

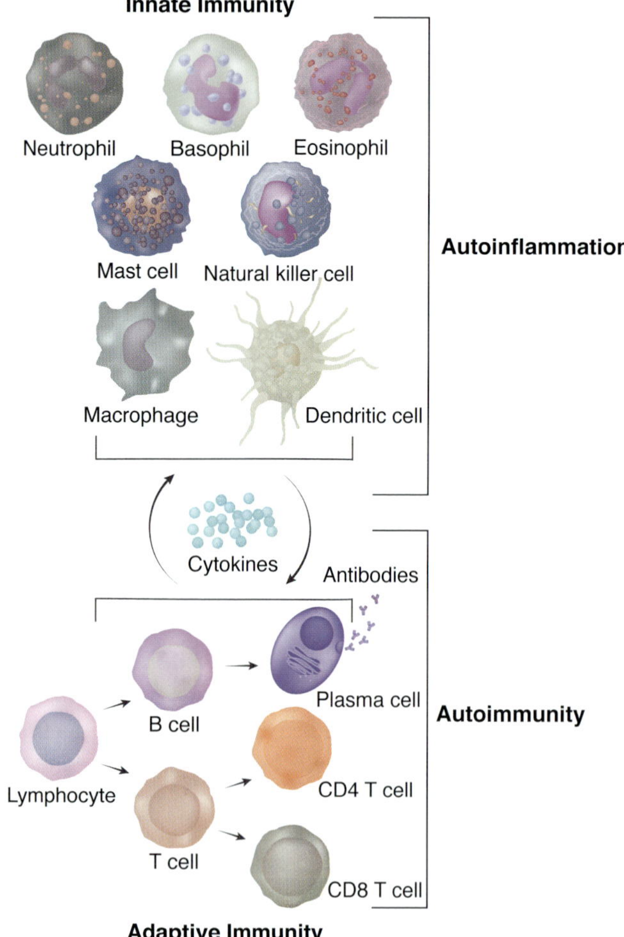

Figure 1-1 Cells of the immune system. *(Original illustration by Jared E. Knickelbein, MD, PhD. Redrawn by Cyndie C. H. Wooley.)*

Neutrophils

Neutrophils possess a multilobed nucleus of varying shapes; hence, they are also called *polymorphonuclear leukocytes* or *polymorphonuclear neutrophils (PMNs).* Neutrophils also feature cytoplasmic granules and lysosomes and are the most abundant granulocytes in the blood. They are efficient phagocytes that readily clear tissues, degrade ingested material, and act as important effector cells through the release of granule products and cytokines.

During the beginning or acute phases of inflammation, neutrophils are one of the first inflammatory cells to migrate from the bloodstream toward the site of inflammation. This process is called *chemotaxis.* Neutrophils dominate the inflammatory infiltrate in experimental models and clinical examples of active bacterial infections of the conjunctiva (conjunctivitis), sclera (scleritis), cornea (keratitis), and vitreous (endophthalmitis). They are also dominant in many types of active viral infections of the cornea (eg, herpes simplex virus keratitis) and retina (eg, herpes simplex virus retinitis).

Eosinophils

Eosinophils are characterized by the presence of a bilobed nucleus and abundant lysosomes and cytoplasmic granules that consist of more basic protein than that found in other polymorphonuclear leukocytes. These basic proteins bind acidic dyes, such as eosin—hence the name eosinophil. Eosinophilic granule products, including major basic protein and ribonucleases, destroy parasites efficiently. Eosinophils accumulate at sites of parasitic infection. They are also important in allergic immune reactions. Eosinophilia in the peripheral blood may occur in both parasitic infections and allergic disease.

Eosinophils are abundant in the conjunctiva and tears in many forms of allergic conjunctivitis, especially atopic and vernal conjunctivitis. They are not considered major effectors for intraocular inflammation, with the notable exception of helminthic infections of the eye, especially toxocariasis.

Basophils and Mast Cells

Basophils are the blood-borne equivalent of the tissue-bound mast cell. There are 2 major types of mast cells, connective tissue and mucosal. Both can release preformed granules and synthesize certain mediators de novo that differ from those of neutrophils and eosinophils. *Connective tissue mast cells* have abundant granules containing histamine and heparin, and they synthesize prostaglandin D_2 upon stimulation. In contrast, *mucosal mast cells* normally contain low levels of histamine and require T-cell–derived growth-promoting cytokines for stimulation. Stimulated mucosal mast cells primarily synthesize leukotrienes, in particular leukotriene C_4. Tissue location can alter the granule type and functional activity, but regulation of these differences is not well understood.

Mast cells act as major effector cells in immunoglobulin (Ig) E–mediated inflammatory reactions, especially of the allergic or immediate hypersensitivity type. They perform this function through their expression of high-affinity Fc receptors for IgE. *Fc* (from "*f*ragment, crystallizable") refers to the constant region of immunoglobulin that binds cell surface receptors (see Chapter 2). Mast cells may also participate in the induction of cell-mediated immunity, wound healing, and other functions not directly related to IgE-mediated degranulation. Other stimuli, such as complement or certain cytokines, may also trigger degranulation.

The healthy human conjunctiva contains numerous mast cells localized in the substantia propria. In certain atopic and allergic disease states, such as vernal conjunctivitis, the number of mast cells increases in the substantia propria and the epithelium, which is usually devoid of mast cells. The uveal tract also contains numerous connective tissue mast cells, whereas the cornea has none.

Monocytes and Macrophages

Monocytes, the circulating cells, and macrophages, the tissue-infiltrating equivalents, are important effectors in innate and adaptive immunity. These mononuclear cells are often detectable in acute ocular infections, even if other cell types, such as neutrophils, are more numerous. Monocytes are relatively large cells (12–20 µm in suspension and up to 40 µm in tissues) that normally travel throughout the body. Most tissues have at least 2 identifiable macrophage populations: tissue resident and blood derived. Although exceptions exist, tissue-resident macrophages are monocytes that migrated into tissue during embryologic development and later acquired tissue-specific properties and cellular markers. Various resident macrophages have tissue-specific names (ie, Kupffer cells in the liver, alveolar macrophages in the lung, and microglia in the brain and retina). Blood-derived macrophages are monocytes that have recently migrated from the blood into a fully developed tissue site.

Macrophages may serve in 3 capacities:

- sentinels that recognize danger signals from pathogens and/or tissue damage
- effectors that induce inflammation and fight pathogens directly
- regulatory/repair cells that conduct tissue repair, regulate the adaptive immune system, and serve as checkpoints during immune cell migration

Various signals can prime resting (immature or quiescent) monocytes for differentiation into efficient antigen-presenting cells (APCs). Upon additional signals, these APCs are activated to become effector cells. Effective activation stimuli include exposure to bacterial products, such as lipopolysaccharide; phagocytosis of antibody-coated or complement-coated pathogens; or exposure to mediators released during inflammation, such as interleukin (IL) 1β or interferon gamma.

Only after full activation do macrophages become most efficient at the synthesis and release of inflammatory mediators and the killing and degradation of phagocytosed pathogens. Activated macrophages may terminally differentiate into epithelioid cells, with larger nuclei, abundant cytoplasm, and indistinct cell borders, resembling squamous epithelium. These epithelioid histiocytes are characteristic of granulomatous inflammation, either in infectious uveitis (ie, tuberculosis, syphilis, herpes, fungal infection, parasitic uveitis) or noninfectious uveitis (ie, sarcoidosis, granulomatosis with polyangiitis). Activated macrophages may also fuse to form *multinucleated giant cells,* which may accompany granulomatous inflammation or occur in the tissue reaction to foreign material.

Dendritic Cells and Langerhans Cells

Dendritic cells (DCs) are terminally differentiated, bone marrow–derived mononuclear cells that are distinct from macrophages and monocytes. These specialized cells bridge the innate and adaptive immune systems but do not directly participate in effector activities. DCs use pattern recognition receptors, such as Toll-like receptors, to recognize pathogens. Activated DCs upregulate costimulatory molecules and produce cytokines to drive T-cell priming and effector differentiation as well as activate various types of immune cells. Interestingly, antigen presentation by nonactivated, steady-state DCs might lead to T-cell unresponsiveness, promoting tolerance.

All human DCs express high levels of human leukocyte antigen (HLA) class II molecules and may be classified by lineage markers as myeloid/classical or plasmacytoid. DCs can also be classified functionally and anatomically, as their function is linked to their location:

- Blood DCs are precursors of tissue and lymphoid organ DCs.
- Migratory or tissue DCs reside in most epithelial tissues, where they acquire antigen and from which they migrate via afferent lymphatics to lymph nodes. In tissue sites, DCs are large (15–30 μm), with cytoplasmic veils that form extensions 2–3 times the diameter of the cell and resemble the dendritic structure of neurons.
- Resident or lymphoid DCs arise in lymph nodes directly from the blood.
- Inflammatory DCs are present in tissues and lymphoid organs during inflammation. Precursors include classical monocytes.

Langerhans cells (LCs) are myeloid cells with DC function that reside in the epidermis and stratified epithelia of the cornea, as well as conjunctival, buccal, gingival, and genital mucosae. LCs are identified by their many dendrites, electron-dense cytoplasm, and Birbeck granules. Interestingly, they originate from primitive hematopoiesis in the yolk sac and form a stable, self-renewing network that does not require bone marrow–derived precursors in the absence of inflammation. At rest, they are not active APCs. On activation, LCs lose their granules and transform to resemble blood and lymphoid DCs. Evidence suggests that LCs migrate along the afferent lymph vessels to the draining lymphoid organs.

LCs are important components of the immune system and play roles in antigen presentation, control of lymphoid cell traffic, differentiation of T lymphocytes, and induction of delayed hypersensitivity. Elimination of LCs from skin before an antigen challenge inhibits induction of the contact hypersensitivity response. In the conjunctiva and limbus, LCs are the only cells that constitutively express HLA class II molecules. LCs are present in the peripheral cornea, and any stimulation of the central cornea results in central migration of the peripheral LCs.

Lymphocytes

Lymphocytes are small (10–20-μm) cells with large, round, and dense nuclei. Like DCs, they are derived from stem cell precursors within the bone marrow; however, unlike other leukocytes, lymphocytes require subsequent maturation in peripheral lymphoid organs.

Three broad categories of lymphocytes are

- T lymphocytes (also called *T cells*)
- B lymphocytes (also called *B cells*)
- non-T, non-B lymphocytes

The expression of specific cell surface proteins (ie, *surface markers*) can be used to further divide lymphocytes. These markers are in turn related to the functional and molecular activity of individual subsets. Two types of lymphocytes participate in the innate immune response, serving as a bridge between innate and adaptive responses: (1) gamma-delta (γδ) T cells or sentinel T cells, also known as *intraepithelial lymphocytes;* and (2) natural killer (NK) cells, a subset of non-T, non-B lymphocytes. Chapter 2 discusses the roles of lymphocytes in adaptive immunity.

Overview of the Innate Immune System

The innate immune system is a relatively broad-acting rapid reaction force that recognizes nonself (foreign) substances, proteins, or lipopolysaccharides. The innate response is immediate and requires no prior exposure to the foreign substance. Innate immune responses are driven by germline-encoded receptors that recognize features common to many pathogens and offending stimuli. The result is the generation of biochemical mediators and cytokines that recruit innate effector cells, especially macrophages and neutrophils, to remove the offending stimulus through phagocytosis or enzymatic degradation. The innate response also alerts the cells of the adaptive immune system to reinforce and refine the attack. For example, in acute endophthalmitis, bacteria-derived toxins or host cell debris stimulates the recruitment of neutrophils and monocytes, leading to the production of inflammatory mediators and phagocytosis of the bacteria.

An array of highly conserved pattern recognition receptors (PRRs) and proteins detect similarly conserved molecular motifs—*pathogen-associated molecular patterns (PAMPs)*—on triggering stimuli. PAMPs include proteins found in bacterial, fungal, and viral nucleic acids. Cell-associated PRRs may be extracellular, endosomal, or cytoplasmic and include Toll-like receptors (TLRs), C-type lectin receptors (CTLRs), nucleotide-binding oligomerization domain-like receptors (NOD-like receptors, or NLRs), and retinoic acid–inducible gene-I-like receptors (RIG-I-like receptors, or RLRs). Since each PRR has evolved to respond to a different PAMP, engagement of a specific PRR subtype conveys information about the type of infection (ie, bacterial, fungal, or viral) and the location (ie, extracellular or intracellular). In humans, there are 10 members of the TLR family. Those that respond to bacterial products (TLR1/2, TLR2/6, TLR4, TLR5) are localized in the plasma membrane of innate immune cells and sense extracellular microbes. The TLRs that detect viral nucleic acids (TLR3, TLR7, TLR9) are located within endosomal compartments and interact with membrane proteins.

Immunity Versus Inflammation

An immune response is the process for removing an offending stimulus. An immune response that becomes clinically evident is termed an *inflammatory response* (see Clinical

CLINICAL EXAMPLE 1-1

Autoinflammatory and Autoimmune Diseases

Dysregulation and overactivity of either innate or adaptive immune responses can lead to clinically evident inflammatory disease. Autoimmune disease results from loss of adaptive immune tolerance to autoantigens (also called *self antigens*) that leads to a dysregulated immune attack on self tissues. Autoreactive B and T cells of the adaptive immune system (discussed further in Chapter 2) are critical to the disease process (see Fig 1-1). An example of a classic autoimmune disease is systemic lupus erythematosus. More recently, the term *autoinflammatory disease* has been used to describe inflammatory conditions driven predominantly by overactivity of the innate immune system in the absence of pathologic B- or T-cell responses. An example of an autoinflammatory disease is juvenile idiopathic arthritis. Most inflammatory diseases likely lie on a spectrum between autoinflammation and autoimmunity. An example of a mixed-spectrum disease is ankylosing spondylitis. The etiology of inflammatory diseases is thought to be multifactorial, with genetic, environmental, and possibly infectious triggers.

Delves PJ, Martin SJ, Burton DR, Roitt IM. *Roitt's Essential Immunology.* 13th ed. Wiley-Blackwell; 2017.

Szekanecz Z, McInnes IB, Schett G, Szamosi S, Benkő S, Szűcs G. Autoinflammation and autoimmunity across rheumatic and musculoskeletal diseases. *Nat Rev Rheumatol.* 2021;17(10):585–595.

Example 1-1). Inflammatory responses typically result in 5 cardinal clinical manifestations: pain, hyperemia, edema, heat, and loss of function. These manifestations are the consequence of 2 physiologic changes within a tissue: cellular recruitment and altered vascular permeability.

The following pathologic findings are typical in inflammation:

- infiltration of effector cells resulting in the release of biochemical and molecular mediators of inflammation, such as cytokines (eg, interleukins and chemokines) and lipid mediators (eg, prostaglandins, leukotrienes, and platelet-activating factors)
- production of oxygen metabolites (eg, superoxide and nitrogen radicals)
- release of granule products as well as catalytic enzymes (eg, proteases, collagenases, and elastases)
- activation of plasma-derived enzyme systems (eg, complement components and fibrin)

These effector processes are described in greater detail later in this chapter.

Immune responses are a constant presence, though usually at a subclinical level. For example, ocular surface allergen exposure, which occurs daily, or the nearly ubiquitous event of bacterial contamination during cataract surgery is usually cleared by immune mechanisms *without* overt inflammation.

Innate Immunity: Triggers and Mechanisms

A variety of triggers and mechanisms are involved in innate immune responses of the eye. Four of the most important triggers are

- bacteria-derived molecules
- damage to nonimmune ocular parenchymal cells by toxins or trauma
- innate mechanisms for the recruitment and activation of neutrophils through the activation of vascular endothelial cells
- innate mechanisms for the recruitment and activation of macrophages

These are discussed in the following sections. Table 1-1 summarizes triggering molecules of innate ocular immune responses.

Bacteria-Derived Molecules That Trigger Innate Immune Responses

Bacterial lipopolysaccharide

Lipopolysaccharide (LPS), also known as *endotoxin,* is an intrinsic component of the cell walls of most gram-negative bacteria. Among the most important triggering molecules of innate immune responses, LPS consists of 3 components: lipid A, O polysaccharide, and core oligosaccharide. Lipid A is the most potent component, capable of activating effector cells at concentrations of a few picograms per milliliter. The exact structures of each component vary among species of bacteria, but all are recognized by the innate immune system. The primary receptors are the TLRs, principally TLR2 and TLR4, which are expressed on macrophages, neutrophils, and DCs, as well as on B cells and T cells.

The effects of LPS include the following:

- activation of monocytes and neutrophils, leading to upregulation of genes for various cytokines (IL-1, IL-6, tumor necrosis factor [TNF])
- degranulation
- activation of complement via the alternative pathway
- activation of vascular endothelial cells

Humans are intermittently exposed to low levels of LPS that the gut releases, especially during episodes of diarrhea and dysentery. Exposure to LPS may play a role in

Table 1-1 Triggering Molecules of Innate Immune Responses in the Eye

Triggering Molecules
Bacteria-derived molecules
Lipopolysaccharide
Other cell wall components
Exotoxins and secreted toxins
Nonspecific soluble molecules (also modulate innate immunity)
Plasma-derived enzymes
Acute-phase reactants
Cytokines produced by parenchymal cells within a tissue site

dysentery-related uveitis, arthritis, and reactive arthritis. LPS is the major cause of shock, fever, and other pathophysiologic responses to bacterial sepsis, making it an important cause of morbidity and mortality during gram-negative bacterial infections. Interestingly, footpad injection of LPS in rodents results in an acute anterior uveitis. This animal model is called *endotoxin-induced uveitis*. See Clinical Example 1-2.

Other bacterial cell wall components

The bacterial cell wall and membrane are complex. They contain numerous polysaccharide, lipid, and protein structures that can initiate an innate immune response independent of adaptive immunity. Killed lysates of many types of gram-positive bacteria or mycobacteria can directly activate macrophages, making them useful as adjuvants. Some of these components have been implicated in various models for arthritis and uveitis. In many cases, the molecular mechanisms might be similar to those of LPS.

CLINICAL EXAMPLE 1-2

Role of Bacterial Toxin Production in the Severity of Endophthalmitis

In experimental models, intraocular injection of lipopolysaccharide (LPS) is highly inflammatory and accounts for much of the enhanced pathogenicity of gram-negative infections of the eye. For example, intravitreal injection of LPS triggers a dose-dependent neutrophilic and monocytic infiltration of the uveal tract, retina, and vitreous. Toll-like receptor 2 (TLR2) recognizes LPS, and binding of LPS by TLR2 on macrophages results in macrophage activation and secretion of a wide array of inflammatory cytokines, including interleukin (IL) 1, IL-6, and tumor necrosis factor α (TNF-α). Degranulation of platelets is among the first histologic changes in LPS-induced uveitis; likely mediators are eicosanoids, platelet-activating factors, and vasoactive amines. The subsequent intraocular generation of several mediators, especially leukotriene B_4, thromboxane B_2, prostaglandin E_2, and IL-6, correlates with the development of the cellular infiltrate and vascular leakage.

Using clinical isolates or bacteria genetically altered to diminish production of the various types of bacterial toxins, investigators have demonstrated that toxin elaboration in gram-positive or gram-negative endophthalmitis greatly influences inflammatory cell infiltration and retinal cytotoxicity. This effect suggests that sterilization through antibiotic therapy alone, in the absence of antitoxin therapy or toxin removal, may not prevent activation of innate immunity, ocular inflammation, and vision loss in eyes infected by toxin-producing strains.

Booth MC, Atkuri RV, Gilmore MS. Toxin production contributes to severity of *Staphylococcus aureus* endophthalmitis. In: Nussenblatt RB, Whitcup SM, Caspi RR, Gery I, eds. *Advances in Ocular Immunology: Proceedings of the 6th International Symposium on the Immunology and Immunopathology of the Eye.* Elsevier; 1994:269–272.

Exotoxins and other secretory products of bacteria

Certain bacteria secrete products known as *exotoxins* into their surrounding microenvironment. Many of these products are enzymes that, although not directly inflammatory, can cause tissue damage and subsequent inflammation and tissue destruction. Examples of these products include

- collagenases
- hemolysins such as streptolysin O, which can kill neutrophils by causing cytoplasmic and extracellular release of their granules
- phospholipases such as the *Clostridium perfringens* α-toxins, which kill cells and cause necrosis by disrupting cell membranes

An intravitreal injection of a purified hemolysin BL toxin derived from *Bacillus cereus* can cause direct necrosis of retinal cells and retinal detachment. In animal studies, as few as 100 *B cereus* organisms can produce enough toxin to cause complete loss of retinal function in 12 hours. In addition to being directly toxic, bacterial exotoxins can be strong triggers of an innate immune response.

Callegan MC, Jett BD, Hancock LE, Gilmore MS. Role of hemolysin BL in the pathogenesis of extraintestinal *Bacillus cereus* infection assessed in an endophthalmitis model. *Infect Immun.* 1999;67(7):3357–3366.

Murphy K, Travers P, Walport M. *Janeway's Immunobiology.* 8th ed. Garland Science; 2012.

Other Triggers or Modulators of Innate Immune Responses

Damage to nonimmune ocular parenchymal cells—especially iris or ciliary body epithelium, retinal pigment epithelium, retinal Müller cells, or corneal or conjunctival epithelium—by toxins or trauma can trigger innate immune responses in the eye. This damage can result in the synthesis of a wide range of mediators, cytokines, and eicosanoids. For example, phagocytosis of staphylococci by corneal epithelium, microtrauma to the ocular surface epithelium by contact lenses, chafing of iris or ciliary epithelium by an intraocular lens, or laser treatment of the retina can stimulate ocular cells to produce mediators that assist in the recruitment of innate effector cells such as neutrophils or macrophages. See Clinical Example 1-3.

CLINICAL EXAMPLE 1-3

Uveitis-Glaucoma-Hyphema Syndrome

One cause of inflammation following cataract surgery, uveitis-glaucoma-hyphema (UGH) syndrome, is related to the physical presence of certain types of intraocular lenses (IOLs). Although UGH syndrome was more common when rigid anterior chamber lenses were used during the early 1980s, it has also been reported with posterior chamber lenses, particularly when a haptic of a 1-piece lens is inadvertently placed in the sulcus. The pathogenesis of UGH syndrome appears related to mechanisms of innate immunity activation. A likely mechanism is cytokine and eicosanoid synthesis triggered by mechanical chafing of or trauma to the iris or ciliary body. Plasma-derived enzymes, especially complement or fibrin, can enter the eye through vascular permeability altered by surgery or trauma and can then be activated by contact with the surface of IOLs. Adherence of bacteria and leukocytes to the surface has also been implicated. Toxicity caused by contaminants on the lens surface during manufacturing is rare. Nevertheless, noninflamed eyes with IOLs can demonstrate histologic evidence of low-grade, foreign-body reactions around the haptics.

Innate Mechanisms for the Recruitment and Activation of Neutrophils

A key part of the innate immune response is the recruitment and activation of neutrophils, which are highly efficient effectors of this response. Neutrophils are categorized as *resting* or *activated,* according to their secretory and cell membrane activity. In the innate immune response, recruitment of resting, circulating neutrophils occurs rapidly in a tightly controlled process consisting of 2 events:

- neutrophil adhesion to the vascular endothelium through cell adhesion molecules (CAMs) on leukocytes as well as on endothelial cells, primarily in postcapillary venules
- transmigration of the neutrophils through the endothelium and its extracellular matrix, mediated by chemotactic factors

Activation of vascular endothelial cells is triggered by various innate immune stimuli, such as LPS, physical injury, thrombin, histamine, or leukotriene release. *Neutrophil rolling*—a process by which neutrophils bind loosely and reversibly to nonactivated endothelial cells—involves molecules from at least 3 sets of CAM families:

- *selectins,* especially E-, L-, and P-selectin
- *integrins,* especially leukocyte function–associated antigen 1 and macrophage-1 antigen
- *immunoglobulin superfamily molecules,* especially intercellular adhesion molecule (ICAM) 1 and ICAM-2

These molecules are expressed on both neutrophils and vascular endothelial cells.

The primary events are mediated largely by members of the selectin family and occur within minutes of stimulation (Fig 1-2). Nonactivated neutrophils express L-selectin, which mediates a weak bond to endothelial cells by binding to specific selectin ligands. Upon exposure to triggering molecules such as LPS, endothelial cells become activated, expressing in turn at least 2 other selectins (E and P) by which they can bind to the neutrophils and help stabilize the interaction in a process called *adhesion.* Subsequently, other factors, such as platelet-activating factor (PAF), various cytokines, and bacterial products can induce upregulation of the β-integrin family. As integrins are expressed, the selectins are shed, and neutrophils then bind firmly to endothelial cells through the immunoglobulin superfamily molecules.

After adhesion, various chemotactic factors are required in order to induce *transmigration* of neutrophils across the endothelial barrier and into the extracellular matrix of

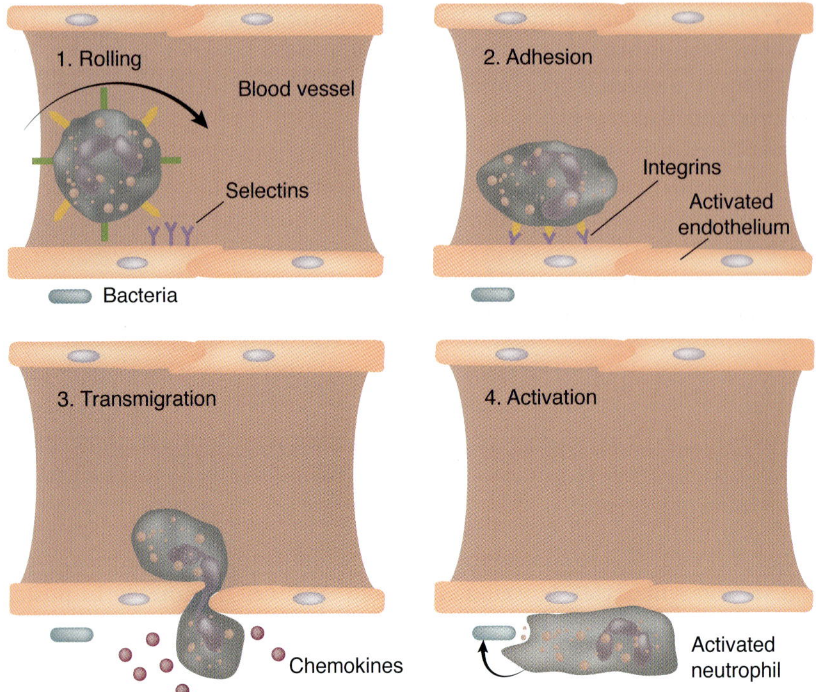

Figure 1-2 Steps of neutrophil migration and activation in infection. **1,** In response to innate immune stimuli, *rolling* neutrophils within the blood vessel bind loosely and reversibly to nonactivated endothelial cells by selectins. **2,** Neutrophil adhesion is mediated by E- and P-selectins, β-integrins, and immunoglobulin superfamily molecules, which are expressed on activated vascular endothelial cells in response to innate activating factors and bacterial products. **3,** Chemotactic factors triggered by the infection induce *transmigration* of neutrophils across the endothelial barrier into the extracellular matrix of the tissue. **4,** Finally, upon stimulation by bacterial toxins and phagocytosis, neutrophils are fully activated, becoming functional effector cells. *(Original illustration by Barb Cousins, modified by Joyce Zavarro; redrawn by Cyndie C. H. Wooley.)*

the tissue. Chemotactic factors are short-range signaling molecules that diffuse in a declining concentration gradient from the source of production within a tissue to the vessel. Neutrophils have receptors for these molecules and are induced to undergo membrane changes that cause migration in the direction of highest concentration. Examples of chemotactic factors include

- complement products, such as the anaphylatoxin C5a
- fibrin split products
- certain neuropeptides, such as substance P
- bacteria-derived formyl tripeptides, such as *N*-formyl-methionyl-leucyl-phenylalanine (fMLP)
- leukotrienes
- α-chemokines, such as IL-8

Activation of neutrophils into functional effector cells begins during adhesion and transmigration but is fully achieved upon neutrophil interaction with specific signals within the site of injury or infection. The most effective activation triggers are bacteria and their toxins, especially LPS. Other innate or adaptive mechanisms (especially complement) and chemical mediators (such as leukotrienes and PAF) also contribute to neutrophil activation. Neutrophils, unlike monocytes or lymphocytes, do not leave a tissue to recirculate but remain and die.

Phagocytosis

Phagocytosis of bacteria and other pathogens is a process mediated by receptors. The 2 most important are *antibody Fc receptors* and *complement receptors.* Pathogens in an immune complex with antibody or activated complement components bind to cell surface membrane–expressed Fc or complement receptors.

The area of membrane bound by the pathogen invaginates and becomes a phagosome. Cytoplasmic granules and lysosomes then fuse with the phagosomes. Phagocytes have multiple means of destroying microorganisms, notably, antimicrobial polypeptides residing within the cytoplasmic granules as well as reactive oxygen and nitrogen radicals. Although these mechanisms primarily destroy pathogens, released contents, such as lysosomal enzymes, may contribute to the amplification of inflammation and tissue damage.

Neutrophil-derived granule products

As mentioned earlier, neutrophils are proficient phagocytes that act as effector cells through the release of granule products and cytokines. Many antimicrobial polypeptides are present in neutrophilic granules. The principal ones are bactericidal/permeability-increasing protein, defensins, lysozyme, lactoferrin, and the serine proteases.

In addition to antimicrobial polypeptides, neutrophils contain numerous other molecules that contribute to inflammation. These compounds include hydrolytic enzymes, elastase, matrix metalloproteinases (MMPs), gelatinase, myeloperoxidase, vitamin B_{12}–binding protein, and cytochrome b_{558}. Granule contents remain inert and membrane bound when the granules are intact and become active and soluble when granules fuse to the phagocytic vesicles or plasma membrane. Collagenase is an example of an MMP found within neutrophilic granules. Various forms of collagenase contribute to corneal injury and liquefaction during bacterial keratitis and scleritis, especially in infections with *Pseudomonas* species. Collagenases also contribute to peripheral corneal melting syndromes secondary to rheumatoid arthritis–associated peripheral keratitis.

Innate Mechanisms for the Recruitment and Activation of Macrophages

Monocyte-derived macrophages are another important type of effector cell for the innate immune response that follows trauma or acute infection. The various molecules involved in monocyte adhesion and transmigration from blood into tissues are probably similar to those for neutrophils, although they have not been studied as thoroughly. The functional activation of macrophages, however, is more complex than that of neutrophils. Macrophages exist in different levels or stages of metabolic and functional activity, each representing different "programs" of gene activation and synthesis of macrophage-derived cytokines and mediators. The categories of macrophages include

- resting (immature or quiescent)
- primed

- activated
- stimulated or reparative (partially activated)

Resting and scavenging macrophages

Phagocytosis removes host cell debris in the process called *scavenging.* Resting macrophages are the classic scavenging cell, capable of phagocytosis and uptake of the following:

- dead cell membranes
- chemically modified extracellular protein (ie, acetylated or oxidized lipoproteins)
- sugar ligands, through mannose receptors
- naked nucleic acids
- bacterial pathogens

Resting monocytes express at least 3 types of scavenging receptors but synthesize very low levels of proinflammatory cytokines. Scavenging can occur in the absence of inflammation. See Clinical Example 1-4.

Primed macrophages

Resting macrophages become primed by exposure to certain cytokines. Upon priming, these cells become positive for HLA class II molecules and capable of functioning as APCs to T lymphocytes (see Chapter 2). Priming involves the following:

- activation of specialized lysosomal enzymes, such as cathepsins D and E, for degrading proteins into peptide fragments
- upregulation of specific genes (ie, major histocompatibility complex class II) and costimulatory molecules (ie, B7.1)
- increased cycling of proteins between endosomes and the cell surface membrane

CLINICAL EXAMPLE 1-4

Phacolytic Uveitis

Mild infiltration of scavenging macrophages centered around retained lens cortex or nucleus fragments occurs in nearly all eyes with lens injury, including those that have undergone routine cataract surgery. This infiltrate is notable for the *absence* of both prominent neutrophil infiltration and substantial nongranulomatous inflammation. An occasional giant cell may be present, but granulomatous changes are not extensive.

Phacolytic uveitis (phacolytic glaucoma) is a variant of scavenging macrophage infiltration in which leakage of lens protein occurs through the intact capsule of a mature or hypermature cataract. Lens protein–engorged scavenging macrophages block the trabecular meshwork outflow channels, resulting in elevated intraocular pressure. Other signs of typical lens-associated uveitis are conspicuously absent. Experimental studies suggest that lens proteins may be chemotactic stimuli for monocytes. See Chapter 8 for further discussion of the clinical presentation of phacolytic uveitis.

Primed macrophages thus resemble DCs. They can exit tissue sites by afferent lymphatic vessels to reenter the lymph node.

Activated and stimulated macrophages

Activated macrophages are classically defined as macrophages that produce the full spectrum of inflammatory and cytotoxic cytokines; thus, they mediate and amplify acute inflammation, tumor killing, and major antibacterial activity. *Epithelioid cells* and *giant cells* represent different terminal differentiations of the activated macrophage.

Activation of macrophages can occur through exposure to innate stimuli or various substances, such as the following:

- cytokines, including chemokines, derived from T lymphocytes and other cell types
- bacterial cell walls or toxins from gram-positive or acid-fast organisms
- complement activated through the alternative pathway
- foreign bodies composed of potentially toxic substances, such as talc or beryllium
- exposure to certain surfaces, such as some plastics

Activation of macrophages is also termed *polarization*. Macrophages can be classified as M1 or M2 based on the observation that certain stimuli produce distinct patterns of gene or protein expression under experimental conditions. For example, exposure to bacterial LPS and interferon gamma typically polarizes macrophages to the M1 phenotype, whereas activation by other innate stimuli in the absence of interferon gamma polarizes toward the M2 phenotype. The activation state seems to be somewhat reversible, suggesting that macrophages may switch between subsets (plasticity), depending on environmental signals. In fact, macrophage research suggests there are at least 9 distinct classes of macrophage activation. Thus, although the M1/M2 model may be oversimplified, it does provide a framework for conceptualizing different levels of macrophage activation in terms of acute inflammation (Fig 1-3).

M1–classically activated macrophage characteristics include

- high production of proinflammatory cytokines (eg, IL-1, IL-6, and TNF-α) and oxygen radicals
- expression of inducible nitric oxide synthase with production of reactive nitrogen intermediates
- promotion of T helper-1 (Th1) response
- strong microbicidal and tumoricidal activity

M2–alternatively activated macrophage characteristics include

- parasite containment
- promotion of tissue remodeling
- promotion of tumor progression
- immunoregulatory functions (eg, arginase and IL-10 secretion)

As noted, macrophages that are partially activated are termed *stimulated* or *reparative* macrophages (M2). Partially activated macrophages contribute to (1) fibrosis and wound healing through the synthesis of mitogens such as platelet-derived growth factors, MMPs,

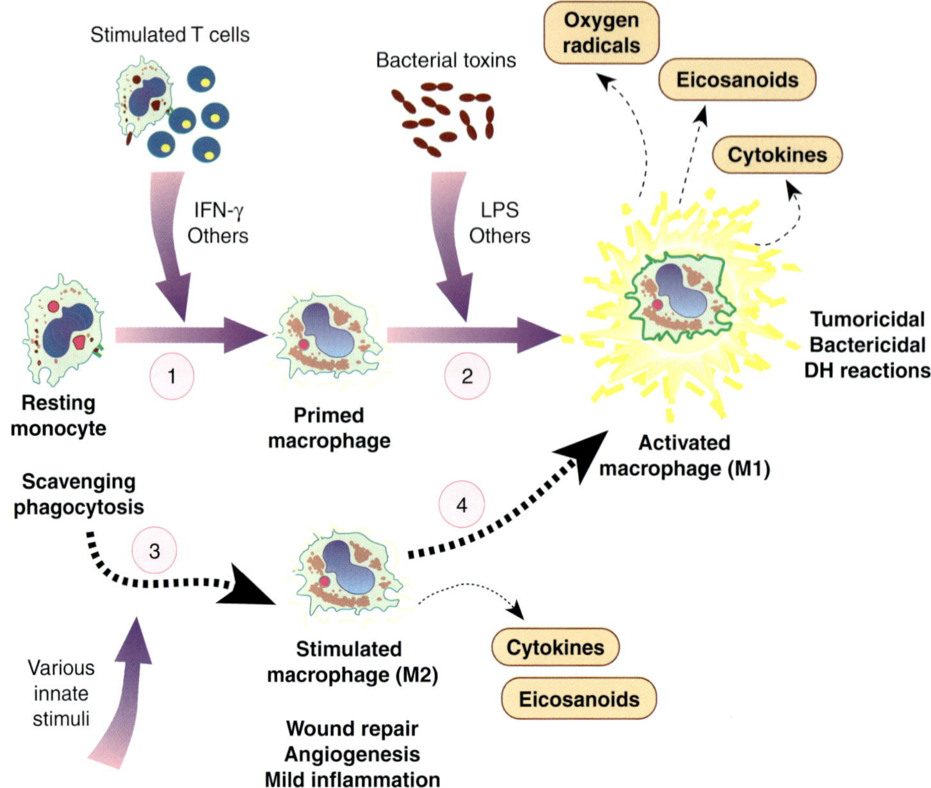

Figure 1-3 Schematic representation of macrophage activation pathway. Classically, *resting monocytes* are thought to be the principal type of noninflammatory scavenging phagocyte. **1,** Upon exposure to low levels of interferon gamma (IFN-γ) from T cells, monocytes become primed, upregulating human leukocyte antigen class II molecules for antigen presentation and performing other functions. **2,** *Fully activated macrophages (M1),* after exposure to bacterial lipopolysaccharide and interferon (classical activation), are bactericidal and tumoricidal and mediate severe inflammation. **3,** *Stimulated macrophages (M2)* result from resting monocyte activation by other innate stimuli, without exposure to IFN-γ (alternative activation). These cells are incompletely activated, producing low levels of cytokines and eicosanoids but not reactive oxygen intermediates. They participate in wound healing and angiogenesis and have immunoregulatory functions. **4,** Macrophages may switch between subsets (plasticity), depending on environmental signals. DH = delayed hypersensitivity; LPS = lipopolysaccharide. *(Illustration by Barb Cousins, modified by Joyce Zavarro.)*

and other matrix degradation factors; and to (2) angiogenesis through synthesis of angiogenic factors such as vascular endothelial growth factor.

Phagocyte Killing Mechanisms

Reactive oxygen intermediates

Under certain conditions, oxygen can undergo chemical modification into highly reactive substances with the potential to damage cellular molecules and inhibit functional properties in pathogens or host cells. Three of the most important oxygen intermediates are the superoxide anion, hydrogen peroxide, and the hydroxyl radical. Oxygen metabolites triggered by immune responses and generated by leukocytes, especially neutrophils and macrophages, are the most important source of free radicals during inflammation. Leukocyte oxygen metabolism can be initiated by a wide variety of stimuli, including

- innate triggers, such as LPS or fMLP
- adaptive effectors, such as complement-fixing antibodies or certain cytokines produced by activated T cells
- other chemical mediator systems, such as C5a, PAF, and leukotrienes

Reactive oxygen intermediates can also be generated as part of noninflammatory cellular biochemical processes, especially by electron transport in the mitochondria, detoxification of certain chemicals, or interactions with environmental light or radiation. These reactive intermediates are highly toxic to living pathogens and damage pathogenic mediators such as exotoxins and lipids.

Reactive nitrogen products

Nitric oxide (NO) is a highly reactive chemical species. Like reactive oxygen intermediates, NO is involved in various important biochemical functions in microorganisms and host cells. At high concentrations, NO has direct cytotoxic effects on pathogens. The formation of NO depends on the enzyme nitric oxide synthetase (NOS), which is in the cytosol and dependent on NADPH (the reduced form of nicotinamide adenine dinucleotide phosphate). Several types of NOS are known, including various forms of constitutive NOS and inducible NOS (iNOS). Activation induces enhanced production of NO in certain cells, especially macrophages, via the calcium-independent, induced synthesis of iNOS. Many innate and adaptive stimuli modulate induction of iNOS, especially cytokines and bacterial toxins.

Mediator Systems That Amplify Immune Responses

Although innate or adaptive effector responses may directly induce inflammation, in most cases this process must be amplified to produce overt clinical manifestations. Molecules generated within the host that induce and amplify inflammation are termed *inflammatory mediators,* and mediator systems include several categories of these molecules (Table 1-2). Most act on target cells through receptor-mediated processes, although some act in enzymatic cascades that interact in a complex fashion.

Table 1-2 Mediator Systems That Amplify Innate and Adaptive Immune Responses

Plasma-derived enzyme systems: complement, kinins, and fibrin
Vasoactive amines: serotonin and histamine
Lipid mediators: eicosanoids and platelet-activating factors
Cytokines
Neutrophil-derived granule products

Plasma-Derived Enzyme Systems

Complement

Complement is an important inflammatory mediator in the eye. Complement components account for approximately 5% of plasma protein and comprise more than 30 different proteins. Complement is activated by 1 of 3 pathways, and this activation generates products that contribute to the inflammatory process (Fig 1-4):

- *Classical pathway.* Activation occurs upon fixation of C1 by antigen–antibody (immune) complexes formed by IgM, IgG1, or IgG3. This pathway results in a connection between innate and adaptive immunity.
- *Alternative pathway.* Activation occurs continuously but is restricted by host complement regulatory proteins.
- *Mannose-binding lectin pathway.* This is activated by certain carbohydrate moieties on the cell wall of microorganisms.

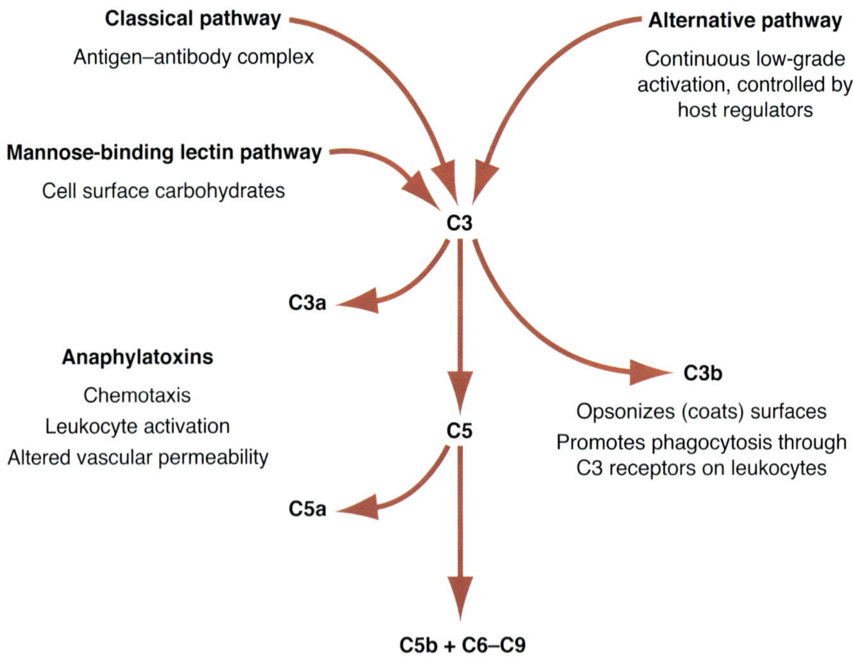

Figure 1-4 Overview of the essential intermediates of the complement pathway. C3a, C3b, C5a, and C5b are complement split products. C5b combines with intact C6, C7, C8, and C9 from the serum.

Complement serves the following 4 basic functions during inflammation:

- coats antigenic or pathogenic surfaces with C3b to enhance phagocytosis (opsonization)
- promotes lysis of cell membranes through pore formation by the membrane attack complex
- recruits neutrophils and induces inflammation through generation of the anaphylatoxins C3a and C5a
- modulates adaptive immune responses (effects on B and T cells)

Anaphylatoxin effects include chemotaxis, changes in cell adhesiveness, and degranulation and release of mediators from mast cells and platelets. C5a stimulates oxidative metabolism and the production and release of toxic oxygen radicals from leukocytes, as well as the extracellular discharge of leukocyte granule contents.

Defendi F, Thielens NM, Clavarino G, Cesbron JY, Dumestre-Pérard C. The immunopathology of complement proteins and innate immunity in autoimmune disease. *Clin Rev Allergy Immunol.* 2020;58(2):229–251.

Walport MJ. Complement. First of two parts. *N Engl J Med.* 2001;344(14):1058–1066.

Walport MJ. Complement. Second of two parts. *N Engl J Med.* 2001;344(15):1140–1144.

Fibrin and other plasma factors

Fibrin is the final deposition product of the coagulation pathway. Its deposition during inflammation promotes hemostasis, fibrosis, angiogenesis, and leukocyte adhesion. Fibrin is released from its circulating zymogen precursor, *fibrinogen,* upon cleavage by thrombin. In situ polymerization of smaller units gives rise to the characteristic fibrin plugs or clots. Fibrin dissolution is mediated by *plasmin.* Plasminogen is converted to its active form (plasmin) after cleavage by a tissue plasminogen activator. Thrombin, which is derived principally from platelet granules, is released after any vascular injury that causes platelet aggregation and release. Fibrin may be observed in severe anterior uveitis (the "plasmoid aqueous"), and it contributes to complications such as synechiae, cyclitic membranes, and traction retinal detachment.

Histamine

Histamine is present in the granules of mast cells and basophils and is actively secreted after exposure to a wide range of stimuli. Histamine acts by binding to 1 of at least 3 known types of receptors that are differentially present on target cells. The best-studied pathway for degranulation is antigen crosslinking of IgE bound to mast cell Fc IgE receptors, but many other inflammatory stimuli can induce histamine secretion, including complement, direct membrane injury, and certain drugs. Classically, histamine release has been associated with allergy. The contribution of histamine to intraocular inflammation remains subject to debate.

Lipid Mediators

Two groups of lipid molecules synthesized by stimulated cells act as powerful mediators and regulators of inflammatory responses: arachidonic acid (AA) metabolites, or

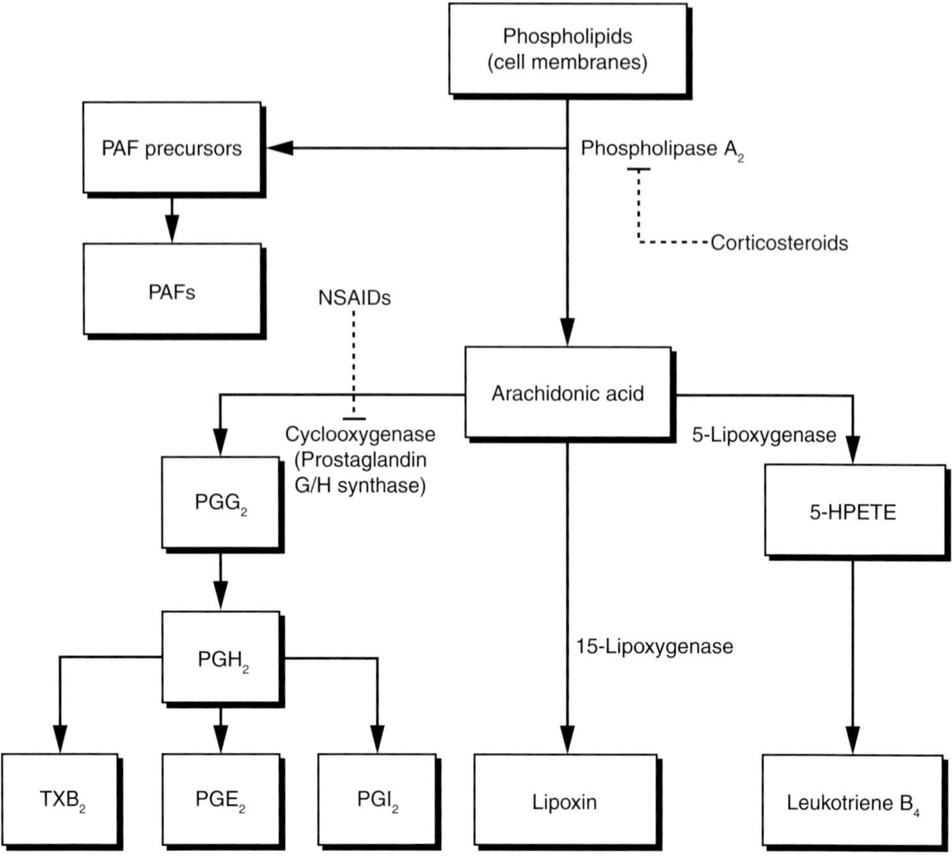

Figure 1-5 Overview of the essential intermediates of the eicosanoid and platelet-activating factor (PAF) pathways. 5-HPETE = 5-hydroperoxyeicosatetraenoic acid; NSAIDs = nonsteroidal anti-inflammatory drugs; PG = prostaglandin; TXB_2 = thromboxane B_2. *(Modified with permission from Pepose JS, Holland GN, Wilhelmus KR, eds.* Ocular Infection and Immunity. *Mosby; 1996.)*

eicosanoids, and acetylated triglycerides, usually called *platelet-activating factors (PAFs).* Both groups of molecules may be rapidly generated from the same lysophospholipid precursors by the enzymatic action of cellular phospholipases such as phospholipase A_2 (Fig 1-5).

Eicosanoids

All eicosanoids are derived from AA. AA is liberated from membrane phospholipids by phospholipase A_2, which is activated by various agonists. AA is oxidized by 2 major pathways to generate the various mediators:

- cyclooxygenase (COX) pathway, which produces prostaglandins, thromboxanes, and prostacyclins
- 5-lipoxygenase pathway, which produces 5-hydroperoxyeicosatetraenoic acid, lipoxins, and leukotrienes

Two forms of COX have been identified. COX-1 is thought to be constitutively expressed by many cells. COX-2 is inducible by various inflammatory stimuli (eg, LPS, PAF, and some cytokines). The COX-derived products are evanescent compounds induced in virtually all cells by a variety of stimuli. In general, they act in the immediate environment of their release to directly mediate many inflammatory activities. These include effects on vascular permeability, cell recruitment, platelet function, and smooth-muscle contraction. Prostaglandins may play a role in uveitic macular edema in association with anterior segment surgery or inflammation. Posterior diffusion of 1 or more of the eicosanoids through the vitreous is assumed to alter the permeability of the perifoveal capillary network, leading to macular edema. Clinical trials in humans suggest that topical treatment with COX inhibitors (eg, nonsteroidal anti-inflammatory drugs [NSAIDs]) reduces the incidence of macular edema after cataract surgery.

Derivatives of 5-lipoxygenase, an enzyme found mainly in granulocytes and some mast cells, have been detected in the brain and retina. Some leukotrienes have 1000 times the effect of histamine on vascular permeability. Another lipoxygenase product, lipoxin, is a potent stimulator of superoxide anion. Because many of the COX-derived prostaglandins downregulate the lipoxygenase pathway, NSAIDs can tilt AA metabolism toward increased production of inflammatory metabolites, leukotrienes, and lipoxins.

Platelet-activating factors

Platelet-activating factors are a family of phospholipid-derived mediators that appear to be important stimuli in the early stage of inflammation. Phospholipase A_2 metabolizes phosphocholine precursors in cell membranes, releasing AA and PAF precursors, which are acetylated into multiple species of PAF. PAF release is stimulated by various innate immune triggers, such as bacterial toxins, trauma, and cytokines. PAFs activate not only platelets but also most leukocytes, which in turn produce and release additional PAFs. PAFs function by binding to 1 or more guanosine triphosphate protein–associated receptors on target cells.

In vitro, PAFs induce an impressive repertoire of responses, including phagocytosis, exocytosis, superoxide production, chemotaxis, aggregation, proliferation, adhesion, eicosanoid generation, degranulation, and calcium mobilization, as well as diverse morphologic changes. PAFs are a major regulator of cell adhesion and vascular permeability in many forms of acute inflammation, trauma, shock, and ischemia. The precise role of PAFs in intraocular inflammation remains unknown, but synergistic interactions probably exist among PAFs, nitric oxide, eicosanoids, and cytokines. However, intravitreal injection of PAFs in animals induces an acute retinitis and photoreceptor toxicity.

Cytokines

Cytokines are soluble polypeptide mediators synthesized and released by cells for the purposes of intercellular signaling and communication, both within the innate immune system and between the innate and adaptive immune systems. Various types of intercellular signaling occur, including *paracrine* (signaling of neighboring cells at the same site), *autocrine* (stimulation of a receptor on its own surface, and *endocrine* (action on a distant site through release into the blood). Table 1-3 lists examples of cytokines associated with ocular inflammation.

Table 1-3 Cytokines of Relevance to Ocular Immunology

Family	Example	Major Cell Source	Major Target Cells	Major General Actions	Specific Ocular Actions/Clinical Relevance
Interleukins (ILs)	IL-1β	Monocytes Macrophages Neutrophils Dendritic cells T cells	Most leukocytes Various ocular cells	Induces cyclooxygenase type 2 leading to fever, vasodilatation, hypotension (shock) Promotes infiltration of inflammatory cells into extravascular space and tissues Promotes angiogenesis Induces IL-6 and IL-17 expression	Altered vascular permeability Neutrophil and macrophage infiltration Langerhans cell migration to central cornea Elevated levels in aqueous and serum in many forms of uveitis
	IL-2	Th0 or Th1 CD4 T lymphocytes	T lymphocytes B lymphocytes NK cells	Activates CD4 and CD8 T lymphocytes Induces Th1	Detectable levels in some forms of uveitis
	IL-4	Th2 CD4 T lymphocytes Basophils, mast cells	T lymphocytes B lymphocytes	Induces Th2, blocks Th1 Induces B lymphocytes to synthesize immunoglobulin E	Role in atopic and vernal conjunctivitis
	IL-5	Th2 CD4 T lymphocytes	Eosinophils	Recruits eosinophils	Role in atopic and vernal conjunctivitis
	IL-6	Monocytes Macrophages T lymphocytes Mast cells Endothelium	Most leukocytes Various ocular cells	Has many actions on B lymphocytes, including enhancement of antibody production Induces T-cell polarization Induces systemic toxicity (fever, shock, production of acute-phase proteins in liver)	Altered vascular permeability Neutrophil infiltration High levels in serum, aqueous, and vitreous in many forms of uveitis and nonuveitic diseases

Family	Example	Major Cell Source	Major Target Cells	Major General Actions	Specific Ocular Actions/Clinical Relevance
	IL-12/23 (IL-12 family)	Macrophages Dendritic cells B lymphocytes (IL-23) Endothelium (IL-23)	Naive CD4 T lymphocytes	Key Th1-inducing cytokine Activates NK cells Mediates chronic inflammation through promotion of Th17 lymphocytes	High expression in aqueous and vitreous from idiopathic uveitis cases High expression in serum in Behçet disease and VKH syndrome
	IL-17A	T lymphocytes (Th17, gamma-delta [γδ]) NK T lymphocytes	Most leukocytes Various ocular cells	Key cytokine of Th17 response, driving inflammation/tissue damage Induces proinflammatory cytokines, chemokines, and adhesion molecules Important driver of autoimmunity	High expression in patients with active uveitis, noninfectious (Behçet disease, birdshot chorioretinopathy, HLA-B27 uveitis, VKH syndrome) and infectious (toxoplasmic retinochoroiditis, viral retinitis) Leads to disruption of outer blood–retina barrier Role in infectious keratitis
α-Chemokines	IL-8/CXCL8	Many cell types	Endothelial cells Neutrophils Many others	Recruits and activates neutrophils Upregulates CAM on endothelium Chemotactic for basophils and T lymphocytes Promotes angiogenesis	High expression in inflamed eye Altered vascular permeability Neutrophil infiltration
β-Chemokines	Macrophage chemotactic protein-1/CCL2	Macrophages Endothelium RPE	Endothelial cells Macrophages T lymphocytes	Recruits and activates macrophages, some T lymphocytes	High expression in noninflamed and inflamed eyes Recruits macrophages and T lymphocytes to eye
Tumor necrosis factors (TNFs)	TNF-α or TNF-β	Macrophages T lymphocytes	Most leukocytes Various ocular cells	Tumor apoptosis Macrophage and neutrophil activation Cell adhesion and chemotaxis Fibrin deposition and vascular injury Systemic toxicity (fever, shock)	Altered vascular permeability Mononuclear cell infiltration

(Continued)

Table 1-3 *(continued)*

Family	Example	Major Cell Source	Major Target Cells	Major General Actions	Specific Ocular Actions/Clinical Relevance
Interferons (IFNs)	IFN-γ	Th1 cells NK cells	Macrophages Dendritic cells	Activates macrophages Facilitates Th1 development Mediates delayed-type hypersensitivity reactions	Neutrophil and macrophage infiltration MHC II upregulation on iris and ciliary epithelium, RPE
	IFN-α	Most leukocytes	Most parenchymal cells	Prevents viral infection of many cells Inhibits hemangioma, conjunctival intraepithelial neoplasia, and other tumors	Innate protection of ocular surface from viral infection Treatment of ocular surface neoplasms
Growth factors	Transforming growth factor β family (TGF-β)	Leukocytes RPE and NPE of ciliary body Pericytes Fibroblasts	Macrophages T lymphocytes RPE Glia Fibroblasts	Regulates immune response, suppresses T-lymphocyte and macrophage inflammatory functions Regulates wound repair: fibrosis	High expression in the noninflamed eye Regulator of immune privilege and ACAID
	Platelet-derived growth factors	Platelets Macrophages RPE	Fibroblasts Glia Many others	Fibroblast proliferation	Role in inflammatory membranes, subretinal fibrosis
	Vascular endothelial growth factor (VEGF) family	Macrophages Platelets Several retinal cells (RPE, astrocytes, Müller cells, vascular endothelium)	Vascular endothelial cells Leukocytes	Neovascularization and vascular permeability Leukocyte recruitment	Role in retinovascular disease (diabetic macular edema, exudative AMD, PDR, retinal vein occlusion, ROP) Corneal neovascularization and nerve growth
Neuropeptides	Substance P	Ocular nerves	Leukocytes Others	Pain Altered vascular permeability	Altered vascular permeability Leukocyte infiltration
	Vasoactive intestinal peptide	Ocular nerves	Leukocytes Others	Suppresses macrophage and T-lymphocyte inflammatory function	Role in ACAID and immune privilege

ACAID = anterior chamber–associated immune deviation; AMD = age-related macular degeneration; CAM = cell adhesion molecules; CCL = chemokine ligand; CXCL = C-X-C motif chemokine ligand; HLA = human leukocyte antigen; MHC = major histocompatibility complex; NK = natural killer; NPE = nonpigmented epithelium; PDR = proliferative diabetic retinopathy; RPE = retinal pigment epithelium; ROP = retinopathy of prematurity; Th = T helper; VKH = Vogt-Koyanagi-Harada.

Traditionally, investigators have divided cytokines into families with related activities, sources, and targets, using terms such as *growth factors, interleukins, lymphokines, interferons, monokines,* and *chemokines.* Thus, *growth factor* traditionally refers to cytokines that mediate cell proliferation and differentiation. The terms *interleukin* and *lymphokine* identify cytokines thought to mediate intercellular communication among lymphocytes or other leukocytes. Interferons are cytokines that limit or interfere with the ability of a virus to infect a cell. Monokines are immunoregulatory cytokines secreted by monocytes and macrophages. Chemokines are chemotactic cytokines. Although some cytokines are specific for particular cell types, most have high degrees of multiplicity and redundancy of source. For example, activated macrophages in an inflammatory site synthesize growth factors, interleukins, interferons, and chemokines.

Both innate and adaptive responses result in the production of cytokines. T lymphocytes are the classic cytokine-producing cell of adaptive immunity, but macrophages, mast cells, and neutrophils also synthesize a wide range of cytokines upon stimulation. Cytokine interactions can be additive, combinatorial, synergistic, or antagonistic. Elimination of the action of a single molecule may have an unpredictable outcome. For example, monoclonal antibodies directed against TNF-α result in substantial suppression of immune responses but also increase susceptibility to multiple sclerosis. Finally, cytokines not only act as mediators and amplifiers of inflammation in innate and adaptive immune responses but also modulate the initiation of immune responses; the function of most leukocytes is altered by preexposure to various cytokines. Thus, for many cytokines, their regulatory role may be as important as their actions as mediators of inflammation.

Targeting cytokines with monoclonal antibodies or soluble receptors has become an important and highly effective therapeutic strategy for combating inflammatory diseases (see Table 1-4 on the following pages). For example, TNF-α is a potent proinflammatory cytokine produced predominantly by activated monocytes, macrophages, and T cells that plays a role in the pathogenesis of several autoimmune diseases. Multiple TNF-α blockers are currently approved by the US Food and Drug Administration for the treatment of a number of inflammatory diseases, including noninfectious intermediate uveitis, posterior uveitis, and panuveitis (also see Chapter 6).

Neutrophils and Their Products

Neutrophils are a source of specialized products that can amplify immune responses. These products are discussed in the section "Neutrophil-derived granule products."

Table 1-4 Clinically Relevant Cytokine Inhibitors

Cytokine Targeted	Drug Examples	Drug Description	Route of Administration	FDA-Approved Indication	Ocular Relevance/Use
IL-1β	Anakinra	IL-1 receptor antagonist	Subcutaneous injection	Rheumatoid arthritis and several rare autoinflammatory conditions	Off-label use in Behçet disease
	Canakinumab	Human monoclonal Ab	Subcutaneous injection	JIA and periodic fever syndromes	Off-label use in Behçet disease
IL-6	Tocilizumab	Humanized monoclonal Ab	IV infusion or subcutaneous injection	Rheumatoid arthritis, giant cell arteritis, JIA, cytokine release syndrome	Off-label use in noninfectious intermediate, posterior, and panuveitis
IL-17A	Secukinumab	Human monoclonal Ab	Subcutaneous injection	Plaque psoriasis and psoriatic arthritis, ankylosing spondylitis	Failed to show efficacy in treatment of noninfectious intermediate, posterior, and panuveitis in randomized clinical trial
TNF-α	Adalimumab	Human monoclonal Ab	Subcutaneous injection	Rheumatoid arthritis; JIA; plaque psoriasis and psoriatic arthritis; ankylosing spondylitis; Crohn disease; ulcerative colitis; hidradenitis suppurativa; noninfectious intermediate, posterior, and panuveitis	On-label use in noninfectious intermediate, posterior, and panuveitis
	Infliximab	Chimeric monoclonal Ab	IV infusion	Crohn disease, ulcerative colitis, rheumatoid arthritis, ankylosing spondylitis, plaque psoriasis, psoriatic arthritis	Off-label use in noninfectious intermediate, posterior, and panuveitis

Cytokine Targeted	Drug Examples	Drug Description	Route of Administration	FDA-Approved Indication	Ocular Relevance/Use
VEGF-A	Bevacizumab	Humanized monoclonal Ab	IV infusion for FDA-approved indications; intravitreal injection for off-label ocular use	Metastatic colorectal cancer and several other cancers	Off-label use in retinovascular disease (neovascular AMD, diabetic retinopathy, diabetic macular edema, ROP, RVO) and refractory uveitic macular edema
	Ranibizumab	Humanized monoclonal Ab	Intravitreal injection	Neovascular AMD, macular edema following RVO, diabetic macular edema	In addition to FDA indications, off-label use in diabetic retinopathy, myopic CNV, refractory uveitic macular edema
	Aflibercept	Fusion protein with human VEGF receptors 1 and 2 fused to human Fc	Intravitreal injection	Neovascular AMD, macular edema following RVO, diabetic macular edema, diabetic retinopathy	In addition to FDA indications, off-label use in refractory uveitic macular edema

Ab = antibody; AMD = age-related macular degeneration; CNV = choroidal neovascularization; Fc = fragment, crystallizable; FDA = Food and Drug Administration; IL = interleukin; IV = intravenous; JIA = juvenile idiopathic arthritis; ROP = retinopathy of prematurity; RVO = retinal vein occlusion; TNF = tumor necrosis factor; VEGF = vascular endothelial growth factor.

CHAPTER 2

Immunization and Adaptive Immunity: The Immune Response Arc and Immune Effectors

Highlights

- Adaptive (or acquired) immunity involves a "learned" response to specific antigens rather than a response to conserved molecular patterns.
- The adaptive immune system continuously samples antigenic epitopes, determines whether they are self or nonself, and then mounts an immune response to eliminate foreign antigens.
- Conversion of an antigenic stimulus to an immune response involves activation of immune cells, particularly T and B lymphocytes, and development of immunologic memory for that specific antigen.
- The adaptive immune response comprises antibody-mediated responses, cell-mediated defense primarily coordinated by T lymphocytes, and combined antibody and cellular mechanisms.
- Cell-mediated responses (particularly T helper [Th]-1, Th2, and Th17 responses) are relevant to the immunopathology of several intraocular inflammatory conditions.

Definitions

The term *antigen* refers to a substance recognized by the immune system. The term *epitope* refers to each specific portion of an antigen to which an antibody molecule can bind. Antigenic epitopes exist on both native self tissues and foreign, or nonself, tissues. A complex, 3-dimensional protein has multiple antigenic epitopes that the immune system can recognize, as well as many other sites that remain unrecognizable and thus invisible to the immune system.

The adaptive immune response, unlike the innate immune response (discussed in Chapter 1), is a learned response to highly variable but specific antigenic epitopes rather

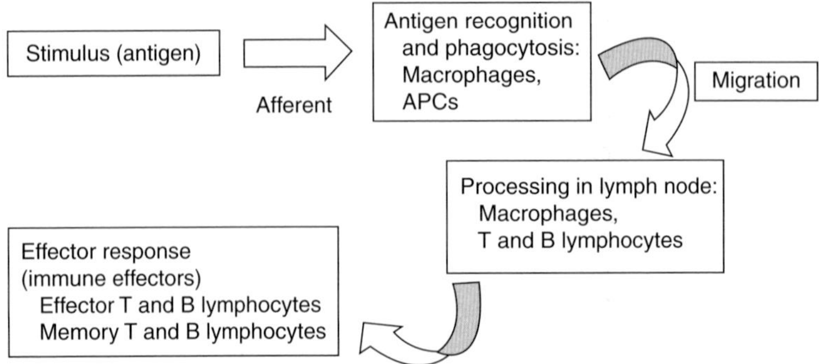

Figure 2-1 The immune response arc. APCs = antigen-presenting cells.

than a response to conserved molecular patterns. The purpose of the adaptive immune system is to continuously sample antigenic epitopes, determine whether they are self or non-self, and then mount an immune response to eliminate foreign antigens. The immune response arc—the interaction between antigen and the adaptive immune system—can be divided into 3 phases: afferent, processing, and effector (Fig 2-1).

Phases of the Immune Response Arc

Afferent Phase

The afferent phase of the immune response arc comprises the initial recognition, transport, and presentation of antigenic substances to the adaptive immune system. Recognition starts with antigen-presenting cells (APCs), specialized cells that bind antigen at a peripheral site. After the APC receives stimulatory signals (ie, complement), phagocytosis of the antigen occurs, as discussed in Chapter 1. Following ingestion of antigen, APCs migrate via afferent lymphatics to regional lymph nodes.

In the APCs, enzymatic digestion of proteins within endocytic vesicles produces antigenic epitope fragments of 7–11 amino acids (Fig 2-2). Each antigenic fragment binds to a groove-shaped human leukocyte antigen (HLA) peptide residing on the APC surface. The combination of antigenic peptide and HLA protein is recognized by the T-lymphocyte receptors CD4 and CD8. HLA molecules differ in their capacity to bind various antigenic peptide fragments within their grooves; thus, the HLA type determines the array of peptide antigens that can be presented to T lymphocytes. Specific HLA alleles are important risk factors for certain forms of uveitis. See Chapter 4 for further discussion of HLA molecules and disease susceptibility.

HLA peptides are part of a family of cell surface glycoproteins called *major histocompatibility complex (MHC) proteins.* In humans, MHC proteins are termed *human leukocyte antigen (HLA) molecules.* HLA class I molecules (ie, HLA-A, -B, and -C) serve as the antigen-presenting platform for $CD8^+$ T lymphocytes, which are essentially cytotoxic T cells (see Fig 2-2A). Class I molecules are present on almost all nucleated cells and generally function to process peptide antigens synthesized by the host cell. If these presented antigens are

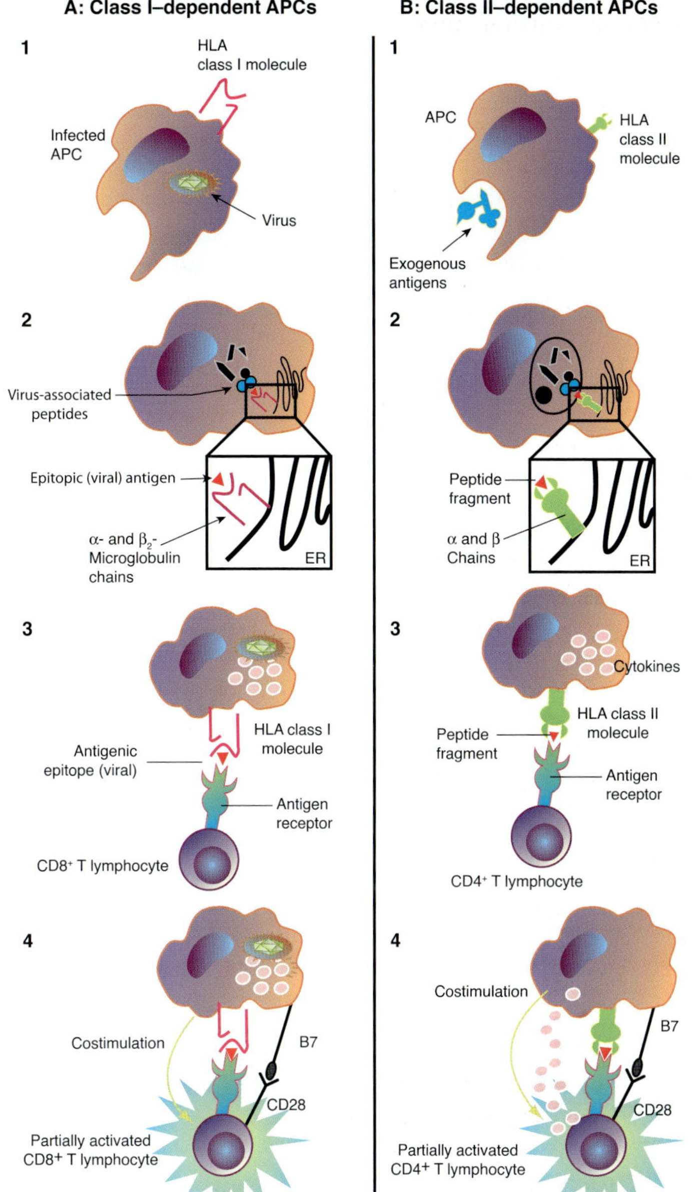

Figure 2-2 **A,** Class I–dependent APCs. **1,** APC is infected by a virus, which causes the cell to synthesize virus-associated peptides that are present in the cytosol. **2,** The viral antigen is transported through specialized transport systems into the endoplasmic reticulum (ER), where the viral antigen encounters human leukocyte antigen (HLA) class I molecules. The antigenic fragment binds to the groove formed by the α chain of the HLA class I molecule. Unlike class II molecules, the second chain, called *β_2-microglobulin,* is constant among all class I molecules. **3,** The CD8 T-lymphocyte receptor recognizes the fragment–class I complex displayed on the cell membrane. **4,** With the help of costimulatory molecules such as CD28-B7 and cytokines, the $CD8^+$ T lymphocyte becomes primed, or partially activated. A similar mechanism is used to recognize tumor antigens that are produced by cells after malignant transformation. **B,** Class II–dependent APCs. **1,** APCs endocytose exogenous antigens into the ER. **2,** In the ER, the antigen is digested, generating peptide fragments that bind to the groove formed by the α and β chains of the HLA class II molecule. **3,** The $CD4^+$ T-lymphocyte receptor recognizes the fragment–class II complex. **4,** With the help of costimulatory molecules such as CD28-B7 and cytokines, the $CD4^+$ T lymphocyte becomes primed, or partially activated. *(Illustration by Barb Cousins, modified by Joyce Zavarro.)*

recognized as self (ie, normal host protein), no immune reaction occurs. However, if there is an alteration of the normal host peptide (termed *altered self*), by tumor or viral peptides after host cell invasion, an immune response is initiated. A viral infection, a neoplasm, or simply a genetic mutation that alters protein structure may induce autoimmunity by stimulating an inappropriate immune response to normal host proteins.

HLA class II molecules (ie, HLA-DR, -DP, and -DQ) serve as the antigen-presenting platform for $CD4^+$, or *helper*, T lymphocytes (see Fig 2-2B). The antigen receptor on the helper T lymphocyte recognizes peptide antigens only if the antigens are presented with class II molecules simultaneously. Only certain cell types express HLA class II molecules. Macrophages and dendritic cells are the most important of these types, although B lymphocytes also may function as class II–dependent APCs, especially within a lymph node. Class II–dependent APCs are considered the most efficient APCs for processing extracellular protein antigens; that is, antigens that have been phagocytosed from the external environment (eg, bacterial or fungal antigens).

Processing Phase

The conversion of an antigenic stimulus into an immunologic response occurs through *priming* of naive B and T lymphocytes (lymphocytes that have not yet encountered their specific antigen) within lymph nodes and the spleen. Processing involves regulation of the interaction between antigen and naive lymphocytes, followed by lymphocyte *activation,* which consists of lymphocyte proliferation and differentiation (Fig 2-3).

Preconditions necessary for processing

The principal cell type for immune processing is the $CD4^+$ T lymphocyte. These lymphocytes have a receptor that detects antigen only upon formation of a trimolecular complex consisting of an HLA class II molecule, a processed antigenic fragment, and a T-lymphocyte antigen receptor (see Fig 2-2B). The $CD4^+$ molecule stabilizes binding and enhances signaling between the HLA complex on the APC and the T-lymphocyte receptor. When helper T lymphocytes recognize their specific antigen, they become primed, or partially activated, acquiring new functional properties, including cell division, cytokine synthesis, and cell membrane expression of *accessory molecules,* such as cell adhesion molecules and costimulatory molecules. The synthesis and release of immune cytokines, especially interleukin (IL)-2, by T lymphocytes is crucial for the progression of initial activation and the functional differentiation of T lymphocytes through autocrine stimulation.

Helper T-lymphocyte differentiation

Prior to priming, $CD4^+$ T lymphocytes are classified as T helper (Th)-0 cells. These cells can differentiate into 1 of at least 4 functional subtypes—Th1, Th2, Th17, or T regulatory (Treg)—based on the pattern of cytokines to which they are exposed (Fig 2-4). Each helper T-cell subtype, in turn, produces a characteristic profile of cytokines that is regulated by the expression of subtype-specific transcription factors.

Th1 cells participate in the elimination of intracellular pathogens as well as in cell-mediated and delayed hypersensitivity reactions. Th1 cells secrete interferon gamma (IFN-γ), IL-2, and tumor necrosis factor α and β (TNF-α, TNF-β).

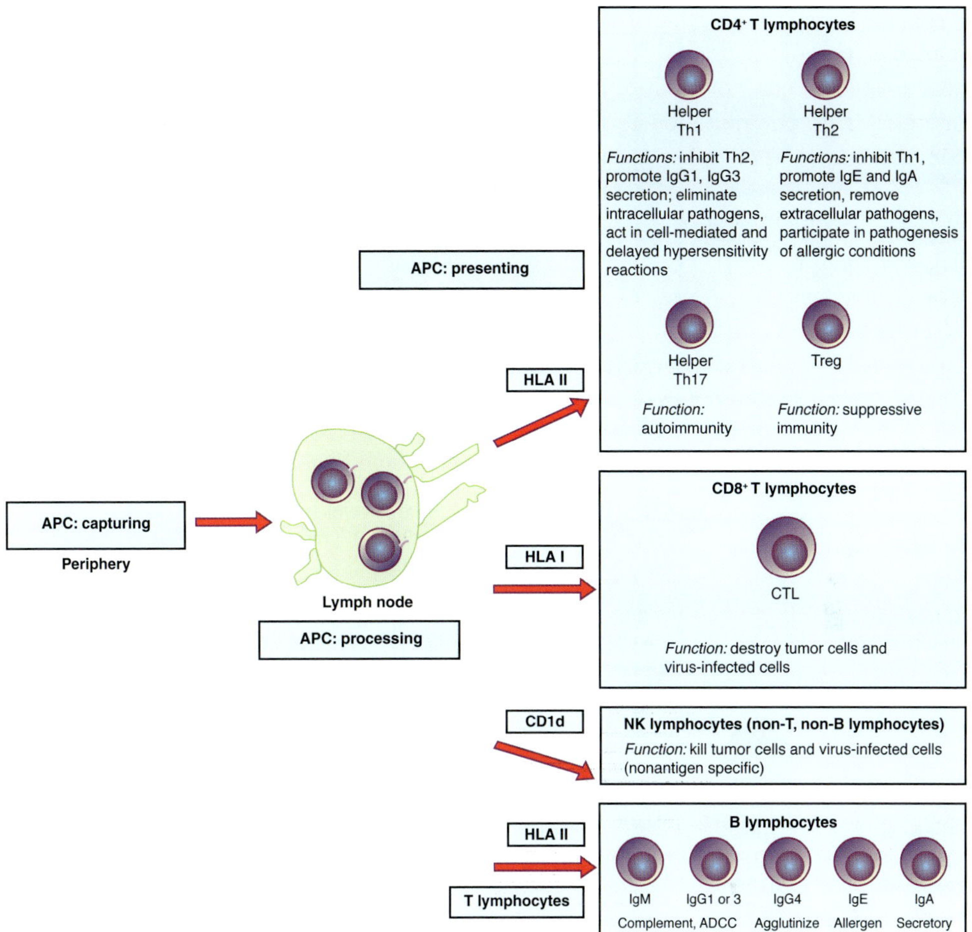

Figure 2-3 Schematic illustration of immune processing of antigen within the lymph node. On exposure to antigen and APCs within the lymph node, the 3 major lymphocyte subsets—B lymphocytes, CD4+ T lymphocytes, and CD8+ T lymphocytes—and natural killer (NK) (non-T, non-B) lymphocytes are activated to release specific cytokines and perform particular activities. Antigen presented by HLA class II molecules stimulates CD4+ T lymphocytes to differentiate into 1 of at least 4 subtypes: T helper (Th)-1, Th2, Th17, or T regulatory (Treg).

Naive CD8+ T cells become cytotoxic T lymphocytes (CTLs), and non-T, non-B lymphocytes become NK lymphocytes. B lymphocytes are stimulated to produce 1 of the various antibody isotypes, whose functions may include complement activation, antibody-dependent cellular cytotoxicity (ADCC), agglutination, allergen recognition, and/or secretory release. Ig = immunoglobulin. *(Illustration by Barb Cousins, modified by Joyce Zavarro.)*

Th2 cells are involved in the clearance of extracellular pathogens and play an important role in the pathogenesis of allergic conditions such as asthma. Th2 cells produce IL-4, IL-5, and IL-13 but not Th1 cytokines.

Th17 cells contribute to immunity against certain extracellular bacteria and fungi and play a role in the defense of mucosal surfaces. Th17 cells produce IL-17, IL-21,

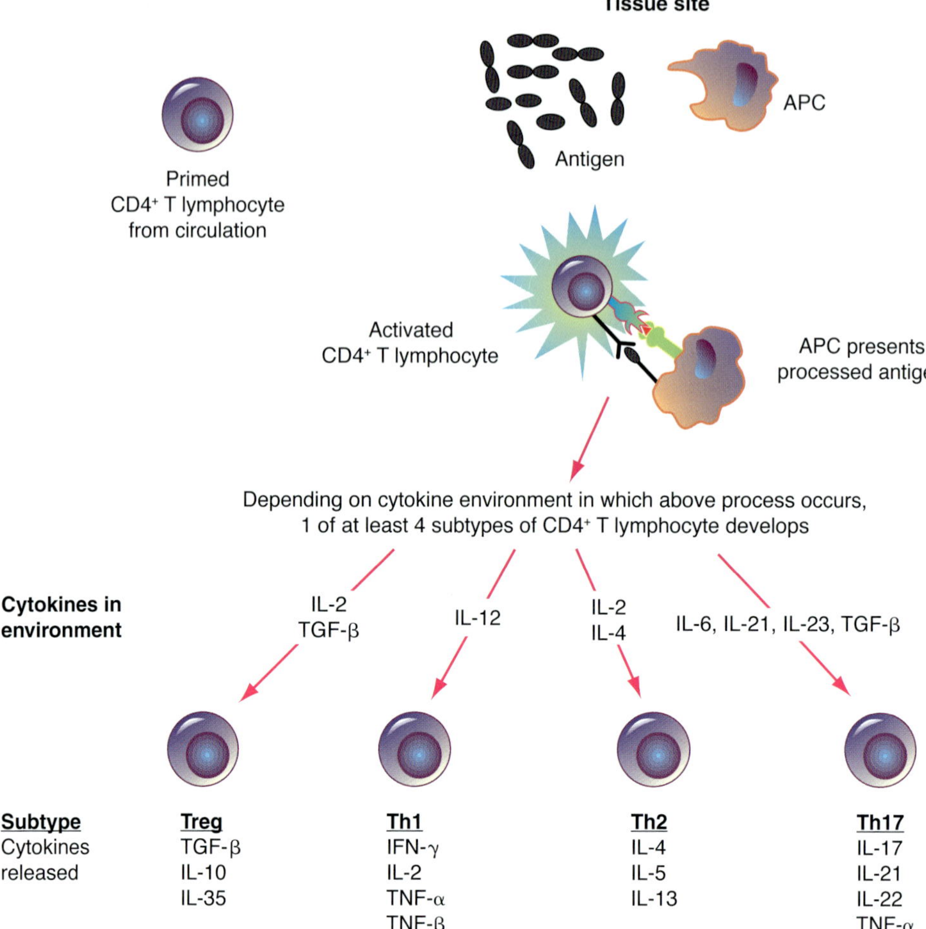

Figure 2-4 Schematic representation of CD4+ T-lymphocyte development. After initial priming in the lymph node, CD4+ T lymphocytes enter the tissue site, where they again encounter APCs containing processed antigen. Upon restimulation and depending on the cytokines present in the local environment at the time of restimulation, CD4+ T lymphocytes become activated into 1 of at least 4 subtypes. Tregs suppress other T-cell responses. Th1 lymphocytes are the classic delayed hypersensitivity effector cells and mediate interferon gamma (IFN-γ)–driven responses. Th2 lymphocytes are thought to be less intensively inflammatory and have been associated with granuloma formation in response to parasite-derived antigens, as well as manifestations of atopic diseases. Th17 lymphocytes mediate and sustain inflammation. IL = interleukin; TGF = transforming growth factor. *(Illustration developed by Russell W. Read, MD, PhD.)*

IL-22, and TNF-α, in association with several transcription factors, including retinoic acid receptor–related orphan receptor-γt and receptor-α (ROR-γt and -α). Dysregulation of Th17 proinflammatory cytokines IL-17 and IL-22 has been implicated in the pathogenesis of systemic inflammatory diseases, such as psoriasis, rheumatoid arthritis, multiple sclerosis, inflammatory bowel disease, Sjögren syndrome, Behçet disease, and systemic lupus erythematosus, as well as in uveitis and scleritis.

Treg cells are essential for maintaining peripheral tolerance to autoantigens (also called *self antigens*), thereby preventing autoimmune diseases and limiting chronic inflammatory diseases. Treg cells suppress excessive immune responses deleterious to the host and downregulate autoreactive T cells. Treg cells are identified by their simultaneous expression of CD4, CD25, and Foxp3. The suppressive cytokines transforming growth factor β and IL-10 have been implicated as active players in the effector function of Treg cells as regulators of inflammation.

An imbalance between regulatory mechanisms that inhibit the immune system and proinflammatory responses is thought to be the underlying cause of uveitis and many other immune-mediated diseases. The cytokine profiles produced by these various helper T-cell subtypes determine subsequent immune processing, B-lymphocyte antibody synthesis, and cell-mediated effector responses. For example, IFN-γ produced by Th1 lymphocytes inhibits the Th2 response, whereas IL-4 produced by Th2 lymphocytes inhibits the Th1 response. The process determining whether a Th1 or a Th2 response develops with exposure to a specific antigen is not entirely understood, but presumed variables include cytokines preexisting in the microenvironment, the nature and amount of antigen encountered, and the type of APC involved. For example, IL-12, which is produced by macrophage APCs, might preferentially induce Th1 responses.

Abbas AK, Lichtman AH, Pillai S. *Cellular and Molecular Immunology*. 9th ed. Elsevier/Saunders; 2018.

Amadi-Obi A, Yu CR, Liu X, et al. Th17 cells contribute to uveitis and scleritis and are expanded by IL-2 and inhibited by IL-27/STAT1. *Nat Med.* 2007;13(6):711–718.

Caspi RR. Understanding autoimmunity in the eye: from animal models to novel therapies. *Discov Med.* 2014;17(93):155–162.

B-lymphocyte activation

A major function of helper T lymphocytes is B-lymphocyte activation. B lymphocytes are responsible for producing antibodies, or immunoglobulin (Ig) molecules (glycoproteins that bind to the specific antigens or epitopes that induced their synthesis). These antibodies contain an epitope-specific binding site, termed *paratope,* on the Fab (*f*ragment, *a*ntigen-*b*inding) portion of the molecule. B lymphocytes begin as naive lymphocytes; IgM and IgD are expressed on their cell surface and serve as B-lymphocyte antigen receptors. Through these surface antibodies, B lymphocytes detect epitopes on intact antigens *without* the requirement of antigen processing by APCs. After appropriate stimulation of the B-lymphocyte antigen receptor, helper T lymphocyte–B lymphocyte interaction occurs, leading to further B-lymphocyte activation and differentiation. B lymphocytes acquire new functional properties, such as cell division, cell surface expression of accessory molecules, and synthesis of large quantities of antibody. The terminal form of B-lymphocyte differentiation is the plasma cell, which secretes antibodies, or immunoglobulins. Activated B lymphocytes acquire the ability to switch their surface IgM antibodies to another immunoglobulin class (eg, IgG, IgA, or IgE). This class shift requires a molecular change in the immunoglobulin heavy chain and is regulated by specific cytokines released by the helper T lymphocyte. For example, the cytokine IFN-γ induces a switch from IgM to IgG1 production in an antigen-primed B lymphocyte, whereas treatment with IL-4 induces a switch from IgM to IgE.

Effector Phase

The elimination or neutralization of foreign antigen, which is the purpose of the adaptive immune response, is accomplished during the effector phase. Antigen-specific effectors exist in 2 major subsets (Fig 2-5):

- T lymphocytes, including delayed hypersensitivity and cytotoxic T lymphocytes
- B lymphocytes and the antibodies produced by their derived plasma cells

A third subset of effector lymphocytes—grouped as non-T, non-B lymphocytes—includes natural killer cells, lymphokine-activated cells, and killer cells (see Fig 2-3).

Effector lymphocytes require 2 exposures to antigen for maximum effectiveness. The initial (*priming* or *activation*) exposure occurs in the lymph node. The second *(restimulation)* exposure occurs in the peripheral tissue from which the antigen originated.

Delayed hypersensitivity T lymphocytes usually express the cell marker CD4 and release IFN-γ and TNF-β. Cytotoxic T lymphocytes express CD8 and kill tumor cells and virus-infected host cells. See the section Lymphocyte-Mediated Effector Responses for further discussion of these cells.

The B-lymphocyte effector response is mediated by antibodies produced by plasma cells. Antibodies are released into the efferent lymph fluid (downstream from lymph nodes), draining into the venous circulation. Once bound to their specific epitope, antibodies

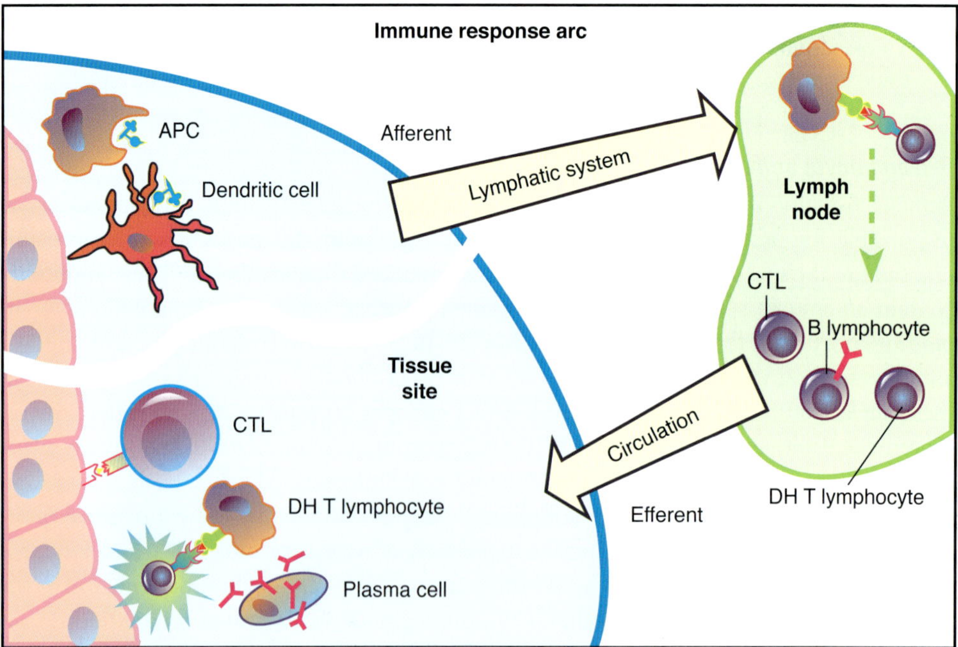

Figure 2-5 Schematic representation of effector mechanisms during the adaptive immune response. The tissue site *(left)* is not only where the immune response is initiated but is also ultimately where the immune response arc is completed—when effectors encounter antigen within tissue after their release from the lymph node *(right)* into the circulation. The 3 most important effector mechanisms of adaptive immunity are CTLs, delayed hypersensitivity (DH) T lymphocytes ($CD4^+$ T lymphocytes), and antibody-producing plasma cells derived from B lymphocytes. *(Illustration by Barb Cousins, modified by Joyce Zavarro.)*

mediate a variety of effector activities, including opsonization for phagocytosis and complement activation via the classical pathway.

The Immune Response Arc and Primary or Secondary Immune Response

Immunologic memory is the most distinctive feature of adaptive immunity. Protective immunization is the prototypical example of this powerful phenomenon.

Differences Between Primary and Secondary Responses

The immune response that occurs on the second or subsequent encounter with an antigen *(anamnestic response)* is regulated differently from that occurring on the first encounter. During the processing phase of the primary response, relatively rare antigen-specific B lymphocytes (perhaps 1 in 100,000 B lymphocytes) and T lymphocytes (perhaps 1 in 10,000 T lymphocytes) must come in contact with appropriately presented antigen. Stimulation of these cells from a completely resting and naive state then occurs, a process that requires days. Following the primary response, various events occur that set the stage for a subsequent rapid and robust secondary response:

- Following stimulation, lymphocytes divide, dramatically increasing the population of antigen-responsive T and B lymphocytes *(clonal expansion),* and migrate to other sites of potential encounter with antigen.
- Upon removal of antigen, T and B lymphocytes activated during the primary response gradually return to a resting state but are no longer naive. They retain the capacity to become reactivated within 12–24 hours of antigen exposure and thus are termed *memory cells.*
- Memory lymphocytes express higher levels of certain cell adhesion molecules, such as integrins, than do naive lymphocytes. Expression of these cell adhesion molecules facilitates *homing,* or migration into target tissues.
- IgM produced during the primary response may be too large to leak passively into a peripheral site. Following antibody-class switching, IgG or other isotypes can leak passively into or be produced at the site; thus, they can immediately bind to antigen and trigger a rapid secondary response.
- In some cases, such as in mycobacterial infection, low doses of antigen may remain in the node or site, producing a chronic, low-level antigenic stimulation of T and B lymphocytes. See Clinical Example 2-1.

CLINICAL EXAMPLE 2-1

Primary and Secondary Response to Tuberculosis

The afferent phase of the primary response begins when alveolar macrophages ingest *Mycobacterium tuberculosis* within the lung and then transport the organisms to the hilar lymph nodes. As T and B lymphocytes

(Continued on next page)

(continued)

are primed, the hilar nodes become enlarged. The effector phase begins when the primed T lymphocytes recirculate and enter the infected lung. The T lymphocytes interact with macrophage-ingested bacteria, and cytokines are released that activate neighboring macrophages to differentiate into epithelioid cells, which fuse to form giant cells, eventually forming caseating granulomas. Meanwhile, some effector T lymphocytes become inactive memory T lymphocytes.

A secondary response in the skin is the basis of the tuberculin skin test used to diagnose tuberculosis (TB). The afferent phase of the secondary response begins when a purified protein derivative (PPD) reagent (antigens purified from nontuberculous mycobacteria) is taken up by dermal macrophages after injection. The secondary processing phase begins when the PPD-stimulated macrophages migrate into the draining lymph node, where they encounter memory T lymphocytes, which then reactivate.

The secondary effector phase commences when the reactivated memory T lymphocytes recirculate and home to the dermis, where they encounter additional antigen and macrophages at the injection site, causing the T lymphocytes to become fully activated and release cytokines. Within 24–72 hours, the cytokines induce infiltration of additional lymphocytes and monocytes as well as fibrin clotting. This process produces the typical indurated dermal lesion of the TB skin test, called the *tuberculin form* of delayed hypersensitivity.

Effector Responses and Mechanisms of Adaptive Immunity

In 1962, Gell and Coombs elaborated on 4 mechanisms of adaptive immune-triggered inflammatory responses, creating a classification of allergic reactions comprising types I through IV:

- anaphylaxis
- antibody-dependent cellular cytotoxicity
- immune complex-mediated reactions
- cell-mediated reactions

Familiarity with Gell and Coombs' classifications is important for understanding older literature. However, it is more accurate to divide the effector responses of adaptive immunity into 3 main categories:

- antibody-mediated effector responses
- lymphocyte-mediated effector responses (delayed hypersensitivity, cytotoxic lymphocytes)
- combined antibody and cellular mechanisms

Delves PJ, Martin SJ, Burton DR, Roitt IM. *Roitt's Essential Immunology.* 13th ed. Wiley-Blackwell; 2017.

Owen JA, Punt J, Stranford SA. *Kuby Immunology.* 7th ed. WH Freeman; 2013.

Antibody-Mediated Effector Responses

Structural and functional properties of antibody molecules

Structural features of immunoglobulins There are 5 major classes or isotypes of immunoglobulins (M, G, A, E, and D). IgG and IgA can be further divided into subclasses (IgG1, IgG2, IgG3, IgG4, IgA1, and IgA2). The basic immunoglobulin structure, referred to as a *monomer,* is composed of 4 covalently bonded glycoprotein chains (Fig 2-6):

- 2 identical light chains, either kappa (κ) or lambda (λ)
- 2 identical heavy chains

Each monomer is approximately 150,000–180,000 Da. The type of heavy chain defines the specific immunoglobulin isotype or subclass. IgM can form pentamers or hexamers in vivo, and IgA can form dimers in secretions, so the in vivo molecular size of these 2 classes is much larger than that of the others.

Antibodies contain regions called *domains* that carry out the specific functions of the antibody molecule. The Fab region (2 of which are present on each molecule) contains the antigen-binding domain, called the *variable region.* The opposite end of the molecule, on the heavy chain portion, contains the attachment site for effector cells (the *Fc* [*f*ragment crystallizable] *portion*). It also contains the site of other effector functions, such as complement fixation (for IgG3) or binding to a secretory component for transportation through epithelia and secretion into tears (for IgA). Table 2-1 summarizes key differences between immunoglobulin isotypes.

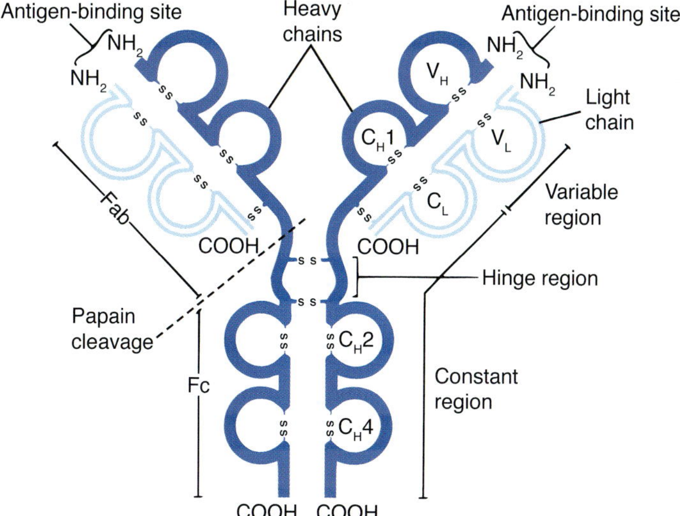

Figure 2-6 Schematic representation of an immunoglobulin molecule. The *solid lines* indicate the 2 identical heavy chains; the *light-blue double lines* indicate the identical light chains; *-ss-* indicates intrachain and interchain covalent disulfide bonds. Fab = *f*ragment, *a*ntigen-*b*inding region; Fc = *f*ragment *c*rystallizable region (attachment site for effector cells). *(Reproduced with permission from* Dorland's Illustrated Medical Dictionary. *32nd ed. Elsevier/Saunders; 2012:921.)*

Table 2-1 Structural and Functional Properties of Immunoglobulin Isotypes

Immunoglobulin (Ig) Isotype	Percentage of Total Serum Immunoglobulins	Structural Features	Functions
IgD	<1%	Mostly on surface of B lymphocytes	B-lymphocyte antigen receptor
IgM	5%	Mostly on surface of B lymphocytes or intravascular	B-lymphocyte antigen receptor, agglutination, neutralization, intravascular cytolysis, classical complement pathway activation
IgG	77%	Intravascular, in tissues; crosses placenta	Cytolysis (IgG1, IgG3), ADCC (IgG2, IgG3), agglutination (IgG3), neutralization (IgG4), classical complement pathway activation (IgG1, IgG3)
IgE	<1%	Mostly in skin or mucosa; bound to mast cells	Mast cell degranulation
IgA	18%	In mucosal secretions, binds secretory component in subepithelial tissues for transepithelial transport and protection from proteolysis	Mucosal immunity, neutralization, alternative complement pathway activation

ADCC = antibody-dependent cellular cytotoxicity.

Functional properties of immunoglobulins Immunoglobulin isotypes differ in how they mediate antibody effector functions. Human IgM and IgG3 are good complement activators, whereas IgG4 is not. Only IgA can bind the secretory component and be actively passed into mucosal secretions. The importance of these differences is that 2 antibodies with identical capacity to bind to an antigen—but of different isotype—will produce different effector and inflammatory outcomes.

Terminology

Clonality Each B cell creates a unique Fab fragment that recognizes a single antigenic configuration. Clonal expansion, or proliferation of an individual B lymphocyte via cell division, results in a population of identical B cells that recognize the same epitope, termed a *monoclonal* population. Biologic drugs such as infliximab, adalimumab, and rituximab are examples of recombinant monoclonal antibodies that specifically target immune system molecules (see Chapter 6). However, the typical immune response is a *polyclonal response* since many individual B cells will recognize various epitopes on the same substance, and each B cell will undergo simultaneous clonal expansion.

Idiotypes Because they are proteins, antibodies themselves can be antigenic. Their antigenic sites are called *idiotopes,* as distinguished from *epitopes,* the antigenic sites on foreign molecules. Anti-idiotypic antibodies may function as feedback mechanisms for immune regulation and have clinical significance for modern biologic therapies. Infliximab, for example, is a monoclonal chimeric (mouse and human) antibody to TNF-α that is used to treat some forms of uveitis. Efficacy of this drug may be limited by the development of anti-idiotypic antibodies that neutralize the antigen-binding site for TNF-α.

Infiltration of B lymphocytes into tissues and local production of antibody

B-lymphocyte infiltration B lymphocytes can infiltrate the site of an immunologic reaction in response to persistent antigenic stimulus. If the process becomes chronic, plasma cell formation occurs, with local production of antibody specific for the inciting antigen(s). Assessment of local antibody production can serve as a diagnostic test (see Clinical Example 2-2) when the antigen is known or suspected, as in the case of a presumed infection.

CLINICAL EXAMPLE 2-2

The Clinical Significance of Local Antibody Production

Distinguishing between local production of antibody and passive leakage of antibody from the blood to the intraocular compartment involves determination of the *Goldmann-Witmer (GW) coefficient.* This is calculated by comparing the ratio of specific IgG antibody present in intraocular fluid to the total IgG level in intraocular fluid versus the ratio of specific IgG level in serum to the total IgG level in serum:

GW Coefficient = (Intraocular Specific IgG/Intraocular Total IgG) / (Serum Specific IgG/Serum Total IgG)

(Continued on next page)

(continued)

Quentin and Reiber used the GW coefficient to demonstrate that aqueous from eyes with Fuchs uveitis syndrome had markedly elevated intraocular IgG titers to rubella virus compared with levels found in controls. The average GW coefficient was 20.6 in patients with Fuchs uveitis syndrome, compared with less than 1.5 in controls.

Quentin CD, Reiber H. Fuchs heterochromic cyclitis: rubella virus antibodies and genome in aqueous humor. *Am J Ophthalmol.* 2004;138(1):46–54.

Local antibody production within a tissue and chronic inflammation Persistence of antigen within a site, coupled with infiltration of specific B lymphocytes and local antibody formation, can produce a chronic inflammatory reaction called the *chronic Arthus reaction.* The histologic pattern often demonstrates lymphocytic infiltration, plasma cell infiltration, and granulomatous features. This type of chronic inflammation may contribute to the pathophysiology of certain chronic autoimmune disorders, such as rheumatoid arthritis, which feature formation of pathogenic antibodies.

Abbas AK, Lichtman AH, Pillai S. *Cellular and Molecular Immunology.* 9th ed. Elsevier/Saunders; 2018.

Mousa HM, Saban DR, Foster CS, Cordero-Coma M, Streilein JW. Allergy and immune-mediated tissue injury. In: Albert DM, Miller JW, Azar DT, Young LH, eds. *Albert and Jakobiec's Principles and Practice of Ophthalmology.* 4th ed. Springer; 2022:837–855.

Lymphocyte-Mediated Effector Responses

Delayed hypersensitivity T lymphocytes

Delayed hypersensitivity (DH) represents the prototypical adaptive immune mechanism for lymphocyte-triggered inflammation. It is especially powerful in secondary immune responses. Previously primed DH $CD4^+$ T lymphocytes leave the lymph node, home to local tissues where antigen persists, and become activated by restimulation with the specific priming antigen and HLA class II–expressing APCs. Fully activated DH T lymphocytes secrete mediators and cytokines (see Fig 2-4), leading to the recruitment and activation of macrophages and/or other nonspecific leukocytes. The term *delayed* for this type of hypersensitivity refers to the fact that the reaction becomes maximal 12–48 hours after antigen exposure.

Just as helper T lymphocytes can be divided into 3 subsets—Th1, Th2, and Th17—according to the spectrum of cytokines they secrete, DH T lymphocytes can also be grouped by the same criteria. Experimentally, Th1 cytokines, especially IFN-γ (also known as *macrophage-activating factor*) and TNF-α, activate macrophages to secrete inflammatory mediators and kill pathogens, thus amplifying inflammation. Th1-mediated DH effector mechanisms, therefore, are thought to produce the following effects:

- the classic DH reaction (eg, the PPD skin reaction)
- immune responses to intracellular infections (eg, to mycobacteria or *Pneumocystis* organisms)

Table 2-2 Ocular Inflammatory Diseases Likely Involving Th1-Mediated Delayed Hypersensitivity Effector Mechanisms

Site	Disease	Presumed Antigen
Conjunctiva	Contact hypersensitivity to contact lens solutions	Thimerosal or other chemicals
	Giant papillary conjunctivitis	Unknown
	Phlyctenulosis	Bacterial antigens
Cornea and sclera	Chronic allograft rejection	Histocompatibility antigens
	Marginal infiltrates of blepharitis	Bacterial antigens
	Disciform keratitis after viral infection	Viral antigens
Anterior uvea	Acute anterior uveitis	Uveal autoantigens, bacterial antigens
	Sarcoidosis-associated uveitis	Unknown
	Idiopathic intermediate uveitis	Unknown
Retina and choroid	Sympathetic ophthalmia	Uveal or retinal autoantigens
	Vogt-Koyanagi-Harada syndrome	Uveal or retinal autoantigens
	Birdshot chorioretinopathy	Retinal or uveal autoantigens
Orbit	Acute thyroid orbitopathy	Probably thyrotropin receptor
	Giant cell arteritis	Unknown

Th = T helper.

- immune responses to fungal infections
- most forms of severe T-lymphocyte–mediated autoimmune diseases
- chronic transplant rejection

Table 2-2 summarizes the ocular inflammatory diseases thought to require a major contribution of Th1-mediated DH effector mechanisms.

The Th2 subset of DH cells secretes IL-4, IL-5, and other cytokines. IL-4 can induce B lymphocytes to synthesize IgE, and IL-5 can recruit and activate eosinophils within a site. IL-4 can also induce granuloma formation in response to parasite-derived antigens. Thus, Th2-mediated DH mechanisms are thought to play a major role in the following:

- response to parasitic infections
- late-phase responses in allergic reactions
- asthma
- atopic dermatitis or other manifestations of atopic diseases

Persistence of certain infectious agents, especially bacteria within intracellular compartments of APCs and certain extracellular parasites, can cause destructive induration with granuloma formation and giant cells, termed the *granulomatous form of DH.* Also, immune complex deposition and innate immune mechanisms in response to heavy metal or foreign-body reactions can cause granulomatous inflammation, in which the inflammatory cascade (resulting in DH) is triggered in the absence of specific T lymphocytes. Unfortunately, for most clinical entities in which T-lymphocyte responses are suspected, especially autoimmune disorders such as multiple sclerosis or rheumatoid arthritis, the precise immunologic mechanisms remain highly speculative. See Clinical Example 2-3.

CLINICAL EXAMPLE 2-3

Toxocara granuloma (Th2 DH) *Toxocara canis* is a nematode parasite that infects up to 2% of all children worldwide. *T canis* infection occasionally produces inflammatory vitreoretinal manifestations (see Chapter 12). Humans become infected through ingestion of viable *T canis* eggs, which subsequently mature into larvae within the intestine. Animal models and immunopathogenesis of human nematode infections at other sites suggest that the primary immune response begins in the gut. The primary processing phase produces a strong Th2 response, leading to a primary effector response with production of IgM, IgG, and IgE antibodies, as well as DH T lymphocytes. Through immune evasion, a few larvae may disseminate hematogenously to the choroid or retina and subsequently invade the retina and/or vitreous. There, a Th2-mediated T-lymphocyte effector response against larva antigens releases Th2 cytokines to induce eosinophil and macrophage infiltration, causing the characteristic eosinophilic granuloma seen in the eye. In addition, antilarval B lymphocytes can infiltrate the eye and are induced to secrete various immunoglobulins, especially IgE. Finally, eosinophils, in part by attachment through Fc receptors, can recognize IgE or IgG bound to parasites and release cytotoxic granules containing the antiparasitic cationic protein directly near the larvae, using a mechanism similar to antibody-dependent cellular cytotoxicity.

Yasuda K, Nakanishi K. Host responses to intestinal nematodes. *Int Immunol.* 2018;30(3):93–102. doi: https://doi.org/10.1093/intimm/dxy002

Sympathetic ophthalmia (Th1 DH) Sympathetic ophthalmia is a bilateral granulomatous panuveitis that develops following penetrating trauma to an eye (see Chapter 10). This disorder represents one of the few human diseases in which autoimmunity can be directly linked to an initiating event. In most cases, penetrating injury activates the afferent phase of the immune response. The precise pathogenesis of sympathetic ophthalmia is unclear, but a leading hypothesis is that the injury causes (1) a de novo primary immunization to autoantigens—perhaps because externalization of previously sequestered uveal antigens through the wound initiates an immune response in the conjunctiva or extraocular sites—and (2) a change in the immunologic microenvironment of the retina, retinal pigment epithelium, and uvea to allow an immune response within the eye to overcome local suppressor mechanisms.

The inflammatory effector response is generally thought to be dominated by a Th1-mediated DH mechanism generated in response to uveal or retinal antigens, with $CD4^+$ T-lymphocyte predominance early in the disease course. Activated macrophages are also numerous in granulomas, and Th1 cytokines have been identified in the vitreous of affected patients. Th1-mediated DH effector mechanisms also are implicated in many other forms of ocular inflammation (see Table 2-2).

Boyd SR, Young S, Lightman S. Immunopathology of the noninfectious posterior and intermediate uveitides. *Surv Ophthalmol.* 2001;46(3):209–233.

Cytotoxic lymphocytes

Cytotoxic T lymphocytes Cytotoxic T lymphocytes (CTLs) are a subset of antigen-specific T lymphocytes bearing the CD8 marker that are especially good at killing tumor cells and virus-infected cells. CTLs can also mediate graft rejection and some types of autoimmunity. In most cases, the ideal antigen for CTLs is an intracellular protein that occurs naturally or is produced because of viral infection. CTLs appear to require assistance from $CD4^+$ helper T-cell signals in order to fully differentiate. Also, local $CD4^+$ T lymphocytes and other accessory costimulatory molecules on the target cell may be required to achieve maximal killing.

CTLs kill cells in 1 of 2 ways: "assassination" or "suicide" induction (Fig 2-7). *Assassination* refers to CTL-mediated lysis of target cells. A specialized pore-forming protein called *perforin* is released that inserts into cell membranes and causes osmotic lysis of the cell. *Suicide induction* refers to the capability of CTLs to stimulate programmed cell death of target cells, called *apoptosis,* using the CD95 ligand (FasL) to activate the CD95 receptor (Fas) on target cells. Alternatively, CTLs can release cytokines such as TNF to induce apoptosis. CTLs produce low-grade lymphocytic infiltrates within tumors or infected tissues and usually kill without causing significant inflammation.

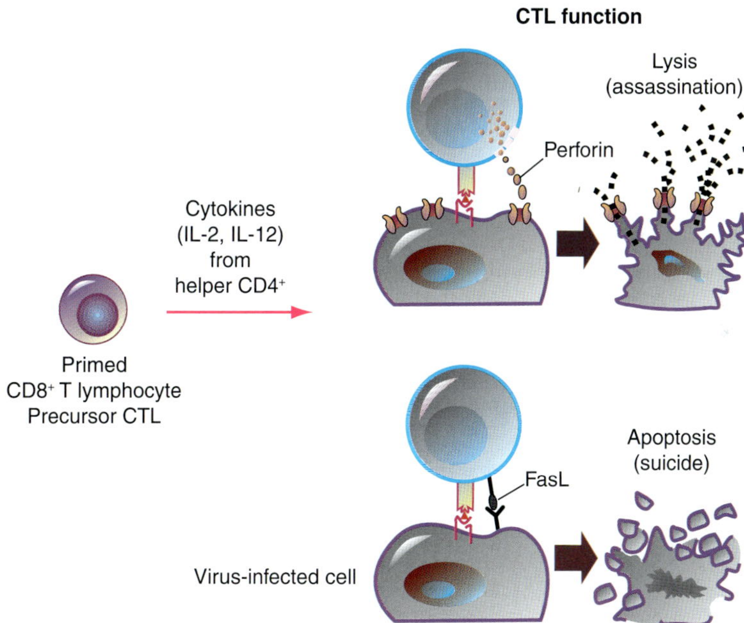

Figure 2-7 Schematic representation of the 2 major mechanisms of $CD8^+$ T-lymphocyte cytotoxicity. $CD8^+$ T lymphocytes, having undergone initial priming in the lymph node, enter the tissue site, where they again encounter antigen in the form of infected target cells. Upon restimulation, usually requiring $CD4^+$ T-cell factors, $CD8^+$ T lymphocytes are activated, fully becoming CTLs. CTLs can kill by lysing the infected cell using a pore-forming protein called *perforin* or by inducing programmed cell death, called *apoptosis,* using either Fas ligand (FasL) or cytokine-mediated mechanisms. *(Illustration by Barb Cousins, modified by Joyce Zavarro.)*

Natural killer cells Natural killer (NK) cells are a subset of non-T, non-B lymphocytes. They kill tumor cells and virus-infected cells using the same molecular mechanisms as CTLs. Unlike CTLs, NK cells do not have a specific antigen receptor and do not require priming or prior activation. Instead, they express multiple activating and inhibitory receptors; the balance of signals from these receptors determines whether NK cells are activated or inhibited. Activating receptors trigger the NK cell to kill target cells that are missing HLA class I molecules or those that display inappropriate molecules. Inhibitory NK receptors prevent NK cells from indiscriminately attacking healthy host tissue by recognizing ligands that ought to be present.

Combined Antibody and Cellular Effector Mechanisms

Antibody-dependent cellular cytotoxicity

An antibody can bind to a cell-associated antigen such as a tumor or viral antigen, but if the antibody is not a member of a subclass that activates complement, the antibody may not directly induce cytotoxicity. However, various leukocytes may recognize the exposed Fc domain of the bound antibody and then activate various leukocyte cytotoxic mechanisms, including degranulation and cytokine production. Classically, *antibody-dependent cellular cytotoxicity (ADCC)* was observed to be mediated by a subset of large granular (non-T, non-B) lymphocytes, called *killer cells,* that induce cell death in a manner similar to CTLs. The killer cell itself is nonspecific but gains antigen specificity through interaction with specific antibody. Macrophages, NK cells, certain T lymphocytes, and neutrophils can also participate in ADCC using other Fc receptor types. An IgE-dependent form of ADCC may also exist for eosinophils.

ADCC is presumed to be important in tumor immune surveillance, antimicrobial host protection, graft rejection, and certain autoimmune diseases, such as cutaneous systemic lupus erythematosus. However, this effector mechanism probably does not play an important role in uveitis, although it might contribute to antiparasitic immunity.

Acute IgE-mediated mast cell degranulation

Mast cells bind IgE antibodies to their surface through a high-affinity Fc receptor specific for IgE molecules, positioning the antigen-recognition site of the bound IgE externally. Combining 2 adjacent IgE antibody molecules with a specific allergen causes degranulation of the mast cell and release of preformed and de novo synthesized mediators within minutes. This acute inflammatory reaction is called *immediate hypersensitivity* (previously called *Gell and Coombs type I,* or *anaphylaxis*).

Preformed mediators include histamine, serotonin, proteoglycans (heparin), neutral proteases (ie, tryptase, chymase), chemotactic factors (eosinophil, neutrophil, or monocyte), and possibly basic fibroblast growth factor. Among the newly generated mediators are the arachidonic acid metabolites prostaglandin D_2, leukotrienes, and thromboxane as well as Th2 cytokines (IL-4, IL-5, IL-13), TNF-α, IL-1, and CCL2.

Releasing these mediators results in vasodilation, increased capillary permeability, contraction of bronchial and gastrointestinal smooth muscle, and increased mucous secretion in mucosal sites. Mast cell–derived cytokines play a role in the late phase of allergic response by activating endothelial cells to recruit eosinophils and other inflammatory cells to the site of hypersensitivity reactions, thus sustaining inflammation. When severe, the immediate hypersensitivity response can produce a systemic reaction, with manifestations ranging from generalized skin lesions, such as erythema, urticaria, or angioedema, to severely altered vascular permeability with plasma leakage into tissues and airway obstruction or hypotensive shock. The use of antihistamine medications such as diphenhydramine to treat acute allergic reactions illustrates the central role of histamine in immediate hypersensitivity reactions.

CHAPTER 3

Ocular Immune Responses

Highlights

- Unique regional immune responses influence ocular pathology.
- Several immunoregulatory mechanisms modulate the intraocular immune environment as part of the immune privilege of the eye.
- Anterior chamber–associated immune deviation is a recognized mechanism of ocular immune privilege.
- Increased understanding of the immune responses of the eye has been valuable to advances in corneal transplantation, retinal gene therapy, and various developing cell-based therapies.

Regional Immunity and Immunologic Microenvironments

Regional immunity is the concept that many organ and tissue sites demonstrate modifications to the classic immune response arc that may affect some or all 3 phases—afferent, processing, and effector. Tissue-specific or organ-specific variation in immune response is determined by differences in the immunologic microenvironments. There are multiple microenvironments within and around the eye (Table 3-1).

Immune privilege encompasses anatomical, physiologic, and immunologic adaptations that limit inflammatory damage to vital structures. Operationally, immune-privileged sites include the central nervous system, eye, testis, ovary, pregnant uterus, hair follicle, and adrenal cortex. *Ocular immune privilege* is a unique feature of the ocular microenvironment. First described in the 1940s, the concept was based on the observation that foreign antigens placed in the anterior chamber did not elicit an inflammatory response. Multiple mechanisms contribute to ocular immune privilege, including the following:

- physical barriers (partial blood–ocular and blood–retina barriers, lack of efferent lymphatics)
- inhibitory ocular microenvironment (cell-bound and soluble immunosuppressive factors)
- anterior chamber–associated immune deviation (ACAID; suppression of foreign antigen–specific inflammation in the eye)

Zhou R, Caspi RR. Ocular immune privilege. *F1000 Biol Rep*. 2010;2:3. doi:10.3410/B2-3

Table 3-1 Comparison of Immune Microenvironments in Various Normal Ocular Sites

	Conjunctiva	Cornea, Sclera	Anterior Chamber, Anterior Uvea, Vitreous	Retina, RPE, Choriocapillaris, Choroid
Anatomical features	Lymphatics, follicles	Lymphatics at limbus, none centrally Macromolecules diffuse through stroma	No well-defined lymphatics, antigen clearance through trabecular meshwork Partial blood–uveal barrier	No lymphatics Blood–retina barrier Permeable uveal circulation
Resident APCs	Dendritic and Langerhans cells, macrophages	Langerhans cells at limbus Rare APCs in central and paracentral cornea No APCs in sclera Epithelium/endothelium can be induced to express HLA class II molecules	Many dendritic cells and macrophages in iris and ciliary body Hyalocytes are macrophage derived	Microglia in the retina Dendritic cells and macrophages in choriocapillaris and choroid RPE expresses TLR and can be induced to express HLA class II molecules
Specialized immune compartments for localized immune processing	Possibly follicles	None	None	None
Resident effector cells	Mast cells, T lymphocytes, B lymphocytes, plasma cells, rare neutrophils	Central cornea—none Sclera—none	Rare to no T lymphocytes or B lymphocytes, rare mast cells	Retina—normally no lymphocytes Choroid—mast cells, some lymphocytes
Resident effector molecules	All antibody isotypes, especially IgE, IgG subclasses; IgA in tears Complement and kininogen precursors present	Peripherally—all immunoglobulins (minimal IgM) Centrally—minimal antibody, some complement present Sclera—low antibody concentration, minimal IgM	Kallikrein but not kininogen precursors Some complement present, but less than in blood Minimal immunoglobulins in iris, some IgG in ciliary body and aqueous humor	Retina—minimal to no immunoglobulins Choroid—IgG and IgM
Immunoregulatory systems	Conjunctival-associated lymphoid tissue	Immune privilege—apoptosis-inducing ligands (Fas ligand, TRAIL, PD-L1), avascularity, lack of central APCs	Immune privilege—ACAID, immunosuppressive factors in aqueous; Fas ligand, TRAIL	Immune privilege—RPE can secrete immunosuppressive molecules (TGF-β2) Complement regulator expression

ACAID = anterior chamber–associated immune deviation; APC = antigen-presenting cell; HLA = human leukocyte antigen; Ig = immunoglobulin; PD-L1 = programmed death ligand; RPE = retinal pigment epithelium; TGF = transforming growth factor; TLR = Toll-like receptors, TRAIL = tumor necrosis factor–related apoptosis-inducing ligand.

Immune Responses of the Conjunctiva

Features of the Immunologic Microenvironment

The conjunctiva shares many of the features that are typical of mucosal sites. It is well vascularized and has good lymphatic drainage to preauricular and submandibular nodes. The tissue contains numerous Langerhans cells, other dendritic cells, and macrophages that serve as potential antigen-presenting cells (APCs). Certain ocular surface infections or inflammation results in enlarged conjunctival follicles that contain T lymphocytes, B lymphocytes, and APCs. By analogy with similar sites, such as Peyer patches of the intestine, these follicles are likely sites for localized immune processing of antigens that permeate through the thin overlying epithelium. See Chapter 10, Figures 10-7 and 10-9 for examples of conjunctival nodules in sarcoidosis.

The conjunctiva, especially the substantia propria, is richly populated with potential effector cells, predominantly mast cells. All antibody isotypes are represented, with immunoglobulin (Ig) A as the most abundant type in the tears. Local antibody production presumably occurs as well as passive leakage. Soluble molecules of the innate immune system, especially complement, are also present. The conjunctiva appears to support most adaptive and innate immune effector responses, especially antibody-mediated and lymphocyte-mediated responses, although IgE-mediated mast cell degranulation is one of the most common and important. See also BCSC Section 8, *External Disease and Cornea,* for further information on conjunctival immune responses.

Immunoregulatory Systems

The conjunctival substantia propria contains *conjunctiva-associated lymphoid tissue (CALT)* and serves as the main T-lymphocyte inductive site of the *ocular mucosal immune system (OMIS),* which also includes the lacrimal gland, conjunctival and corneal epithelia, and draining lymph nodes. CALT and OMIS are part of the mucosal immune system, which is anatomically and functionally distinct from the systemic (primarily bloodborne) immune compartment. The mucosal immune system utilizes innate and adaptive immune responses to maintain the homeostasis of mucosal surfaces. The OMIS can be divided into mucosal inductive sites and mucosal effector sites. APCs take up and process antigens (pathogens and allergens) and then present them to T lymphocytes at mucosal inductive sites, usually in local (cervical, preauricular, and submandibular) lymph nodes. Antigen-specific T lymphocytes are induced in these lymph nodes and then return to ocular mucosal effector sites, where they carry out their immune functions.

Within the mucosal immune system, certain sites may elicit a more far-reaching distal mucosal immune response than others. Due to the nasolacrimal drainage system, there is direct anatomical communication between the OMIS and the *nasal-associated lymphoid tissue (NALT),* which are thought to be immunologically connected and interdependent. For example, intranasal immunization induces IgA within the nose and salivary glands as well as on the ocular surface and may elicit more tear IgA antibody responses than does direct ocular exposure. Increased understanding of the integrated nature of the OMIS and NALT systems has influenced the development of intranasally administered immunotherapeutic agents against inflammatory dry eye disease.

Farid M, Agrawal A, Fremgen D, et al. Age-related defects in ocular and nasal mucosal immune system and the immunopathology of dry eye disease. *Ocul Immunol Inflamm.* 2016;24(3):327–347.

Immune Responses of the Cornea

Features of the Immunologic Microenvironment

The cornea is unique among ocular tissues because the peripheral and central portions of the tissue represent distinctly different immunologic microenvironments. In normal eyes, only the limbus is vascularized and richly invested with Langerhans cells. The avascular paracentral and central cornea are mostly devoid of APCs. Various stimuli, such as mild trauma, certain cytokines (eg, interleukin 1), or infection, can recruit APCs to the central cornea. Immune-mediated corneal changes such as marginal keratitis often occur adjacent to the vascularized limbus.

Plasma-derived proteins (eg, complement and IgG) are present in moderate concentrations in the periphery, but only low levels of IgM are present centrally. Corneal cells also synthesize various antimicrobial and immunoregulatory proteins. Localized immune processing probably does not occur in the cornea, and effector cells are scarce or absent; however, neutrophils, monocytes, and lymphocytes can readily migrate through the stroma if appropriate chemotactic stimuli are activated. These immune cells can also adhere to the endothelial surface during inflammation, giving rise to keratic precipitates or the classic Khodadoust line of endothelial rejection (Fig 3-1). See also BCSC Section 8, *External Disease and Cornea.*

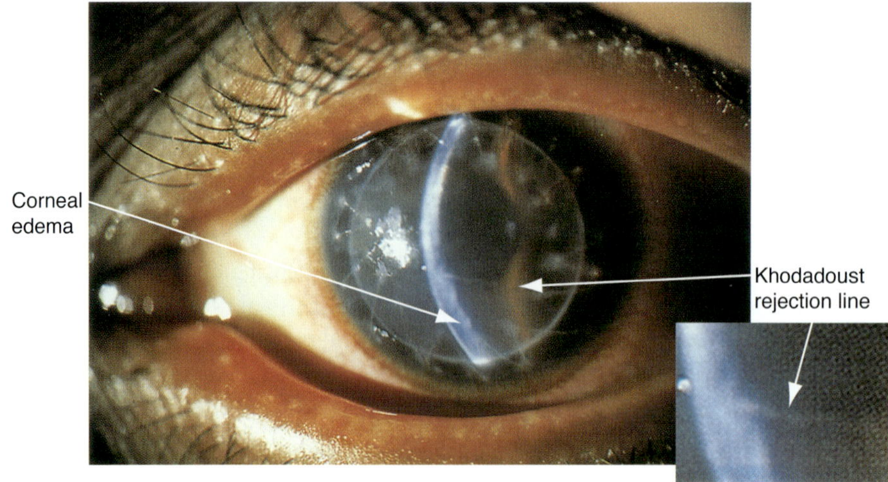

Figure 3-1 Endothelial graft rejection with stromal and epithelial edema on the trailing aspect of the migrating Khodadoust line *(inset).*

Immunoregulatory Systems

Immune privilege of the cornea is multifactorial. Normal limbal physiology is a major component, especially the maintenance of avascularity and the scarcity of APCs in the paracentral and central cornea. The lack of APCs and lymphatic channels partially inhibits the afferent response in the central cornea. The absence of postcapillary venules centrally can limit the efficiency of effector recruitment, although effector cells and molecules can infiltrate even avascular cornea. The corneal endothelium is exposed to anti-inflammatory and immunosuppressive molecules in the aqueous humor such as transforming growth factor β, α-melanocyte–stimulating hormone, macrophage migration inhibitory factor, and vasoactive intestinal peptide. In addition, corneal epithelial and endothelial cells have cell membrane–bound molecules such as Fas ligand (FasL) that resist immunologic attack by inducing apoptosis of infiltrating neutrophils and lymphocytes that express the FasL receptor. (See Clinical Example 3-1.)

CLINICAL EXAMPLE 3-1

Corneal Allograft Rejection

Penetrating keratoplasty, or the transplantation of corneal allografts, has an extremely high success rate (>90%) even in the absence of systemic immunomodulation. This rate is substantially superior to acceptance rates after transplantation of other donor tissues. Corneal allograft survival has been attributed to the mechanisms of immune privilege, including suppression of the immune response against allograft antigens, generation of regulatory T (Treg) lymphocytes that can suppress the destructive alloimmune reaction, and induction of apoptosis of inflammatory cells at the graft–host interface. Experimental models and clinical studies show that factors contributing to rejection include the following:

- stimuli for corneal vascularization that also induce ingrowth of lymphatic vessels and infiltration of dendritic cells
- induction of stromal human leukocyte antigen (HLA) molecule expression (normally low)
- contamination of the donor graft with donor-derived APCs prior to the transplant
- loss of immune privilege via maneuvers (eg, splenectomy) that prevent induction of ACAID

Changes in host immune status may influence graft rejection as well. Graft rejection has been reported in association with systemic checkpoint inhibitor treatment, SARS-CoV-2 infection, and recent vaccination; however, isolated case reports are not necessarily evidence of causality.

Niederkorn JY. The eye sees eye to eye with the immune system: the 2019 Proctor Lecture. *Invest Ophthalmol Vis Sci.* 2019;60(13):4489–4495.

Yin J. Advances in corneal graft rejection. *Curr Opin Ophthalmol.* 2021;32(4):331–337.

Immune Responses of the Anterior Chamber, Anterior Uvea, and Vitreous

Features of the Immunologic Microenvironment

The anterior chamber is a fluid-filled cavity; circulating aqueous humor provides a unique medium for intercellular communication among immune cells and resident tissue cells of the iris, ciliary body, and corneal endothelium. Although aqueous humor is relatively protein depleted compared with serum (containing about 0.1%–1.0% of the total serum protein concentration), even normal aqueous humor contains a complex mixture of biological factors, such as immunomodulatory cytokines, neuropeptides, and complement inhibitors, that influence immunologic events within the eye.

A partial blood–ocular barrier is present in the anterior chamber: fenestrated capillaries in the ciliary body allow a size-dependent concentration gradient of plasma macromolecules to permeate the interstitial tissue. Smaller plasma-derived molecules are present in higher concentration than larger molecules. The tight junctions between the pigmented and nonpigmented ciliary epithelium provide a more exclusive barrier, preventing interstitial macromolecules from permeating directly through the ciliary body into the aqueous humor. Nevertheless, a small number of plasma macromolecules bypass the nonpigmented epithelium barrier and enter the anterior chamber by diffusion directly through the anterior iris surface.

A few resident T lymphocytes and mast cells are present in the normal anterior uvea; B lymphocytes, eosinophils, and neutrophils are usually absent. Very low concentrations of IgG and complement components occur in normal aqueous humor. The iris and ciliary body contain significant numbers of macrophages and dendritic cells that serve as APCs and possible effector cells, but immune processing is unlikely to occur locally. Since the inner eye does not contain well-defined lymphatic channels, clearance of soluble substances depends on aqueous humor outflow channels. Nevertheless, antigen inoculation into the anterior chamber results in efficient communication with the systemic immune system. Particulates can be removed via endocytosis by trabecular meshwork endothelial cells or macrophages. Intact soluble antigens can enter the venous circulation that transports them to the spleen.

The vitreous has not been studied as extensively as the anterior chamber. Studies employing proteomics reveal the vitreous as a physiologically active, complex tissue containing diverse proteins originating from inside and outside the eye. An important source of these inflammatory mediators is the retina. The vitreous gel can electrostatically bind charged protein substances to serve as an antigen depot as well as a substrate for leukocyte cell adhesion. The vitreous may also serve as an autoantigen because of the presence of collagen type II, which has been implicated in the pathogenesis of rheumatoid arthritis. Hyalocytes, which are modified resident macrophages, are important in vitreal immunoregulation/modulation and frequently act as APCs. They also respond to different cytokines, playing a role in the immunopathogenesis of several disorders, including proliferative vitreoretinopathy.

Immunoregulatory Systems

Relatively mild inflammation that would be harmless in the skin can cause severe vision loss in the eye. Fortunately, a variety of immunoregulatory mechanisms modulate intraocular immune responses, including in the anterior chamber, anterior uvea, and vitreous.

Ocular immune privilege has been observed with various antigens, including alloantigens (eg, transplant antigens), tumor antigens, haptens, soluble proteins, autoantigens, bacteria, and viruses. The best-studied mechanism of immune privilege in the eye is ACAID. Although subcutaneous inoculation of antigen elicits a strong, delayed hypersensitivity (DH) reaction, anterior chamber inoculation with the identical antigen results in a robust antibody response but a virtual absence of DH. In fact, preexisting DH can be suppressed by ACAID.

ACAID represents an attenuated effector arc in which cell-mediated immune responses such as DH and cytotoxic T-lymphocyte responses are suppressed by regulatory T (Treg) cells. ACAID blocks T helper-1 (Th1) immune responses and blunts Th2-mediated inflammatory disease. ACAID also shifts the antibody responses to preferential production of non-complement-fixing antibodies, thus reducing the likelihood of antibody-mediated ocular tissue injury from activation of the complement cascade.

Note that the immunoregulatory environment can still be overcome by sufficient immune stimulation.

Boneva SK, Wolf J, Rosmus DD, et al. Transcriptional profiling uncovers human hyalocytes as a unique innate immune cell population. *Front Immunol.* 2020;11:567274. doi:10.3389/fimmu.2020.567274

Niederkorn JY. The induction of anterior chamber–associated immune deviation. *Chem Immunol Allergy.* 2007;92:27–35.

Sen HN. Elements of the immune system and concepts of intraocular inflammatory disease pathogenesis. In: Whitcup SM, Sen HN, eds. *Whitcup and Nussenblatt's Uveitis.* 5th ed. Elsevier Health Sciences; 2022:1–28.

Skeie JM, Roybal CN, Mahajan VB. Proteomic insight into the molecular function of the vitreous. *PLoS One.* 2015;10(5):e0127567.

Immune Responses of the Retina, Retinal Pigment Epithelium, Choriocapillaris, and Choroid

Features of the Immunologic Microenvironment

The immunologic microenvironments of the retina, retinal pigment epithelium (RPE), choriocapillaris, and choroid have not been well characterized. An inner blood–ocular barrier is formed by tight junctions between the endothelial cells of the retinal vasculature, while tight junctions between the cells of the RPE provide an outer barrier between the choroid and the retina. The vessels of the choriocapillaris are highly permeable to macromolecules and allow transudation of most plasma macromolecules into the extravascular spaces of the choroid and choriocapillaris. Well-developed lymphatic channels are absent, although both the retina and the choroid have abundant potential APCs. In the retina, resident microglia (bone marrow–derived cells related to dendritic cells) are interspersed between the ganglion cell and outer plexiform layers and can undergo physical changes and migrate in response to various stimuli. The choriocapillaris and choroid contain an abundance of certain potential APCs, especially macrophages and dendritic cells.

The RPE can be induced to express human leukocyte antigen (HLA) class II molecules, suggesting that the RPE may interact with T lymphocytes in some circumstances. The presence of T lymphocytes or B lymphocytes within the normal posterior segment is not well characterized, but effector cells appear to be absent from the normal retina. Local immune processing does not seem to occur, either. Similar to macrophages, RPE cells also express Toll-like receptors. These special pattern recognition receptors are critical in the detection of pathogens and in the initiation of innate and adaptive immune responses, forming an initial line of defense against invading microorganisms.

A moderate density of mast cells is present in the choroid, especially around the arterioles, but lymphocytes are present only in very low numbers. Eosinophils and neutrophils appear to be absent. However, under various clinical or experimental conditions, a large number of T lymphocytes, B lymphocytes, macrophages, and neutrophils can infiltrate the choroid, choriocapillaris, and retina. The choroid can function as a repository for immunoreactive cells, manifesting clinically as lymphoid hyperplasia. It is hypothesized that the concentration of mast cells in the choroid may facilitate the spread of immunoreactive cells to other parts of the eye. The RPE and various cell types within the retina and choroid (eg, pericytes) can synthesize many different cytokines (eg, transforming growth factor β2) that may alter the subsequent immune response. See also BCSC Section 12, *Retina and Vitreous.*

McMenamin PG, Saban DR, Dando SJ. Immune cells in the retina and choroid: two different tissue environments that require different defenses and surveillance. *Prog Retin Eye Res.* 2019;70:85–98. doi:10.1016/j.preteyeres.2018.12.002

Taylor AW, Hsu S, Ng TF. The role of retinal pigment epithelial cells in regulation of macrophages/microglial cells in retinal immunobiology. *Front Immunol.* 2021;12:724601. doi:10.3389/fimmu.2021.724601

Immunoregulatory Systems

A mechanism of immune privilege, likely similar to ACAID, is present after subretinal injection of antigen. Iris, ciliary body, and RPE cells all contribute to immune homeostasis that is mediated by soluble or membrane-bound molecules. For example, soluble factors secreted by RPE cells can suppress APC and effector T-lymphocyte activation and induce Treg and myeloid-derived suppressor cell activity. These observations may be important because of growing interest in retinal transplantation, stem cell therapies, and gene therapy. (See Clinical Example 3-2.) The capacity of the choriocapillaris and choroid to

CLINICAL EXAMPLE 3-2

Retinal Gene Therapy

Retinal gene therapy is the transfection of neural retina cells or RPE with a replication-defective virus that has been genetically altered to carry a replacement gene. This gene becomes expressed in any cell infected by the virus. Immune clearance of the virus can cause loss of expression of the transferred gene in other body sites. In 2017, the US Food and Drug

Administration approved the first gene replacement therapy for biallelic *RPE65* mutation–associated retinal dystrophy (Leber congenital amaurosis). The agent, voretigene neparvovec-rzyl, uses an adeno-associated viral (AAV) vector to replace defective *RPE65*. It is administered via subretinal injection. Studies are currently under way to investigate gene therapy utilizing AAV for various inherited retinal dystrophies, such as achromatopsia, choroideremia, Leber hereditary optic neuropathy, X-linked retinoschisis, and X-linked retinitis pigmentosa. See also BCSC Section 12, *Retina and Vitreous*.

Despite the relative immune privilege of the eye, immunogenicity of viral vectors is an ongoing area of investigation. In animal models, intravitreal viral vector delivery has led to a humoral response, whereas subretinal delivery has not. Intraocular inflammation was observed in approximately 5% of patients receiving voretigene neparvovec-rzyl; therefore, systemic corticosteroids are started 3 days before injection of this agent.

Hassall MM, Barnard AR, MacLaren RE. Gene therapy for color blindness. *Yale J Biol Med.* 2017;90(4):543–551.

Moore NA, Morral N, Ciulla TA, Bracha P. Gene therapy for inherited retinal and optic nerve degenerations. *Expert Opin Biol Ther.* 2018;18(1):37–49.

function as unique environments for the afferent or effector phases of the immune response has not yet been evaluated.

Lee RW, Nicholson LB, Sen HN, et al. Autoimmune and autoinflammatory mechanisms in uveitis. *Semin Immunopathol.* 2014;36(5):581–594.

Mochizuki M, Sugita S, Kamoi K. Immunological homeostasis of the eye. *Prog Retin Eye Res.* 2013;33:10–27.

Vogt SD, Barnum SR, Curcio CA, Read RW. Distribution of complement anaphylatoxin receptors and membrane-bound regulators in normal human retina. *Exp Eye Res.* 2006;83(4):834–840.

CHAPTER 4

Special Topics in Ocular Immunology

Highlights

- Experimental autoimmune uveoretinitis is an animal model of human uveitis that can be induced by immunization with ocular-specific antigens such as S-antigen and interphotoreceptor retinoid-binding protein. One of the most important observations from animal models is the dominant role of T lymphocytes in ocular inflammation.
- A family of cell surface glycoproteins called *major histocompatibility complex (MHC) proteins* is expressed in all animals with white blood cells. In humans, MHC proteins are called *human leukocyte antigen (HLA) molecules.*
- The presence of many different HLA alleles within a population should ensure that the collective adaptive immune system will be able to respond to a wide range of potential pathogens. However, some individuals might be at increased risk for immunologic diseases.

Animal Models of Human Uveitis

Our understanding of the pathogenesis of inflammatory eye disease has been significantly influenced by research involving animals. Animal models of human uveitis use a variety of species, antigens, adjuvants, and protocols to produce disease ranging from transient to persistent and mild to severe. Although none of these models are an exact corollary to human disease, they have contributed substantially to our understanding of ocular immunology. One of the most important observations is the dominant role of T lymphocytes in ocular inflammation.

The most widely used and well-studied animal model of human uveitis is *experimental autoimmune uveoretinitis (EAU),* which can be induced in experimental animals of several different species that are immunized with ocular-specific antigens such as purified arrestin (also called *S-antigen*). EAU is most commonly induced in mice by immunization with interphotoreceptor retinoid-binding protein (IRBP), a molecule whose role is to transport vitamin A derivatives between the photoreceptors and the retinal pigment epithelium. Within 2 weeks of immunization, clinical and histologic evidence of anterior segment, vitreous, and choroidal inflammation develops. Of note, there is similarity between the histologic changes in mouse EAU and those in human ocular sarcoidosis, specifically, subretinal exudate and retinal detachment.

Other concepts elucidated by various uveitis animal models (noted in parentheses) include the following:

- the dynamics of leukocyte function in the anterior chamber (endotoxin-induced uveitis)
- the presence of autoantibodies and autoreactive T lymphocytes (equine recurrent uveitis)
- the role of the transcription factor *autoimmune regulator (AIRE)* in the development of self tolerance in the thymus (AIRE-deficient mice)
- the promotion of inflammation by ocular resident cells with increased expression of class II antigens (EAU)
- the presence of retina-specific regulatory T lymphocytes that resolve inflammation and maintain remission (EAU)

Chen J, Qian H, Horai R, Chan CC, Caspi RR. Mouse models of experimental autoimmune uveitis: comparative analysis of adjuvant-induced vs spontaneous models of uveitis. *Curr Mol Med.* 2015;15(6):550–557.

Forrester JV, Klaska IP, Yu T, Kuffova L. Uveitis in mouse and man. *Int Rev Immunol.* 2013;32(1):76–96.

Sen HN. Elements of the immune system and concepts of intraocular inflammatory disease pathogenesis. In: Whitcup SM, Sen HN, eds. *Whitcup and Nussenblatt's Uveitis.* 5th ed. Elsevier Health Sciences; 2022:1–28.

Human Leukocyte Antigen Associations and Disease

Major Histocompatibility Complex and Human Leukocyte Antigen Molecules

The major histocompatibility complex (MHC) is a genomic region that includes many genes responsible for coordinating the immune response via cell surface glycoproteins. MHC proteins are expressed in all animals with white blood cells. In humans, the MHC genes are located on chromosome 6; the proteins encoded by these genes are called *human leukocyte antigen (HLA) molecules.* These molecules play a crucial role in the ability of the antigen-presenting cell to bind and present peptide fragments, thus determining T-lymphocyte immune responsiveness. See Chapter 2 for further discussion of the important role that HLA molecules play in immunologic function.

The MHC is divided into 3 genomic regions termed *classes.* Initially, 6 gene families comprising classes I and II were identified:

- MHC class I: *HLA-A, -B, -C*
- MHC class II: *HLA-DR, -DP, -DQ*

The original 6 gene families are called "classic genes" because additional genes with distinctly different gene products, as well as pseudogenes, were subsequently identified in each class. For example, in the class II region, a nonclassic gene encodes HLA-DM, a molecule that serves as a peptide editor and plays a critical role in peptide loading of HLA class II molecules. Class III, located between classes I and II, contains immune and non-immune-related genes, including some that encode complement components and other proteins that play a role in inflammation (ie, tumor necrosis factor).

Allelic Variation

Within the human population, many alleles exist for each of the HLA genes. An individual has 2 alleles for every HLA gene. One set of alleles (called a *haplotype*) is inherited from the mother, and the other haplotype is from the father. Siblings have a 50% chance of sharing a haplotype. Thus, except for identical twins, it is rare for all potential haplotypes to match between 2 individuals. See Figure 4-1.

Allelic diversity provides protection through *population-wide immunity.* Each HLA haplotype covers a theoretical set of antigens that an individual's immune system may recognize. The presence of many different HLA alleles within a population, therefore, should ensure that the collective adaptive immune system can respond to a wide range of potential pathogens. The converse also holds true: some individuals may be at increased risk for immunologic diseases due to an aberrantly strong immune response to a benign pathogen or inappropriate recognition of host peptides if an HLA molecule is misidentified as foreign. See Clinical Example 4-1.

Clinical detection and classification of different alleles

Initially, the HLA haplotype was determined by antisera reactions. Current methods utilize molecular techniques to identify the nucleic acid sequence of the HLA gene alleles. HLA molecules are composed of 2 chains: the α chain and the β_2-microglobulin chain for class I,

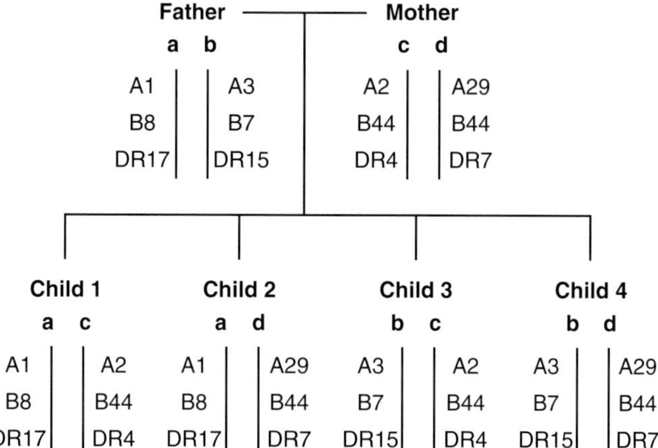

Figure 4-1 Human leukocyte antigen (HLA) inheritance. Each child inherits 1 haplotype from each parent. There are 4 possible HLA haplotype combinations in offspring. A sibling has a 50% chance of sharing 1 haplotype with another sibling. Two siblings have a 25% chance of having the same HLA haplotypes and a 25% chance of sharing no HLA haplotypes. *(Redrawn with permission from Choo SY. The HLA system: genetics, immunology, clinical testing, and clinical implications.* Yonsei Med J. *2007;48(1):11–23, Figure 2.)*

CLINICAL EXAMPLE 4-1

HLA-B27–Associated Acute Anterior Uveitis

Depending on the ethnic population, the prevalence of HLA-B27 ranges from 19% to 88% in patients with acute anterior uveitis. Many of these patients also have other immunologic disorders, such as reactive arthritis, ankylosing spondylitis, inflammatory bowel disease–related arthropathy, and psoriatic arthritis (see Chapter 8). Although the immunopathogenesis of HLA-B27–associated acute anterior uveitis remains unknown, various animal models permit informed speculation. Many cases of uveitis or reactive arthritis in humans follow gram-negative gastroenteritis or chlamydial infection. (Chapter 1 discusses the possible role of bacterial lipopolysaccharide and innate mechanisms.) Experiments in rats and mice genetically altered to express human HLA-B27 molecules suggest that bacterial infection of the gut predisposes rats to arthritis and a reactive arthritis–like syndrome, although uveitis is uncommon.

Wakefield D, Clarke D, McCluskey P. Recent developments in HLA B27 anterior uveitis. *Front Immunol.* 2021;11:608134. doi:10.3389/fimmu.2020.608134

and the α chain and β chain for class II. Genotyping specifies the chain, major genetic type, and specific minor molecular variant subtype. For example, genotype DRB1*04:08 refers to the HLA-DR4 molecule β chain with the "–08" minor variant subtype. Haplotypes currently recognized as a single group will continue to be subdivided into new categories or new subtypes as research progresses.

Disease Associations

In 1973, the first association between an HLA haplotype and a disease—ankylosing spondylitis—was identified. Since then, more than 100 other disease associations have been established, including several for ocular inflammatory diseases (Table 4-1). An HLA–disease association is established when there is a statistically significant increase in frequency of an HLA haplotype in persons with that disease compared with the frequency in a disease-free population. The ratio of the probability of the disease occurring in individuals with the HLA haplotype to individuals without the haplotype is termed *relative risk.* A relative risk of 1 denotes no difference in risk, <1 indicates a reduced risk, and >1 indicates an increased risk. Several points are important when considering HLA–disease associations:

- The HLA association identifies individuals at risk, but it is not a diagnostic marker. The associated haplotype is not necessarily present in all people with the disease, nor does its presence in a person ensure the associated diagnosis.
- The association depends on the validity of the haplotyping. Older literature often reflects associations based on HLA classifications (some provisional) that might have changed.
- The association is only as strong as the clinical diagnosis. Diseases that are difficult to diagnose on the basis of clinical features may obscure real associations.

Table 4-1 HLA Associations and Ocular Inflammatory Disease

Disease	HLA Association	Relative Risk (RR), Other Associations
Uveitic diseases with strong HLA associations		
Tubulointerstitial nephritis and uveitis syndrome	HLA-DRB1*01:02	RR = 167
Birdshot chorioretinopathy	HLA-A29, A29.2	RR up to 224 for North American and European individuals
Reactive arthritis	HLA-B27	RR = 60
Acute anterior uveitis	HLA-B27	RR = 8
Uveitic diseases with weaker HLA associations		
Juvenile idiopathic arthritis	HLA-A2, DR5, DR8, DR11, DP2.1	Acute systemic disease
Behçet disease	HLA-B51, A26	RR = 4–6; Japanese and Middle Eastern individuals HLA-A26 associated with ocular disease
Intermediate uveitis	HLA-B8, B51, DR2, DRB1*15 (part of DR15 haplotype)	RR = 6, possibly the DRB1*15:01 allele
Sympathetic ophthalmia	HLA-DR4	Unknown
Vogt-Koyanagi-Harada syndrome	HLA-DR4, DRB1*04	RR = 2, Japanese and North American individuals RR = 5.3, Mexican Mestizo individuals
Sarcoidosis	HLA-B8 HLA-B13	Acute systemic disease Chronic systemic disease but not for eye
Multiple sclerosis	HLA-B7, DR2, DRB1*15 (part of DR15 haplotype), DQB1*06:02	RR = 3 (DR15)
Retinal vasculitis	HLA-B44	British individuals

HLA = human leukocyte antigen.

- The concept of *linkage disequilibrium* proposes that if 2 genes are physically close together on a chromosome, they are likely to be inherited together rather than undergo genetic randomization in a population. Thus, HLA genes may be coinherited with a separate gene that confers the actual risk. Sometimes 2 HLA haplotypes can occur together more frequently than predicted by their independent frequencies in the population.

The ocular inflammatory disease with the strongest HLA association is birdshot chorioretinopathy (BCR); nearly all patients with BCR are HLA-A29 positive. However, although approximately 8% of the White population in the United States has the HLA-A29 allele, fewer than 1 in 10,000 US residents have this ocular disease. Thus, most individuals who are HLA-A29 positive will never develop BCR, indicating the likely involvement of additional genetic and environmental factors in the pathogenesis of this disease. For example, genome-wide association studies of BCR have identified endoplasmic reticulum aminopeptidase (ERAP) genes, which encode aminopeptidases involved in the processing of HLA class I ligands. See Chapter 5, Tables 5-10 and 5-11, for examples of how HLA haplotyping may be used in the clinical workup of uveitis.

Several mechanisms have been proposed for HLA–disease associations. The most direct theory postulates that HLA molecules act as peptide-binding molecules for pathogenic antigens or infectious agents. Thus, individuals bearing a specific HLA molecule may show a predisposition to processing certain antigens, such as an infectious agent that cross-reacts with an autoantigen (also called *self antigen*). Specific variations or mutations in the peptide-binding region would greatly influence this mechanism; only molecular typing can detect these variations. Preliminary data supporting this theory are available for type 1 diabetes.

A second theory proposes molecular mimicry between bacterial antigens and an epitope on the HLA molecule (ie, an antigenic site on the molecule itself). An appropriate antibacterial effector response might inappropriately initiate a cross-reactive effector response with an epitope of the HLA molecule.

A third theory suggests that the T-lymphocyte antigen receptor (gene) might be the true susceptibility factor. Because each T-lymphocyte receptor uses a specific HLA haplotype, a strong correlation would exist between an HLA molecule and the T-lymphocyte antigen receptor repertoire. See Chapter 2 for further discussion about HLA molecules and T-lymphocyte antigen receptors.

Kuiper J, Rothova A, de Boer J, Radstake T. The immunopathogenesis of birdshot chorioretinopathy; a bird of many feathers. *Prog Retin Eye Res*. 2015;44:99–110.

Takeuchi M, Mizuki N, Ohno S. Pathogenesis of non-infectious uveitis elucidated by recent genetic findings. *Front Immunol.* 2021;12:640473. doi:10.3389/fimmu.2021.640473

CHAPTER 5

Diagnostic Considerations in Uveitis

This chapter includes related videos. Go to www.aao.org/bcscvideo_section09 or scan the QR codes in the text to access this content.

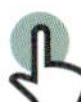

This chapter also includes a related activity. Go to www.aao.org/bcscactivity_section09 or scan the QR code in the text to access this content.

Highlights

- Uveitis refers to a heterogeneous set of diseases characterized by intraocular inflammation that may be infectious or noninfectious in origin and may be associated with a systemic disease or limited to the eye. Worldwide, uveitis is a leading cause of vision loss and visual impairment.
- Ocular inflammatory diseases with similar clinical features may differ in terms of treatment and prognosis, so accurate diagnosis is crucial.
- A formalized uveitis nomenclature uses clinical and anatomical features to describe, categorize, and grade intraocular inflammation.
- The differential diagnosis of uveitis is generated from the patient history, review of systems, and targeted systemic examination in combination with characteristics of the ocular inflammation.
- Laboratory workup and other ancillary testing for uveitis are tailored to the patient and the disease characteristics.

Overview

The uvea (also called the *uveal tract*) is a pigmented and vascular layer of the eye that includes the iris, ciliary body, and choroid. The dark purple choroid resembles a grape; hence, the term *uvea* was derived from the Latin word *uva,* meaning grape. Although the technical definition of *uveitis* is inflammation of the uvea, the clinical manifestation of uveitic diseases is intraocular inflammation that may include non-uveal ocular structures such as the vitreous, optic nerve, and retina. One of the hallmarks of intraocular inflammation is the presence of visible cells in the aqueous and/or vitreous humor. Other manifestations of intraocular inflammation, such as retinal vasculitis and macular edema, may require ophthalmic imaging for detection. Inflammation can also involve other structures of the eye, such as the cornea (keratitis), sclera (scleritis), extraocular muscles (myositis), and orbit (orbital inflammation or orbital pseudotumor). The evaluation and treatment of *non-uveitic* ocular inflammatory disease (eg, scleritis) shares similarities with the approach for uveitis.

The term *uveitis* does not indicate etiology. Uveitis refers to a heterogeneous set of diseases that may be noninfectious (presumed to have an autoimmune or autoinflammatory origin), or that may be caused by infectious organisms. In addition, infectious and noninfectious uveitis can be isolated or associated with systemic disease. Uveitis that is isolated to the eye and noninfectious is considered an autoimmune disease that affects only the eye(s) and may be called *undifferentiated,* or *idiopathic,* uveitis.

When uveitis is suspected, the initial patient evaluation includes careful assessment of the anatomical location and characteristics of the ocular inflammation. Multimodal ophthalmic imaging has an important role in characterizing intraocular inflammation. A detailed patient history and review of systems are essential for gathering evidence of possible associated systemic disease. Limited examination of pertinent nonocular organ systems might be indicated by the review of systems or uveitis differential diagnosis. Further investigations should be guided by the ophthalmic findings in the context of the history and systemic signs or symptoms. Laboratory studies can help determine the etiology of intraocular inflammation; however, they are never a substitute for a thorough history and review of systems. An incomplete or inappropriate workup can delay diagnosis, lead to incorrect treatment, and have disastrous effects on ophthalmic and systemic prognoses. See Chapter 6 for an extensive discussion of uveitis treatment options.

Epidemiology

Uveitis is responsible for approximately 10% of blindness in the United States and Europe and up to 25% of blindness worldwide. The prevalence of uveitis is 58–121 cases per 100,000 people in the United States and reaches 730 cases per 100,000 people in the developing world. Anterior uveitis is the most common type of uveitis, representing 70%–80% of cases, followed by panuveitis, posterior uveitis, and intermediate uveitis. Women have slightly higher rates of uveitis overall. Although most surveys show that the incidence of uveitis peaks in people between 20 and 60 years of age, recent data suggest that the risk of uveitis is also increased in people older than 65 years. In general, the prevalence of uveitis is about five- to tenfold lower in children than in adults. Developing countries have higher rates of infectious uveitis, posterior uveitis, and panuveitis than industrialized nations. Certain types of uveitis are also associated with geographic region or origin, such as birdshot chorioretinopathy in western Europe, Behçet disease in Turkey and China, and tuberculosis-associated uveitis in India.

Acharya NR, Tham VM, Esterberg E, et al. Incidence and prevalence of uveitis: results from the Pacific Ocular Inflammation Study. *JAMA Ophthalmol.* 2013;131(11):1405–1412.

Gritz DC, Wong IG. Incidence and prevalence of uveitis in Northern California: the Northern California Epidemiology of Uveitis Study. *Ophthalmology.* 2004;111(3):491–500.

Rathinam SR, Krishnadas R, Ramakrishnan R, et al; Aravind Comprehensive Eye Survey Research Group. Population-based prevalence of uveitis in Southern India. *Br J Ophthalmol.* 2011;95(4):463–467.

Rim TH, Kim SS, Ham D, Yu S, Chung EJ, Lee SC; Korean Uveitis Society. Incidence and prevalence of uveitis in South Korea: a nationwide cohort study. *Br J Ophthalmol.* 2018;102(1):79–83.

Thorne JE, Suhler E, Skup M, et al. Prevalence of noninfectious uveitis in the United States: a claims-based analysis. *JAMA Ophthalmol.* 2016;134(11):1237–1245.

Classification of Uveitis

In 2005, several international societies developed a universal method for describing uveitis, called the *Standardization of Uveitis Nomenclature (SUN)* system. This classification system, which is based on the anatomical location of inflammation and specific descriptors of its onset, duration, and course, has since been accepted by uveitis specialists worldwide. As mentioned in the overview, uveitis is divided into noninfectious (autoimmune/autoinflammatory) and infectious conditions, and by the presence or absence of associated systemic manifestations. Uveitis is classified anatomically by the SUN system, which includes 4 subcategories: (1) anterior uveitis, (2) intermediate uveitis, (3) posterior uveitis, and (4) panuveitis. Table 5-1 reviews these 4 groups. Of note, if both anterior chamber and vitreous inflammatory cells are present but the amount of vitreous inflammation is more than expected for an isolated anterior uveitis, the classification should be "anterior and intermediate uveitis" and not "panuveitis." Posterior uveitis or panuveitis must include choroidal and/or retinal lesions.

The SUN system further refines the anatomical classification of uveitis with descriptors based on clinical onset, duration, and course (Table 5-2). Terminology for grading and monitoring uveitic activity was also developed (Table 5-3). In 2021, the SUN system established additional criteria for classifying 25 specific types of uveitis, which are discussed elsewhere in Section 9.

Table 5-1 Anatomical Classification of Uveitis Based on Standardization of Uveitis Nomenclature (SUN) Criteria

Type	Primary Site of Inflammation	Includes
Anterior uveitis	Anterior chamber	Iritis Iridocyclitis Anterior cyclitis
Intermediate uveitis	Vitreous	Pars planitis Posterior cyclitis Hyalitis
Posterior uveitis	Retina or choroid	Focal, multifocal, or diffuse choroiditis Chorioretinitis Retinochoroiditis Retinitis Neuroretinitis
Panuveitis	Anterior chamber, vitreous, and retina or choroid	

Reproduced with permission from Jabs DA, Nussenblatt RB, Rosenbaum JT; Standardization of Uveitis Nomenclature (SUN) Working Group. Standardization of nomenclature for reporting clinical data: results of the First International Workshop. *Am J Ophthalmol.* 2005;140(3):510.

Table 5-2 Descriptors of Uveitis Based on Standardization of Uveitis Nomenclature (SUN) Criteria

Category	Descriptor	Comment
Onset	Sudden	
	Insidious	
Duration	Limited	≤3 months' duration
	Persistent	>3 months' duration
Course	Acute	Episode characterized by sudden onset and limited duration
	Recurrent	Repeated episodes separated by periods of inactivity without treatment ≥3 months in duration
	Chronic	Persistent uveitis with relapse in <3 months after discontinuing treatment

Reproduced with permission from Jabs DA, Nussenblatt RB, Rosenbaum JT; Standardization of Uveitis Nomenclature (SUN) Working Group. Standardization of nomenclature for reporting clinical data: results of the First International Workshop. *Am J Ophthalmol.* 2005;140(3):511.

Table 5-3 Uveitis Terminology Based on Standardization of Uveitis Nomenclature (SUN) Criteria

Term	Definition
Inactive	Grade 0 cells (anterior chamber)
Worsening activity	Two-step increase in level of inflammation (eg, anterior chamber cells, vitreous haze) or increase from grade 3+ to 4+
Improved activity	Two-step decrease in level of inflammation (eg, anterior chamber cells, vitreous haze) or decrease to grade 0
Remission	Inactive disease for ≥3 months after discontinuing all treatments for eye disease

Reproduced with permission from Jabs DA, Nussenblatt RB, Rosenbaum JT; Standardization of Uveitis Nomenclature (SUN) Working Group. Standardization of nomenclature for reporting clinical data: results of the First International Workshop. *Am J Ophthalmol.* 2005;140(3):513.

Jabs DA, Nussenblatt RB, Rosenbaum JT; Standardization of Uveitis Nomenclature (SUN) Working Group. Standardization of uveitis nomenclature for reporting clinical data: results of the First International Workshop. *Am J Ophthalmol.* 2005;140(3):509–516.

Anatomical Classification

Anterior uveitis

Anterior uveitis produces inflammatory signs predominantly in the anterior chamber as a result of inflammation of the iris and ciliary body. Inflammation confined to the anterior chamber is also called *iritis;* when there are cells in the retrolental (anterior vitreous) space, it can be called *iridocyclitis.* When more than one ocular structure is involved, the convention is to name the primary site of inflammation first; for example, *sclerokeratitis* is keratitis that develops in association with scleritis. Inflammatory processes that originate in the cornea with secondary involvement of the anterior chamber are called *keratouveitis.* An inflammatory reaction that involves the sclera and uveal tract is called *sclerouveitis.*

Severe or chronic anterior uveitis may produce secondary structural complications such as corneal edema, band keratopathy, iris abnormalities, cataract, uveitic macular edema, and optic disc swelling. These complications are not part of the formal classification system but may facilitate disease recognition and therapy decisions. It is important to understand that the presence of posterior segment complications such as macular edema does *not* indicate that the anatomical classification is posterior uveitis or panuveitis; as discussed previously, inflammatory lesions must be present in the choroid or retina in posterior uveitis or panuveitis. Chapter 8 discusses anterior uveitis in greater detail.

Intermediate uveitis

In intermediate uveitis, inflammation is most prominent in the vitreous cavity. Vitritis results from inflammation of the ciliary body, retinal vasculature, pars plana, and/or peripheral retina. Clinical signs include vitreous haze and cellular debris that is often associated with peripheral or diffuse retinal vascular leakage. Macular edema is the most common structural complication of intermediate uveitis; severe or chronic disease may cause peripheral exudative or tractional detachments, retinal neovascularization, cataract, or retrolental membrane formation. The diagnostic term *pars planitis* refers to a subset of intermediate uveitis in which there are peripheral preretinal collections of exudative and inflammatory debris in the absence of an associated infection or systemic disease. See Chapter 8 for further discussion of intermediate uveitis.

Posterior uveitis

Posterior uveitis is defined as intraocular inflammation involving primarily the retina and/or choroid. Inflammatory cells may be observed diffusely throughout the vitreous cavity, overlying foci of active chorioretinal inflammation, or on the posterior vitreous face. Ophthalmoscopy reveals focal, multifocal, or diffuse areas of retinitis and/or choroiditis, often with retinal vasculitis. Different types of posterior uveitis may have a similar clinical appearance, although some clinical patterns of disease are nearly pathognomonic for diagnosis. Structural complications such as macular edema, epiretinal membrane, and retinal or choroidal neovascularization are not sufficient for the anatomical classification of posterior uveitis. Chapters 9–12 discuss noninfectious and infectious posterior uveitis in greater detail.

Panuveitis

In panuveitis, inflammation is present in all anatomical divisions of the eye without a predominantly affected site. The inflammation may be associated with an infectious or noninfectious systemic disease. See also Chapters 10–12, which discuss noninfectious and infectious panuveitis, and Chapter 14, which covers endophthalmitis.

Retinal vasculitis

Retinal vasculitis is defined by the presence of retinal vascular changes in association with ocular inflammation. The term *retinal vasculitis* is used in distinction to *vasculopathy,* in which there are vessel changes but no visible evidence of inflammation. On fluorescein angiography studies, retinal vasculitis encompasses perivascular sheathing, vascular leakage, or occlusion. Peripheral vascular sheathing may be observed in intermediate uveitis, but it is not sufficient for the anatomical classification of posterior uveitis/panuveitis. Retinal vasculitis is not

Table 5-4 Diseases With Retinal Vasculitis

Primarily Arteritis	Primarily Phlebitis	Arteritis and Phlebitis
Systemic lupus erythematosus	Sarcoidosis	Ocular toxoplasmosis
Polyarteritis nodosa	Multiple sclerosis	Relapsing polychondritis
Syphilis	Behçet disease	Granulomatosis with polyangiitis
HSV, VZV (ARN/BARN)	Birdshot chorioretinopathy	Crohn disease
HSV, VZV (PORN)	HIV paraviral syndrome	Frosted branch angiitis
IRVAN	Eales disease	
Churg-Strauss syndrome		
Susac syndrome		

ARN = acute retinal necrosis; BARN = bilateral acute retinal necrosis; HSV = herpes simplex virus; IRVAN = idiopathic retinal vasculitis, aneurysms, and neuroretinitis; PORN = progressive outer retinal necrosis; VZV = varicella-zoster virus.

Adapted from Foster CS, Vitale AT. *Diagnosis and Treatment of Uveitis.* 2nd ed. Jaypee Brothers Medical Publishers; 2012:123–128.

considered a defining feature for the anatomical classification of any type of uveitis. Table 5-4 summarizes diseases associated with retinal vasculitis.

Classification by Clinical Features

Certain types of uveitis have stereotyped clinical patterns; recognizing and labeling these patterns can aid in obtaining the correct uveitis diagnosis. The SUN system is useful for describing onset, duration, and course of uveitis, as summarized in Table 5-2. The severity of the inflammation may also influence categorization and prognosis. For example, the inflammatory process may occur in one or both eyes, or it may alternate between them. The clinical appearance, size, and distribution of lesions—especially chorioretinal lesions and keratic precipitates—are also used to describe uveitis. Naming conventions for descriptive terms are discussed in the Signs of Uveitis section that follows.

Uveitis can be clinically described as granulomatous or nongranulomatous; however, these descriptions do not necessarily correlate with the *histologic* appearance and may be influenced by the disease stage, the amount of antigen at presentation, or the treatment stage (eg, after initiation of corticosteroid treatment). In addition, uveitis may present with granulomatous features that eventually appear nongranulomatous with chronicity or treatment. Histologically, *granulomatous* inflammation is characterized by epithelioid and giant cells; clinically, granulomatous uveitis may include large, predominantly inferior, clumped keratic precipitates or nodular or creamy deposits in the iris, vitreous, optic nerve, and/or choroid. In contrast, *nongranulomatous* inflammation typically has a lymphocytic and plasma cell infiltrate; clinically, nongranulomatous uveitis is characterized by smaller keratic precipitates that are distributed diffusely, but uveal deposits are absent.

Discrete histologic granulomas are characteristic of sarcoidosis and tuberculosis, and diffuse clinical granulomatous inflammation appears in Vogt-Koyanagi-Harada syndrome and sympathetic ophthalmia. Viral anterior uveitis may present with a granulomatous or nongranulomatous appearance. Zonal histologic granulomatous disease can be observed in lens-induced uveitis.

Symptoms of Uveitis

Symptoms produced by uveitis depend on the site of uveal tract inflammation, the rapidity of onset, the duration of the disease, the course of the disease, and sometimes the underlying etiology.

Depending on the etiology and severity of inflammation, the presentation of anterior uveitis may range from an asymptomatic white eye to an extremely painful red eye. Sudden-onset anterior uveitis usually causes acute eye pain and redness, photophobia, and blurred vision. Pain results from ciliary spasm associated with iris inflammation and may radiate over the larger area served by the fifth cranial nerve (the trigeminal nerve). Intraocular pressure (IOP) elevation due to angle closure or trabeculitis can also cause pain.

In contrast, in patients with juvenile idiopathic arthritis, chronic anterior uveitis may not be associated with any symptoms at all. Even when patients are initially asymptomatic, however, chronic or severe anterior uveitis can cause blurred vision because of structural complications such as calcific band keratopathy, cataract, or macular edema.

Isolated intermediate uveitis presents with a white, quiet eye and produces symptoms of floaters and blurred vision. Floaters result from the shadows cast by vitreous cells and debris on the retina. Blurred vision can result from macular edema or vitreous opacities in the visual axis.

In patients with posterior uveitis, presenting symptoms include painless blurred vision, floaters, photopsias, scotomas, metamorphopsia, nyctalopia, or a combination of these symptoms. The blurred vision is caused primarily by retinitis and/or choroiditis directly affecting macular function or secondarily by complications of inflammation such as macular edema. Table 5-5 summarizes the symptoms of uveitis.

Signs of Uveitis

The chemical mediators involved in inflammation (see Chapter 1) result in vascular dilation (ciliary flush), increased vascular permeability causing migration of proteins into the eye (aqueous flare in the anterior segment), and chemotaxis of inflammatory cells into the eye (aqueous and vitreous cellular reaction). Table 5-6 summarizes the ocular findings that may be seen in uveitis.

Table 5-5 Symptoms of Uveitis

Acute Anterior Segment Inflammation	Posterior Segment Inflammation
Redness	Floaters
Pain	Photopsias
Photophobia	Scotomas (central or peripheral)
Epiphora	Metamorphopsia
Blurred vision[a]	Nyctalopia
	Blurred vision[a]

[a] Blurred vision may occur because of refractive shift; blockage from inflammatory cells; cataract; calcific band keratopathy; macular edema; retinochoroiditis; or corneal, macular, or optic disc edema.
Note: Some subsets of uveitis may have no symptoms.

Table 5-6 Findings Associated With Uveitis

Eyelid and skin
- Vitiligo
- Nodules
- Ptosis/eyelid edema

Conjunctiva or sclera
- Injection
  - Perilimbal (ciliary flush)
  - Diffuse or sectoral
  - Episcleral or scleral
- Nodules
- Scleral thinning

Corneal endothelium
- Keratic (cellular) precipitates (diffuse or inferior cornea)
- Fibrin
- Pigment (nonspecific)

Anterior chamber
- Cells
- Aqueous flare (proteinaceous influx)
- Pigment (nonspecific)

Iris
- Nodules
- Posterior synechiae
- Atrophy
- Heterochromia

Angle
- Peripheral anterior synechiae
- Nodules
- Vascularization

Intraocular pressure
- Hypotony
- High pressure
- Trabeculitis or secondary glaucoma

Vitreous
- Cells (single or clumped)
- Haze (proteinaceous influx)
- Traction bands

Pars plana
- Snowbanks

Retina
- Thickening and/or whitening (retinitis, infiltrate, ischemia, necrosis)
- Inflammatory cuffing of vessels (sheathing)
- Neovascularization
- Edema
- Macular edema
- Epiretinal membranes
- Subretinal fluid
- Retinal pigment epithelium: hypertrophy, clumping, or loss

Choroid
- Inflammatory infiltrate/thickening
- Atrophy
- Neovascularization

Optic nerve
- Edema (nonspecific)
- Neovascularization
- Pallor

Anterior Segment

Signs of uveitis and structural complications in the anterior portion of the eye include

- inflammatory cells (Fig 5-1)
- aqueous flare (Fig 5-2)
- hypopyon
- fibrin in the anterior chamber
- keratic precipitates (Figs 5-3, 5-4)
- iris nodules (Fig 5-5)
- iris atrophy or heterochromia
- pupillary miosis
- synechiae, anterior and posterior (Fig 5-6)
- pigment dispersion
- cataract (more likely in chronic uveitis than in acute disease)
- band keratopathy (more likely in chronic uveitis than in acute disease)

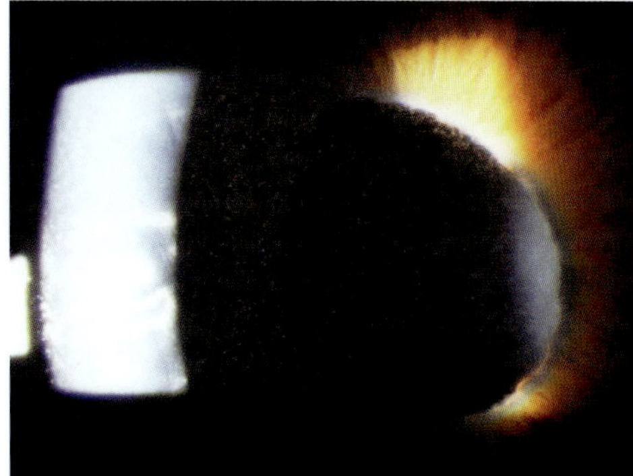

Figure 5-1 Inflammatory cells in the anterior chamber (grade 4+) of a patient with anterior uveitis. *(Courtesy of Emmett T. Cunningham Jr, MD, PhD, MPH.)*

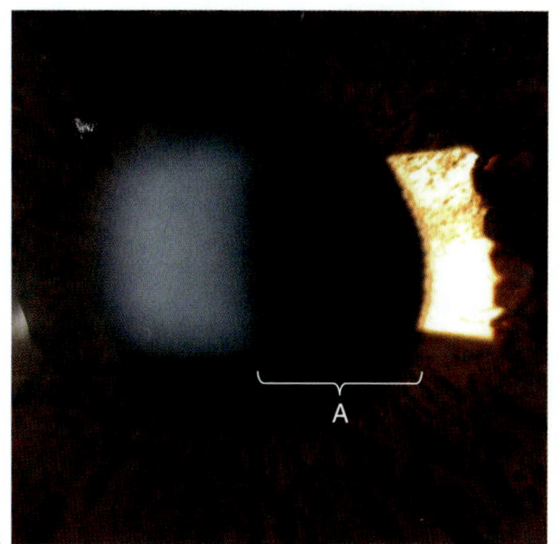

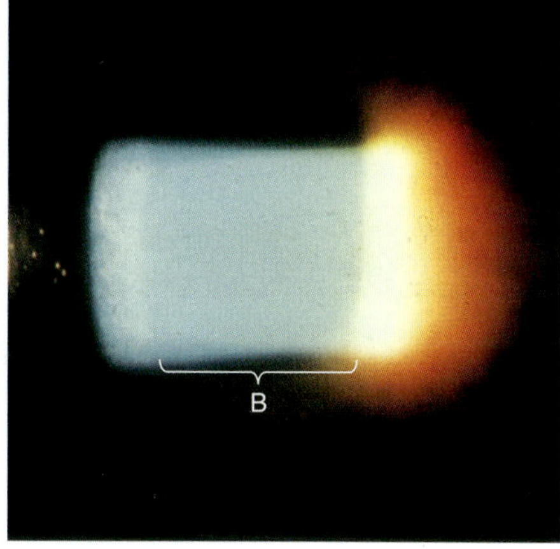

Figure 5-2 Appearance of the slit-lamp beam when grading aqueous flare. **A,** In a healthy eye with no aqueous flare, the anterior chamber is optically empty, creating an interrupted appearance of the light beam. **B,** In a severely inflamed eye, aqueous proteins scatter light, creating a continuous appearance of the beam (4+ flare). *(Part A courtesy of Zachary A. Koretz, MD, MPH.)*

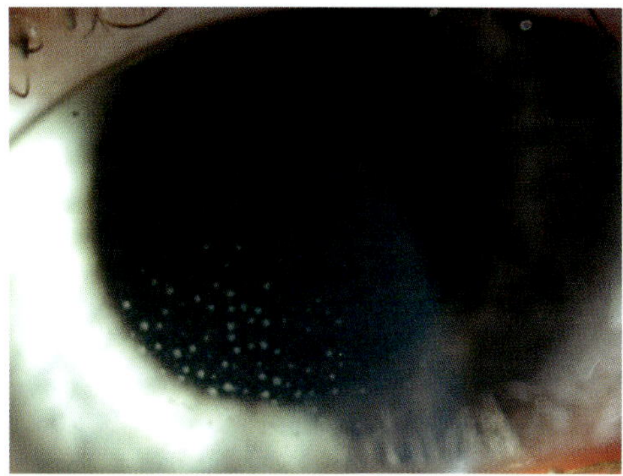

Figure 5-3 Keratic precipitates (medium and small). *(Courtesy of Debra A. Goldstein, MD.)*

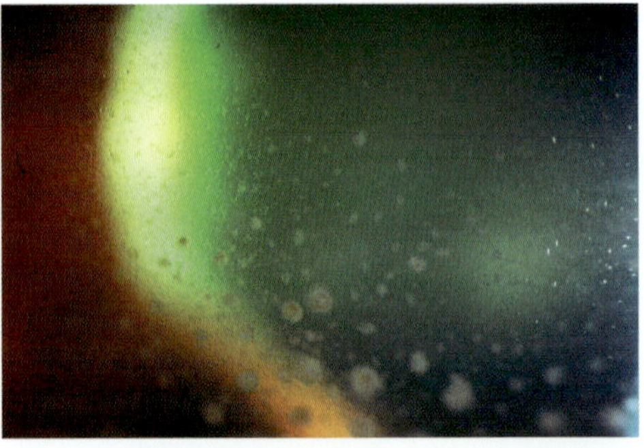

Figure 5-4 Large "mutton-fat" keratic precipitates in a patient with sarcoidosis. Large keratic precipitates such as these may be associated with a granulomatous disease process. *(Courtesy of Debra A. Goldstein, MD.)*

A B

C

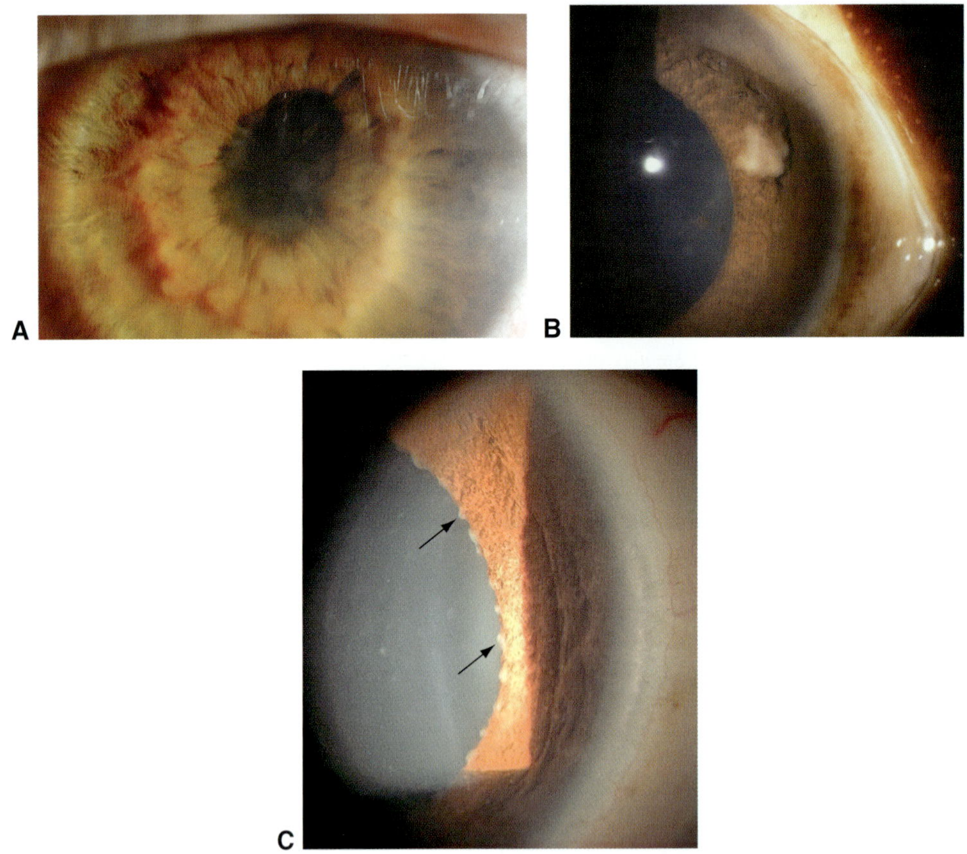

Figure 5-5 **A, B** Mid-iris nodules (Busacca nodules) in two patients with sarcoidosis. **C,** Nodules on pupil margin (Koeppe nodules; *arrows highlight 2 of them*) in another patient with sarcoidosis. *(Part A courtesy of Debra A. Goldstein, MD; part B courtesy of Wendy M. Smith, MD; and part C courtesy of Sam S. Dahr, MD, MS.)*

The major finding in anterior uveitis is the presence of inflammatory cells and flare in the anterior chamber, but there may be many additional sequelae (see the preceding list). The SUN system grades anterior chamber cells according to the number of inflammatory cells observed on slit-lamp examination in a field defined as a 1×1-mm high-power

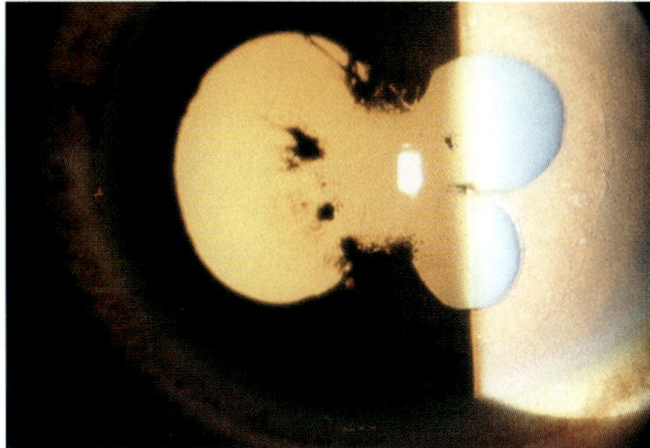

Figure 5-6 Multiple posterior synechiae preventing complete dilation of the pupil. *(Courtesy of David Forster, MD.)*

Table 5-7 Grading Scheme for Anterior Chamber Cells and Flare Based on Standardization of Uveitis Nomenclature (SUN) Criteria

Grade	Number of Cells (High-Intensity 1 × 1-mm Slit Beam)	Flare
0	<1	None
0.5+	1–5	Not applicable
1+	6–15	Faint
2+	16–25	Moderate (clear iris details)
3+	26–50	Marked (hazy iris details)
4+	>50	Intense (fibrin or plasmoid aqueous)

Reproduced with permission from Jabs DA, Nussenblatt RB, Rosenbaum JT; Standardization of Uveitis Nomenclature (SUN) Working Group. Standardization of nomenclature for reporting clinical data: results of the First International Workshop. *Am J Ophthalmol.* 2005;140(3):512.

(16×–20×) beam at full intensity at a 45°–60° angle in a dark room. For the cell grade of 0.5+, there must be at least 1 cell per high-power field in each of the 4 anterior chamber quadrants. Flare is defined by the visibility of the slit-lamp beam in the anterior chamber. The SUN system adopted the flare grading method described previously by Hogan and colleagues (Table 5-7).

The anterior chamber reaction can be described as follows:

- serous (aqueous flare caused by proteinaceous influx)
- purulent (polymorphonuclear leukocytes and necrotic debris causing hypopyon)
- fibrinous (plasmoid or intense fibrinous exudate)
- sanguinoid (inflammatory cells with erythrocytes, as manifested by hypopyon mixed with hyphema)

Keratic precipitates (KPs), collections of inflammatory cells on the corneal endothelium, are described by

- size: small, medium, or large
- morphology: fine, round, nummular, stellate, granulomatous, mutton-fat
- distribution: diffusely over entire corneal endothelium, settled in a gravity-dependent triangular pattern in the inferior cornea *(Arlt triangle)*, or focal and associated with corneal inflammation

Newly formed KPs tend to be white and smoothly rounded, later becoming crenated (shrunken), pigmented, or glassy in nature. Large, yellowish KPs are called *mutton-fat KPs* and are usually associated with granulomatous types of inflammation. Small stellate KPs distributed diffusely on the cornea are usually associated with Fuchs uveitis syndrome or herpetic anterior uveitis. Associated corneal edema may also be present. Band keratopathy is seen in chronic uveitis (especially juvenile idiopathic arthritis associated).

Iris involvement may manifest as either anterior or posterior synechiae, iris nodules (Koeppe nodules at the pupillary border, Busacca nodules within the iris stroma [see Fig 5-5], and Berlin nodules in the angle), iris granulomas, heterochromia (eg, Fuchs uveitis syndrome), or stromal atrophy (eg, herpetic uveitis).

With uveitic involvement of the ciliary body and trabecular meshwork, IOP is often low, secondary to decreased aqueous production or increased uveoscleral outflow; however, IOP may increase precipitously if the meshwork becomes clogged by inflammatory cells or debris or if the trabecular meshwork itself is the site of inflammation (ie, trabeculitis, characteristically in herpetic uveitis). Pupillary block with iris bombé and secondary angle closure may also lead to an acute rise in IOP.

Hogan MJ, Kimura SJ, Thygeson P. Signs and symptoms of uveitis: I. Anterior uveitis. *Am J Ophthalmol.* 1959;47(5, part 2):155–170.

Intermediate Segment

Signs of uveitis and structural complications in the intermediate portion of the eye include

- inflammatory cells in vitreous
- vitreous haze (Fig 5-7)
- snowballs (clumped inflammatory cells in vitreous)
- snowbanks (exudate over pars plana)
- ciliary body detachment
- retrolental membrane
- vitreous strands or traction band

The hallmark of intermediate uveitis is vitreous cells and haze. Cells may be clumped or individual. Vitreous haze is due to proteinaceous vitreous debris. Vitreous cells can be present without haze.

The physician typically grades vitreous cells on a 0–4 numeric scale by observing the retrolental space in a dilated eye using the slit-lamp biomicroscope and a 1 × 0.5-mm beam (Fig 5-8). The consensus is that cells in the vitreous strands are old, and cells in the syneretic areas are most likely new. Of note, the SUN system does not specify a grading system for vitreous cells. Table 5-8 shows the vitreous cell grading scale used in the Multicenter Uveitis Steroid Treatment Trial (MUST).

Vitreous haze may be a better indicator of disease activity than cell counts alone. The grading of vitreous haze is based on the clarity of view of the posterior segment on ophthalmoscopic examination using an indirect ophthalmoscope and a 20 D lens. The National Institutes of Health grading system for vitreous haze, adopted by the SUN system, uses a standardized set of fundus photographs that defines vitreous haze on a 0–4 scale (see Fig 5-7).

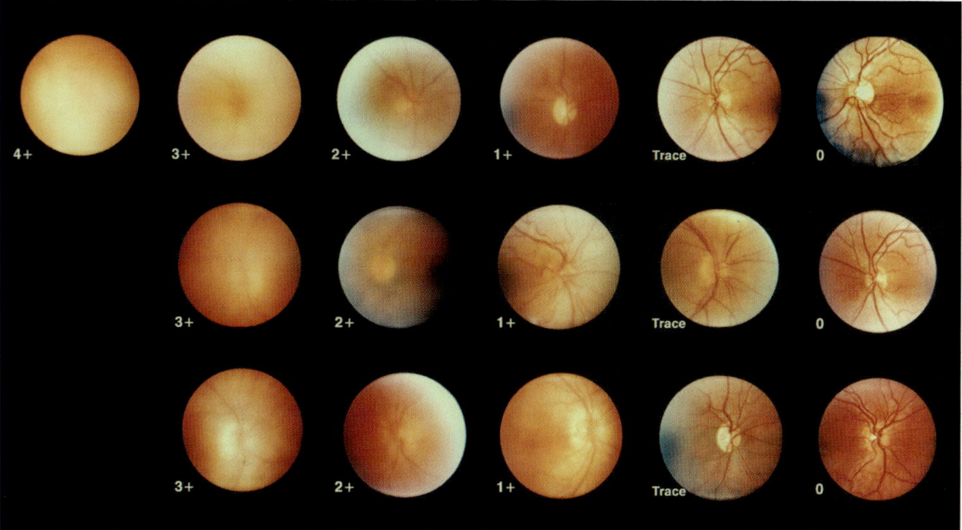

Figure 5-7 Grading scale for vitreous haze: representative standard images. Grade 4: Dense opacity obscuring optic nerve head. Grade 3: Optic nerve visible, borders blurred, no retinal vessels seen. Grade 2: Optic nerve and retinal vessels substantially blurred but still visible. Grade 1: Few opacities, mild blurring of optic nerve and retinal vessels. Trace (0.5+): Trace. Grade 0: Clear. *(Courtesy of National Eye Institute; originally published in Nussenblatt RB, Palestine AG, Chan CC, et al. Standardization of vitreal inflammatory activity in intermediate and posterior uveitis.* Ophthalmology. *1985;92(4):467–471.)*

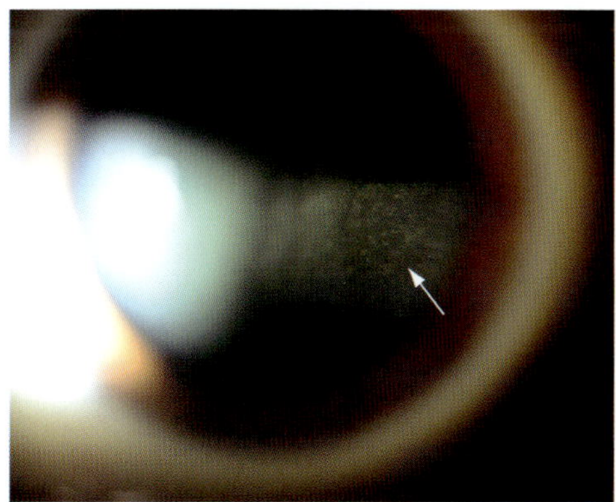

Figure 5-8 Slit-lamp photograph of vitreous cells *(arrow)* in the retrolental space of an inflamed eye. *(Courtesy of Emilio M. Dodds, MD.)*

Table 5-8 Grading Scheme for Vitreous Chamber Cells and Haze

Grade	Number of Cells in Retrolental Space (High-Intensity 1 × 0.5-mm Slit Beam)	Vitreous Haze
0	0	Clear view of fundus
0.5+	1–5	Not applicable
1+	6–10	Faint
2+	11–20	Moderate (clear optic nerve details)
3+	21–50	Marked (hazy optic nerve details)
4+	>50	Intense (minimal/no optic nerve detail)

Vitreous haze has been used as inclusion criteria in clinical trials for uveitis, and a 2-step improvement in haze has been used as a principal outcome measure.

Additional signs of inflammation in the vitreous include *snowball opacities* (clumps of inflammatory cells in the vitreous) and *snowbanks* (exudates over the pars plana, especially prominent inferiorly). Active snowbanks have a fluffy or shaggy appearance. As pars planitis becomes inactive, the pars plana appears gliotic or fibrotic and smooth; thus, these changes are not referred to as *snowbanks.* Vitreous strands and snowballs may also vary in clinical appearance by disease type. Chronic intermediate uveitis may be associated with cyclitic membrane formation, secondary ciliary body detachment, and hypotony.

Posterior Segment

Signs of uveitis and structural complications in the posterior segment of the eye include the following:

- retinal or choroidal inflammatory infiltrates
- inflammatory sheathing of arteries or veins
- perivascular hemorrhage
- exudative, tractional, or rhegmatogenous retinal detachment
- retinal pigment epithelial hypertrophy or atrophy
- atrophy or swelling of the retina, choroid, or optic nerve head
- preretinal or subretinal fibrosis
- retinal or choroidal neovascularization

Posterior segment inflammation is a result of inflammatory or infectious infiltration of the retina and choroid. Retinal and choroidal signs may be unifocal, multifocal, or diffuse. Lesions are described by size, color, morphology, and anatomical relationship to posterior pole landmarks. Some active lesions may exhibit blurred margins, transitioning to sharply defined and/or pigmented borders when inactive.

Chorioretinal lesion morphology may be described as follows:

- punched out: round with well-demarcated borders
- placoid: large, flat, gray-white lesions with patchy distribution and indistinct margins
- serpentine: lesions with sharply defined wavy borders

Altaweel MM, Gangaputra SS, Thorne JE, et al. Morphological assessment of the retina in uveitis. *J Ophthalmic Inflamm Infect.* 2016;6(1):33. doi:10.1186/s12348-016-0103-2

Nussenblatt RB, Palestine AG, Chan CC, Roberge F. Standardization of vitreal inflammatory activity in intermediate and posterior uveitis. *Ophthalmology.* 1985;92(4):467–471.

Review of the Patient's Health and Other Associated Factors

When uveitis is suspected, a comprehensive patient history and review of systems help to narrow the differential diagnosis and guide ancillary testing and treatment options. The patient's personal characteristics, medical history, and social history can help in the

Table 5-9 Patient Factors in the Diagnosis of Uveitis

Patient Characteristics	Family and Social History	Additional Modifying Factors
Age Sex Genetic traits, and sometimes race, ethnicity and/or country of origin	Family or personal history of autoimmune disease/ endemic infection Intravenous drug use Tobacco exposure Occupation Sexual practices Eating habits Animal exposures	Immunization history Immune system status Systemic medications Trauma history Travel history Hospital admissions/surgery Indwelling lines/instrumentation Review of systems and existing medical conditions

classification and identification of uveitis (Table 5-9). Immunocompromise, sexual practices, use of intravenous drugs, hyperalimentation, and certain occupations are some examples of the risk factors that can direct the investigation. In this regard, the diagnostic survey for uveitis shown in Appendix A may be very helpful.

Although ocular inflammation can be an isolated process involving only the eye, it can also be associated with a systemic condition. However, uveitis frequently does not correlate with inflammatory activity elsewhere in the body and may precede the development of inflammation at other body sites.

Differential Diagnosis of Uveitis

The differential diagnosis of uveitis includes infectious diseases due to a variety of agents (viruses, bacteria, fungi, protozoa, and helminths), noninfectious entities of presumed immunologic origin, and unknown causes (called *idiopathic* or *undifferentiated uveitis*). In addition, masquerade syndromes such as vitreoretinal lymphoma, retinoblastoma, leukemia, choroidal metastases, and malignant melanoma may be mistaken for uveitis. Other relevant masquerade syndromes include juvenile xanthogranuloma, pigment dispersion syndrome, retinal detachment, vitreous hemorrhage, retinitis pigmentosa, and ocular ischemic syndrome. Each of these masquerade syndromes should be considered in the differential diagnosis of uveitis. See Chapter 15 for further discussion of masquerade syndromes.

A careful patient history and accurate description of ophthalmoscopic findings are extremely helpful in narrowing the differential diagnosis, as certain presentations are characteristic for specific diseases. However, many patients do not present with the classic signs and symptoms of uveitis, or their clinical appearance may evolve with time and treatment. In these cases, the clinician should still rely on the tools of classification based on anatomical location and associated factors (eg, acute versus chronic, unilateral versus bilateral, adult versus child) to narrow the differential to the uveitic entities that share the patient's characteristics. See Table 5-10 for a simplified version of one system for narrowing the differential diagnosis. Activity 5-1 provides a decision-tree algorithm for the evaluation of a patient with uveitis.

Table 5-10 Simplified Scheme for Patient Evaluation in Uveitis

Type of Inflammation	Possible Associated Factors	Suspected Disease[a]	Ancillary Tests and Consultations
Anterior Uveitis			
Acute/sudden onset, severe with or without fibrin membrane or hypopyon	Arthritis, back pain, GI/GU symptoms	Seronegative spondyloarthropathies (ankylosing spondylitis, reactive arthritis, inflammatory bowel disease, psoriatic arthritis)	HLA-B27; sacroiliac films; rheumatology, gastroenterology referrals
	Oral and genital ulcers, skin findings	Behçet disease	Clinical diagnosis, screen for other organ involvement; rheumatology referral
	Febrile illness, flank or abdominal pain	TINU syndrome	Renal function tests, urinalysis, urine β_2-microglobulin; nephrology referral
	Postsurgical or penetrating eye trauma or systemic indwelling lines/instrumentation/infection	Infectious endophthalmitis, toxic anterior segment syndrome	B-scan for vitritis, consider vitreous culture, vitrectomy For endogenous endophthalmitis, consider blood cultures and systemic infectious workup
	None	Undifferentiated (idiopathic)	HLA-B27
Moderate severity (red, painful)	Shortness of breath, skin findings, granulomatous inflammation	Sarcoidosis	ACE, lysozyme; CXR/chest CT; biopsy
	Blunt eye trauma	Traumatic iritis	
	Increased IOP	Glaucomatocyclitic crisis, herpetic iritis If pseudophakic, uveitis-glaucoma-hyphema syndrome	Clinical diagnosis; PCR of intraocular fluid[b] optional
	Poor response to steroids	Syphilis	Syphilis IgG or FTA-ABS or MHA-TP followed by RPR or VDRL test
	Postsurgical	Low-grade endophthalmitis (eg, *Cutibacterium acnes*); IOL related	Consider vitrectomy, capsulectomy with culture

Type of Inflammation	Possible Associated Factors	Suspected Disease[a]	Ancillary Tests and Consultations
Anterior Uveitis *(continued)*			
Chronic (minimal redness, pain)	Child, especially with arthritis	JIA-associated anterior uveitis	ANA, ESR, RF; rheumatology referral
	Heterochromia or small nodules, diffuse KPs, unilateral	Fuchs uveitis syndrome	Clinical diagnosis
	Postsurgical	Low-grade endophthalmitis (eg, *C acnes*); IOL related	Consider vitrectomy, capsulectomy with culture
	None	Undifferentiated	
Intermediate Uveitis			
Mild to moderate	Shortness of breath, skin findings, granulomatous inflammation	Sarcoidosis	ACE, lysozyme; CXR/chest CT; biopsy
	Tick exposure, erythema chronicum migrans rash, endemic area	Lyme disease (may also be anterior uveitis, posterior/ panuveitis)	ELISA, Western blot for confirmation
	Neurologic symptoms	Multiple sclerosis	MRI of brain and C-spine; LP for oligoclonal bands; neurology referral
	Older than 50 years	Vitreoretinal lymphoma	Vitrectomy; chorioretinal biopsy; cytology; IL-10:IL-6 ratio[b]; *MYD88* mutation, genotyping studies; brain MRI, LP
	None	Pars planitis	
Posterior Uveitis			
Chorioretinitis with vitritis			
Focal	Adjacent scar; ingestion of raw meat, unwashed vegetables, endemic area	Toxoplasmosis	Clinical diagnosis; negative serology to rule out the diagnosis; PCR of intraocular fluid[b] optional
	Child; history of geophagia	Toxocariasis	Clinical diagnosis; ELISA, complete blood count with differential
	HIV infection or immunosuppressed	CMV retinitis (variable vitritis)	PCR of intraocular fluid[b]
Multifocal	Shortness of breath, skin findings	Sarcoidosis	ACE, lysozyme; CXR/chest CT; biopsy
	TB-endemic area	TB	IGRA or PPD, CXR/chest CT
	Peripheral retinal necrosis with occlusive arteriolar vasculitis	ARN	PCR of intraocular fluid[b]; possibly vitrectomy/retinal biopsy

(Continued)

Table 5-10 *(continued)*

Type of Inflammation	Possible Associated Factors	Suspected Disease[a]	Ancillary Tests and Consultations
Posterior Uveitis *(continued)*			
	HIV infection or immunosuppressed	Syphilis, toxoplasmosis	Syphilis IgG or FTA-ABS or MHA-TP and RPR or VDRL test; *Toxoplasma* serology
	IV drug use, indwelling lines	*Candida, Aspergillus* infection	Blood, vitreous cultures
	Visible intraocular parasite, patient origin from Africa or Central/South America	Cysticercosis	ELISA, brain MRI
		Onchocerciasis	Skin snip
	Older than 50 years	Vitreoretinal lymphoma	Vitrectomy; chorioretinal biopsy cytology; IL-10:IL-6 ratio[b]; *MYD88* mutation, genotyping studies; brain MRI, LP
	None	Birdshot chorioretinopathy	Clinical diagnosis; HLA-A29
		Multifocal choroiditis with panuveitis	Rule out TB, sarcoidosis, syphilis
Diffuse	Dermatologic/CNS symptoms; serous retinal disease; no history of ocular surgery or penetrating ocular trauma	Vogt-Koyanagi-Harada syndrome	Clinical diagnosis; LP to document CSF pleocytosis; consider audiology referral
	Postsurgical/traumatic, bilateral, serous retinal disease	Sympathetic ophthalmia	
	Postsurgical/traumatic, unilateral	Infectious endophthalmitis	Consider vitrectomy, culture
	Child; history of geophagia	Toxocariasis	ELISA; complete blood count with differential
Unilateral	Warm climate; host animal exposures	DUSN: early disease has gray, clustered lesions and vitritis; late findings are diffuse RPE degeneration, waxy disc pallor, attenuated arterioles	Clinical diagnosis; visualization of nematode

Type of Inflammation	Possible Associated Factors	Suspected Disease[a]	Ancillary Tests and Consultations
Posterior Uveitis *(continued)*			
Chorioretinitis *without* vitritis			
Focal	None; history of carcinoma	Neoplastic masquerade	Metastatic workup
Multifocal	Ohio/Mississippi Valley	Ocular histoplasmosis	Clinical diagnosis
	Lesions confined to posterior pole	White dot syndromes (eg, APMPPE, MEWDS, PIC)	Clinical diagnosis
	Serpentine or maplike pattern of scars	Serpiginous choroiditis	IGRA or PPD; CXR
Diffuse	From Africa, Central/South America	Onchocerciasis	Skin snip
	Severe immunocompromise (eg, AIDS)	Progressive outer retinal necrosis	Same as for ARN
Vasculitis			
	Aphthous ulcers, hypopyon	Behçet disease	Clinical diagnosis, screen for other organ involvement; rheumatology referral
	Malar rash, female, arthralgias	Systemic lupus erythematosus	ANA, anti-dsDNA, C3, C4; rheumatology referral
	Chronic sinusitis with hemorrhagic rhinorrhea, dyspnea, renal insufficiency, purpura	Granulomatosis with polyangiitis	c-ANCA (anti–proteinase 3); rheumatology referral
Panuveitis			
See entities described earlier in the table: sarcoidosis, Vogt-Koyanagi-Harada syndrome, sympathetic ophthalmia, Behçet disease, syphilis, toxoplasmosis, endophthalmitis, toxocariasis, and cysticercosis.			

ACE = angiotensin-converting enzyme; ANA = antinuclear antibody; anti-dsDNA = anti–double-stranded DNA antibody; APMPPE = acute posterior multifocal placoid pigment epitheliopathy; ARN = acute retinal necrosis; c-ANCA = cytoplasmic antineutrophil cytoplasmic antibody; CMV = cytomegalovirus; CNS = central nervous system; CSF = cerebrospinal fluid; CT = computed tomography; CXR = chest x-ray; DUSN = diffuse unilateral subacute neuroretinitis; ELISA = enzyme-linked immunosorbent assay; ESR = erythrocyte sedimentation rate; FTA-ABS = fluorescent treponemal antibody absorption test; GI = gastrointestinal; GU = genitourinary; HLA = human leukocyte antigen; IgG = immunoglobulin G; IGRA = interferon-gamma release assay; IL = interleukin; IOL = intraocular lens; IOP = intraocular pressure; IV = intravenous; JIA = juvenile idiopathic arthritis; KP = keratic precipitate; LP = lumbar puncture; MEWDS = multiple evanescent white dot syndrome; MHA-TP = microhemagglutination assay–*Treponema pallidum;* MRI = magnetic resonance imaging; PCR = polymerase chain reaction; PIC = punctate inner choroidopathy; PPD = purified protein derivative; RF = rheumatoid factor; RPE = retinal pigment epithelium; RPR = rapid plasma reagin; TB = tuberculosis; TINU = tubulointerstitial nephritis and uveitis.

[a] Syphilis may present as any type of uveitis and should be considered in all patients.

[b] Testing where available.

ACTIVITY 5-1 Flowchart for clinical diagnosis and treatment of uveitis: simplified interactive tool.
Activity developed by Thellea K. Leveque, MD, MPH.

Ancillary Testing

Medical history, review of systems, thorough ophthalmologic and general physical examinations, and formulation of a working differential diagnosis are cornerstones of the workup of a patient with uveitis. Once a list of differential diagnoses has been compiled on the basis of anatomical location and clinical characteristics of the inflammation, the ophthalmologist can order appropriate laboratory tests. A "shotgun" approach to a uveitis workup (eg, ordering laboratory tests without consideration of a reasonable differential) is expensive and may yield confusing results, which may not be related to the uveitis but will still require further evaluation to rule out clinical significance. Laboratory testing is not a substitute for a thorough, hands-on clinical evaluation.

Regarding ancillary testing, *no standardized battery of tests is appropriate for all patients with uveitis.* Rather, a tailored testing approach should be based on the most likely causes of ocular inflammation in each case. Many patients will require only a few diagnostic tests.

Most uveitis specialists do recommend syphilis testing for all patients with uveitis because syphilis can present as any form of ocular inflammation and systemic infection is often undiagnosed. In addition, if a patient with occult syphilis infection is treated with only corticosteroids, the systemic and ophthalmic outcomes can be disastrous. In the appropriate clinical scenario or when systemic immunomodulatory therapy will be used, most uveitis specialists also recommend testing for tuberculosis. A chest radiograph can also screen for sarcoidosis, which is a common cause of uveitis with protean manifestations. Table 5-11 lists some of the laboratory tests and imaging studies used in uveitis evaluations, as well as their indications. Later chapters also discuss these tests according to types of uveitis.

CLINICAL PEARL

There is no accepted "uveitis workup" or standard workup that is appropriate for all of the various types of uveitis. Use the review of systems and the examination findings to define the differential diagnosis. Based on the differential, select diagnostic testing and imaging to rule in or rule out diagnoses. A "shotgun" approach to a uveitis workup (eg, ordering laboratory tests without consideration of a reasonable differential) is expensive and may yield confusing results that are not related to the uveitis but still require further evaluation to confirm the lack of clinical significance.

It is important to use caution not only when ordering laboratory tests but also when interpreting their results, as even very sensitive and specific tests can yield misleading results if the likelihood of disease in a particular patient is low. In other words, when a large group of patients are tested for a very rare disease, a positive test result may not represent the true presence of disease. The Bayes theorem, a statistical calculation used to determine

Table 5-11 Laboratory Tests and Imaging Studies Used in Uveitis Evaluations or Medication Monitoring

Test	Indications and/or Potential Diagnoses
Hematologic blood tests	
Complete blood count with differential	Baseline or monitoring for IMT and select antibiotics/antivirals Leukemia, lymphoma, immune status (eg, neutropenia)
Erythrocyte sedimentation rate	Giant cell arteritis, nonspecific systemic inflammation
Interferon-gamma release assay	Latent and active tuberculosis
T-cell subsets	Opportunistic infection, HIV
Serologic tests	
Liver function tests (ALT, AST)	IMT monitoring (antimetabolites) Sarcoidosis, hepatitis
Serum urea nitrogen, creatinine	IMT monitoring (T-cell inhibitors) Interstitial nephritis
Angiotensin-converting enzyme, lysozyme, calcium	Sarcoidosis
Antinuclear antibody	Connective tissue disease, juvenile idiopathic arthritis
Antiphospholipid antibodies	Vasculitis, vascular occlusion
Rheumatoid factor, anti-citrullinated protein antibody	Rheumatoid arthritis, juvenile idiopathic arthritis
HLA testing	
HLA-B27	Spondyloarthropathy, acute anterior uveitis
HLA-A29	Birdshot chorioretinopathy
HLA-B51 (rarely obtained and of limited value)	Behçet disease (*not* required for diagnosis)
HLA-DRB1*01:02	TINU syndrome
ANCA testing—c-ANCA (proteinase 3) and p-ANCA (myeloperoxidase)	Systemic vasculitides
Syphilis IgG/FTA-ABS/MHA-TP (treponemal tests); followed by reflex VDRL/RPR (nontreponemal tests)	Syphilis
Lyme disease serology	Lyme disease
Brucella species serology	Brucellosis
Toxoplasma gondii serology	Toxoplasmosis
Fungal serology (complement fixation), (1→3)-β-D-glucan assay	Coccidioidomycosis, typically not obtained for presumed ocular histoplasmosis; nonspecific fungal infection
Bartonella quintana and *Bartonella henselae* serology	Cat-scratch disease
EBV, HSV, VZV, CMV serology	Viral uveitis (little benefit unless negative)
HIV serology/Western blot	HIV/AIDS, opportunistic infections, vascular occlusions

(Continued)

Table 5-11 *(continued)*

Test	Indications and/or Potential Diagnoses
CSF studies	
Protein, glucose, cell counts/cytology, cultures, Gram stain, CSF VDRL, oligoclonal bands	APMPPE (if magnetic resonance imaging evidence of central nervous system vasculitis), VKH syndrome, syphilis and other infection, malignancy, vitreoretinal lymphoma, multiple sclerosis
Urine studies	
Urinalysis for hematuria, proteinuria, and casts; urinary β_2-microglobulin	IMT monitoring (cyclophosphamide toxicity) ANCA-associated vasculitides, TINU syndrome
Radiographic studies	
Chest radiography	Tuberculosis, sarcoidosis, granulomatosis with polyangiitis
Sacroiliac joint x-rays	Spondyloarthropathy
Computed tomography of chest	Tuberculosis, sarcoidosis, granulomatosis with polyangiitis
Computed tomography/magnetic resonance imaging of brain and orbits	Sarcoidosis, central nervous system lymphoma, toxoplasmosis, APMPPE, multiple sclerosis
Intraocular fluid analysis and tissue biopsy	
Polymerase chain reaction	Viridae: HSV-1, HSV-2, VZV, CMV, EBV, Ebola, Zika, West Nile, rubella Bacteria: universal 16S subunit for pan bacteria; individual polymerase chain reaction primers available for many individual bacteria, varies by laboratory Protozoa: *Toxoplasma gondii* Fungi: universal 18S or 28S subunit for pan fungi: *Candida albicans, Aspergillus* species (28S rRNA gene) Vitreoretinal lymphoma (IgH, TCR, *MYD88,* others)
Endoretinal, subretinal, choroidal biopsy	Necrotizing retinitis, neoplasia (vitreoretinal lymphoma, metastasis)
Skin, conjunctival, lacrimal biopsy	Sarcoidosis, infection, lymphoma, amyloidosis
Stool for detection of pathogenic microorganisms	Parasitic diseases; viruses, bacteria, fungi

ALT = alanine aminotransferase; ANCA = antineutrophil cytoplasmic antibody; APMPPE = acute posterior multifocal placoid pigment epitheliopathy; AST = aspartate aminotransferase; c-ANCA = cytoplasmic ANCA; CMV = cytomegalovirus; CSF = cerebrospinal fluid; EBV = Epstein-Barr virus; FTA-ABS = fluorescent treponemal antibody absorption test; HLA = human leukocyte antigen; HSV = herpes simplex virus; IgG = immunoglobulin G; IgH = immunoglobulin heavy locus; IMT = immunomodulatory therapy; MHA-TP = microhemagglutination assay–*Treponema pallidum;* p-ANCA = perinuclear ANCA; RPR = rapid plasma reagin; rRNA = ribosomal ribonucleic acid; TCR = T-cell receptor; TINU = tubulointerstitial nephritis and uveitis syndrome; VDRL = venereal disease research laboratory; VKH = Vogt-Koyanagi-Harada; VZV = varicella-zoster virus.

the probability of an event based on prior knowledge of conditions that may be related to the event, describes this concept. See BCSC Section 1, *Update on General Medicine.*

McKay KM, Lim LL, Van Gelder RN. Rational laboratory testing in uveitis: a Bayesian analysis. *Surv Ophthalmol.* 2021;66(5):802–825.

Ophthalmic Imaging and Functional Tests

Ophthalmic imaging and functional testing are useful for diagnosis of uveitis as well as for monitoring the patient's response to therapy. In addition, these tests can provide information not obtainable from biomicroscopic or fundus examination. The use of combined imaging modalities, called *multimodal imaging,* can be complementary and additive in these tasks. For discussion of ophthalmic imaging modalities and electroretinography, see BCSC Section 12, *Retina and Vitreous.*

Kawali A, Pichi F, Avadhani K, Invernizzi A, Hashimoto Y, Mahendradas P. Multimodal imaging of the normal eye. *Ocul Immunol Inflamm.* 2017;25(5):721–731.

Van Gelder RN. Diagnostic testing in uveitis. *Focal Points: Clinical Modules for Ophthalmologists.* American Academy of Ophthalmology; 2013, module 4.

Optical coherence tomography

Optical coherence tomography (OCT), a noncontact imaging technique that produces a series of high-resolution cross-sectional images of the retina and choroid, is used to identify morphologic changes in eyes with uveitis. In addition, OCT has become the reference standard for objective measurement of uveitic macular edema (Fig 5-9), retinal thickening, subretinal and intraretinal fluid associated with choroidal neovascularization, serous retinal detachments, and chorioretinal lesions. Although OCT can be surprisingly useful in evaluating the macula in eyes with nondilating pupils, media opacity can limit its clarity. In addition, OCT is valuable in monitoring the nerve fiber layer in patients with uveitic glaucoma, and anterior segment OCT may be useful in evaluating an eye for retained lens fragments or intraocular lens (IOL) chafing in those with persistent postoperative uveitis. Efforts to develop objective OCT-based grading of intraocular cells/inflammation are also ongoing.

Enhanced depth imaging OCT (Fig 5-10) provides deeper tissue penetration than standard OCT. This technique allows visualization of the choroid, which can undergo structural alterations in several uveitic diseases, notably Vogt-Koyanagi-Harada syndrome, sympathetic ophthalmia, and birdshot chorioretinopathy.

OCT angiography (OCTA) provides repeated high-resolution scans of the same area to assess differences in blood flow, producing structural images of perfused vessels in ocular tissues. OCTA can be useful in distinguishing between inflammatory lesions and choroidal neovascularization in the inflammatory retinochoroidopathies of unknown etiology (the *white dot syndromes*). Case reports and case series describing OCTA characteristics of active and inactive chorioretinal lesions are emerging. Over time, these may have increasing implications for the diagnosis and treatment of posterior uveitis entities.

Kim J, Knickelbein JE, Jaworski L, et al. Enhanced depth imaging optical coherence tomography in uveitis: an intravisit and interobserver reproducibility study. *Am J Ophthalmol.* 2016;164:49–56.

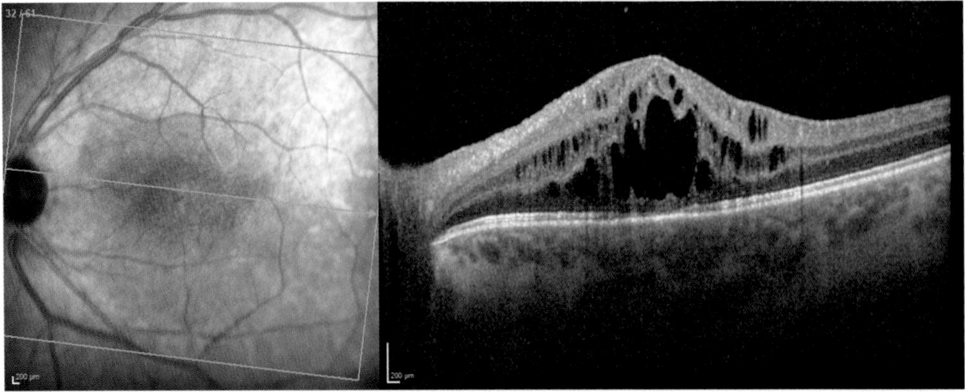

Figure 5-9 Optical coherence tomography (OCT) image of uveitic macular edema in a patient with juvenile idiopathic arthritis–associated uveitis. *(Courtesy of Thellea K. Leveque, MD, MPH.)*

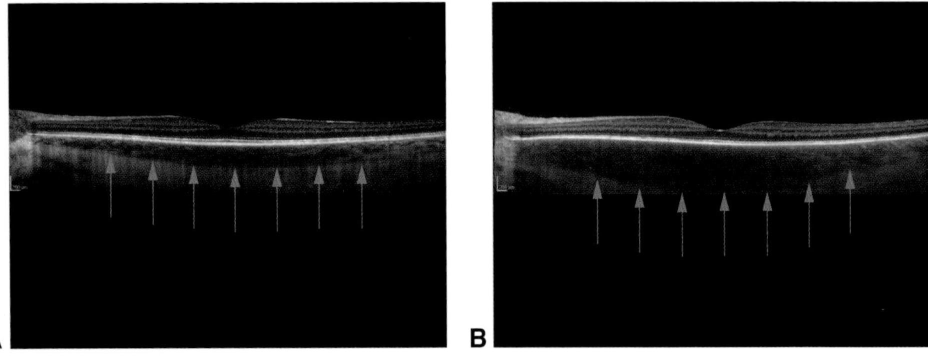

Figure 5-10 Enhanced depth imaging OCT in a patient with Vogt-Koyanagi-Harada syndrome. **A,** Relatively normal choroidal thickness *(arrows)* during quiescence. **B,** Massive, diffuse choroidal thickening *(arrows)* during active uveitis. *(Courtesy of Thellea K. Leveque, MD, MPH.)*

Pichi F, Sarraf D, Arepalli S, et al. The application of optical coherence tomography angiography in uveitis and inflammatory eye diseases. *Prog Retin Eye Res.* 2017;59:178–201.

Fluorescein angiography

Fluorescein angiography (FA) is an essential imaging modality for evaluating chorioretinal disease and structural complications caused by posterior uveitis. After intravenous injection of fluorescein sodium, a series of filtered posterior segment images provides functional and structural views of retinal (and to some degree choroidal) vasculature and anatomy. FA can also detect macular edema (Fig 5-11); retinal vasculitis; secondary choroidal or retinal neovascularization; and areas of optic nerve, retinal, and choroidal inflammation. In addition, several of the white dot syndromes have characteristic appearances on FA. Wide-field FA can identify retinal vascular pathology not visible on clinical examination.

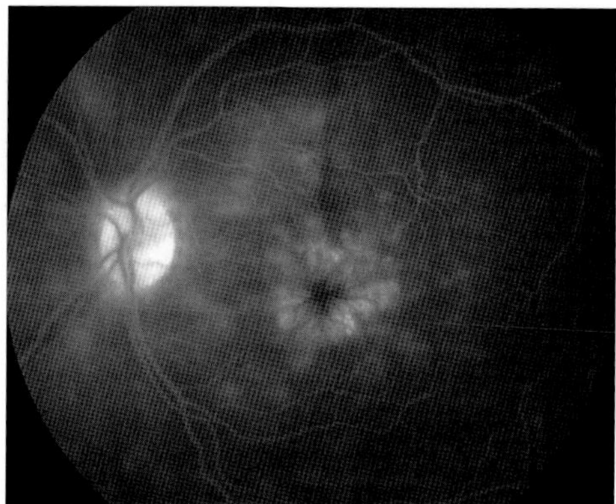

Figure 5-11 Late transit phase fluorescein angiogram of the left eye of a patient with sarcoidosis-associated anterior uveitis showing the petalloid pattern typical of uveitic macular edema. *(Courtesy of Ramana S. Moorthy, MD.)*

Laovirojjanakul W, Acharya N, Gonzales JA. Ultra-widefield fluorescein angiography in intermediate uveitis. *Ocul Immunol Inflamm.* 2019;27(3):356–361.

Color photography

Color photographs of the anterior or posterior segment can document lesion size, color, location, and morphologic characteristics and can be used to assess clinical progression or regression of disease, often in combination with other imaging modalities. These images can help establish a baseline when a relapsing and remitting inflammatory process is being assessed (eg, the presence of new posterior synechiae in anterior uveitis or transitory posterior segment inflammation characteristic of Behçet disease).

Fundus autofluorescence

Fundus autofluorescence imaging, another noninvasive technique for analyzing the posterior segment, maps the fluorescent property of lipofuscin, a breakdown product of retinal proteins, within the retinal pigment epithelium (RPE). This technique is useful in evaluating patients with posterior uveitis that involves the outer retina, RPE, and inner choroid. Hyperautofluorescence corresponds to increased metabolic activity of the RPE or window defect due to the loss of photoreceptors, whereas hypoautofluorescence occurs with loss or blockage of RPE cells. Although autofluorescence patterns vary between the different types of uveitis, in many cases, hyperautofluorescence occurs with increased disease activity and resolves or evolves to hypoautofluorescence as the inflammation subsides.

Indocyanine green angiography

Like FA, indocyanine green angiography (ICGA) uses an intravenous injection coupled with serial retinal images to provide data about vasculature and anatomy of the posterior segment; the properties of ICGA allow for specialized imaging of the choroidal circulation. In inflammatory diseases involving the outer retina and choroid, findings on ICGA often exceed those visible on either ophthalmoscopy or FA, which may have diagnostic and therapeutic implications. ICGA is especially beneficial in the evaluation of choroidal neovascular membrane as well as white dot syndromes (Fig 5-12), Vogt-Koyanagi-Harada syndrome, sympathetic ophthalmia, and posterior segment sarcoidosis (see Chapters 9 and 10).

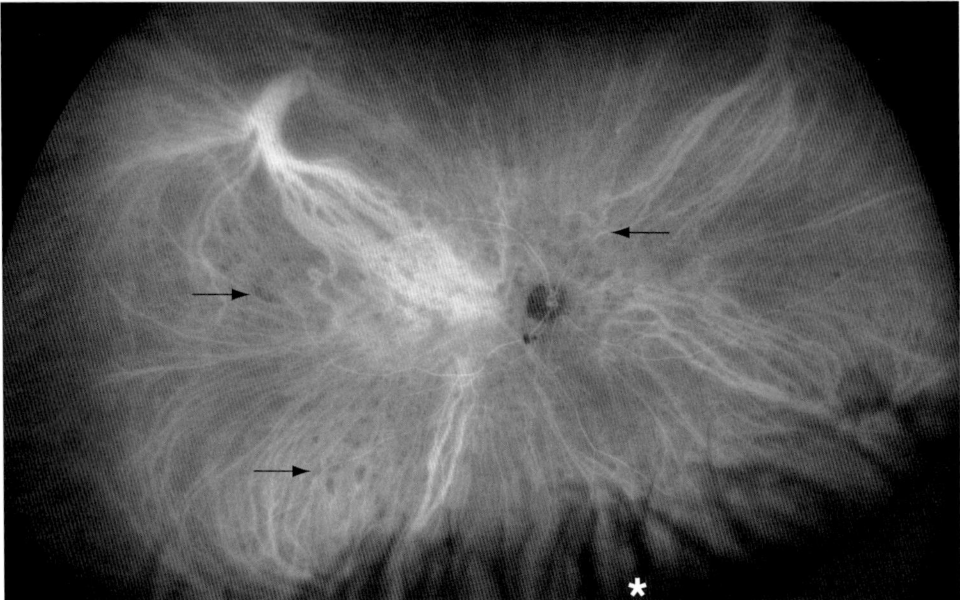

Figure 5-12 Wide-field image of late-phase indocyanine green angiography demonstrating numerous scattered hypocyanescent spots *(arrows)* in a patient with birdshot chorioretinitis. Eyelash artifact *(asterisk)* is also shown. *(Courtesy of Thellea K. Leveque, MD, MPH.)*

Ultrasonography

Anterior segment ultrasound biomicroscopy (UBM) can be useful in diagnosing pathology of the ciliary body, iris, and iridocorneal angle in uveitis. B-scan ultrasonography of the posterior segment can demonstrate vitreous opacities, choroidal thickening or elevation, retinal detachment, and cyclitic membrane formation, as well as rule out occult foreign bodies, particularly when media opacities preclude a view of the posterior segment. Retained crystalline lens fragments may be visualized in the anterior or posterior segment with either form of ultrasonography, whereas malposition of an IOL haptic can be demonstrated with anterior segment UBM. Findings on B-scan ultrasonography may be diagnostic for posterior scleritis (see Chapter 7).

Electroretinography

Full-field electroretinography can be used to monitor progression of birdshot chorioretinopathy and diagnose acute zonal occult outer retinopathy (AZOOR) complex diseases and autoimmune retinopathy. During uveitis workup, electroretinogram findings may help to distinguish retinal dystrophy from posterior uveitis.

Visual field testing (perimetry)

Kinetic and static perimetry are used to monitor progression and response to treatment of birdshot chorioretinopathy and AZOOR complex diseases. These tests are also used to monitor visual field defects in uveitic glaucoma and inflammatory optic neuritis. Microperimetry may be helpful in diseases involving the macula, such as punctate inner choroiditis.

Ocular Fluid and Tissue Sampling

Polymerase chain reaction testing of aqueous and vitreous humor

Polymerase chain reaction (PCR) testing is highly sensitive and specific for the diagnosis of infectious uveitis. For example, it can directly amplify the DNA of a suspected pathogen from a small volume of intraocular fluid, making it ideal for evaluation of ophthalmic disease. PCR-based techniques can also be very useful for vitreous genomic testing in suspected cases of vitreoretinal lymphoma.

Anterior chamber paracentesis is generally safer and easier to perform than vitreous sampling. Fortunately, viral PCR testing has high sensitivity and specificity for both aqueous and vitreous samples, but the diagnostic yield is affected by the clinical presentation. In cases of herpetic posterior uveitis or panuveitis (ie, acute retinal necrosis), aqueous and vitreous PCR results are nearly equally informative. In contrast, aqueous PCR may not be diagnostic in a patient with suspected viral anterior uveitis, especially if there is minimal inflammation when the aqueous is sampled. For *Toxoplasma* infection, aqueous PCR testing may also be less informative than vitreous testing unless the patient is immunocompromised or the retinochoroiditis lesions are large and/or multifocal.

Until recently, PCR analysis was not practical for the diagnosis of bacterial and fungal uveitis because of the need to specify the selected pathogen of interest for amplification. Due to the presence of conserved genetic subunits within bacteria (16S) and fungi (5.8S/18S/28S), pan-bacterial and pan-fungal PCR tests can be used to screen ocular specimens for these pathogens. The diagnostic yield of PCR assessments is equal or superior to that of intraocular fluid cultures.

When PCR testing of intraocular fluid is negative for a given infectious organism but clinical suspicion for the pathogen is still high, aqueous or vitreous biopsy may be repeated when inflammation is high grade or after antimicrobial treatment is discontinued. Disadvantages of PCR testing are cost, inability to test for multiple entities due to small sample size, risk of improper amplification of a contaminant, and risk of a false-negative result when there is a paucity of cellular material.

Doan T, Acharya N, Pinsky BA, et al. Metagenomic DNA sequencing for the diagnosis of intraocular infections. *Ophthalmology.* 2017;124(8):1247–1248.

Harper TW, Miller D, Schiffman JC, Davis JL. Polymerase chain reaction analysis of aqueous and vitreous specimens in the diagnosis of posterior segment infectious uveitis. *Am J Ophthalmol.* 2009;147(1):140–147.

Rothova A, de Boer JH, Ten Dam-van Loon NH, et al. Usefulness of aqueous humor analysis for the diagnosis of posterior uveitis. *Ophthalmology.* 2008;115(2):306–311.

Sowmya P, Madhavan HN. Diagnostic utility of polymerase chain reaction on intraocular specimens to establish the etiology of infectious endophthalmitis. *Eur J Ophthalmol.* 2009;19(5):812–817.

Taravati P, Lam D, Van Gelder RN. Role of molecular diagnostics in ocular microbiology. *Curr Ophthalmol Rep.* 2013;1(4):10.1007/s40135-013-0025-1.

Culture and vital staining

Cell culture and bacterial and fungal staining are useful in cases of suspected bacterial or fungal endophthalmitis. Isolation is time consuming, however, and may lack sensitivity when the pathogen load in an ocular sample is small. Nevertheless, the technique remains the traditional first-line test for suspected infections, in part because it is widely available and inexpensive to perform.

Cytology and Pathology

Cytology studies of aqueous humor may be diagnostic in ocular diseases involving the anterior and sometimes the posterior segment (eg, leukemia or lymphoma). When there is clinical suspicion for vitreoretinal lymphoma, an undiluted vitreous biopsy specimen can be sent for cytology and flow cytometry analysis with gene rearrangement studies and cytokine analysis.

Although chorioretinal biopsy is technically challenging and requires an experienced vitreoretinal surgeon, it may be useful in rapidly progressive, vision-threatening types of posterior uveitis when other investigations have failed to identify an etiology and response to empiric treatment has been poor. Another indication for chorioretinal biopsy is suspected subretinal infiltration of vitreoretinal lymphoma in the absence of substantial vitreous cells or after a negative result from vitreous biopsy.

Directed conjunctival biopsy of visible lesions can be useful in lymphoma, cicatricial pemphigoid, and sarcoidosis. In rare cases, scleral biopsy may be indicated if suspicion is high for an infectious etiology (see Chapter 7).

In general, when the suspected disease involves nonocular organ systems, yield may be higher and morbidity lower with biopsy of a nonocular site versus a vitreous or chorioretinal biopsy.

Anterior chamber paracentesis technique

Paracentesis is performed using sterile technique at the slit lamp or with the patient supine on a treatment gurney or chair. Topical anesthetic drops are instilled, the eye is prepared with topical povidone-iodine solution, and an eyelid speculum can be placed. A tuberculin (1-mL) syringe is attached to a sterile 30-gauge needle, which is then advanced under direct or slit-lamp visualization into the anterior chamber through the temporal limbus or clear cornea, parallel to the iris plane. As much aqueous is aspirated as is safely possible (usually 0.1–0.2 mL), avoiding needle contact with the iris and lens. Possible complications include iris hemorrhage and hyphema, wound leak, infection, and injury to the iris or lens. Video 5-1 shows the anterior chamber paracentesis technique.

VIDEO 5-1 Anterior chamber paracentesis technique.
Courtesy of Thellea K. Leveque, MD, MPH.

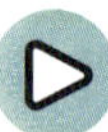

Vitreous biopsy technique

The most common indications for vitreous biopsy include suspected vitreoretinal lymphoma or other intraocular malignancy, infectious posterior segment inflammation, and chronic uveitis with atypical presentation or inadequate response to therapy. (Endophthalmitis is discussed in detail in Chapter 14, and vitreoretinal lymphoma in Chapter 15.)

Vitreous specimens can be obtained via the pars plana either with a needle or a vitrectomy instrument. If only a small sample is required, a vitreous needle tap can be performed with the patient partially reclining in an examination room chair. Topical and subconjunctival anesthesia are administered; the eye is then prepared with topical povidone-iodine solution, and an eyelid speculum is placed. Typically, a 25-gauge, 1-inch needle on a 3-mL syringe (to provide greater vacuum) is introduced through the pars plana, directed toward the mid-vitreous cavity, and used to aspirate the vitreous sample, usually 0.2–0.5 mL. A diagnostic vitrectomy is performed via a standard 3-port pars plana vitrectomy (see BCSC Section 12, *Retina and Vitreous*). Testing usually requires undiluted vitreous specimens. It is possible to obtain 0.5–1.0 mL of undiluted vitreous using standard vitrectomy techniques.

Complications of diagnostic vitrectomy in uveitic eyes may include retinal tears or detachment, suprachoroidal or vitreous hemorrhage, worsening of cataract or inflammation, and in rare cases, sympathetic ophthalmia. Although vitreous surgery can be therapeutic and diagnostic in cases of uveitis, the pharmacokinetics of intravitreal drugs are markedly altered in vitrectomized eyes; for example, the half-life of intravitreal corticosteroids is significantly reduced.

Chorioretinal biopsy technique

Video 5-2 demonstrates chorioretinal biopsy.

VIDEO 5-2 Chorioretinal biopsy.
Courtesy of P. Kumar Rao, MD.

CHAPTER 6

Therapy for Uveitis

This chapter includes a related video. Go to www.aao.org/bcscvideo_section09 or scan the QR code in the text to access this content.

Highlights

- Therapy for uveitis consists of local (ocular) or systemic administration of anti-inflammatory and/or antimicrobial agents. Ocular medications may be delivered topically, by ocular injection, or via surgical implantation.
- The goal of uveitis treatment is to prevent vision loss from uncontrolled inflammation while minimizing the ocular and systemic adverse effects of therapy.
- Infectious causes of uveitis must be investigated and treated before corticosteroids, especially the periocular and intravitreal forms, are administered.

Introduction

Therapy for uveitis ranges from observation to complex medical and/or surgical intervention. In cases of suspected chronic or vision-threatening uveitis, uveitis specialists can help confirm the diagnosis and determine a therapeutic regimen. Factors influencing therapy decisions include the risk of morbidity from ocular inflammation as well as the potential adverse effects of the treatments. Management may require coordination with rheumatologists and other medical or surgical subspecialists; in general, early involvement of subspecialists can improve prognosis.

Medical Management of Uveitis

The goals of management of uveitis and other forms of ocular inflammation are to control disease activity and to reduce the risk of vision loss from structural complications of inflammation. It is critical to determine whether the uveitis is related to a systemic or ocular infection, as anti-inflammatory therapy may severely exacerbate an untreated infection. Once infection is properly addressed, residual inflammation may be cautiously treated with adjuvant anti-inflammatory therapy, as many types of infectious uveitis have a significant inflammatory component. Some diseases, such as multiple evanescent white dot syndrome or acute posterior multifocal placoid pigment epitheliopathy, are self-limited and usually resolve without treatment. Other diseases, such as Fuchs uveitis syndrome and mild pars planitis, are chronic but do not require treatment. However, the majority of patients with chronic ocular inflammation will benefit from sustained suppression of inflammation.

Corticosteroids are the most effective agents to control ocular inflammation quickly. Drug route and dose are tailored to each patient depending on disease severity and the duration of and response to therapy. Additional factors to consider when choosing a corticosteroid are the presence of systemic disease and the patient's age, weight, immune status, and tolerance of adverse effects. It is common practice to use systemic immunomodulatory therapy (IMT) to decrease or stop corticosteroids. In the appropriate clinical scenario, cycloplegic agents, nonsteroidal anti-inflammatory drugs (NSAIDs), fibrinolytic agents, and carbonic anhydrase inhibitors may also be used as adjunctive therapy.

The remainder of this chapter offers a detailed discussion of corticosteroids and systemic IMT for the management of uveitis.

TREATMENT OF NONINFECTIOUS OCULAR INFLAMMATORY DISEASE

The basic principles of treatment of noninfectious ocular inflammatory disease are summarized as follows:

1. The absence of infection should be confirmed.
2. The inflammation is quieted with some form of corticosteroids. If inflammation worsens, an infectious etiology should be reconsidered.
3. Corticosteroids are slowly tapered off completely or down to a medically safe dose.*
4. If inflammation recurs upon corticosteroid taper, a longer-acting or stronger option is indicated:
   - For example, if topical corticosteroids are being used, a periocular, intravitreal, or systemic formulation can be considered.
   - When corticosteroids are maximized or cannot be continued, systemic corticosteroid-sparing immunomodulatory therapy (IMT) may be added.
5. Antimetabolites have historically been considered first-line treatment. In certain cases, a biologic agent (usually a tumor necrosis factor inhibitor) or, less likely, an alkylating agent, may be used first.
6. IMT takes time to achieve a therapeutic effect, and not every agent works in every situation. These factors should be considered in assessing efficacy. Adding or switching to another agent may be necessary. When effective and well tolerated, IMT is maintained for at least 1–3 years.
7. For certain ocular inflammatory diseases, especially those with systemic manifestations, IMT may be indicated as first-line treatment.

* A maximum of 7.5 mg/day oral prednisone, or a topical drug at a dose low enough to avoid ocular side effects.

Corticosteroids

Corticosteroids are often the first-line treatment for all forms of ocular inflammation as well as for complications such as macular edema. They may be administered locally (eg, as topical eyedrops or as periocular or intraocular injections) or systemically (eg, orally, intravenously, or less frequently, intramuscularly).

The corticosteroid dose, duration of therapy, and route of administration must be individualized. For maximum effect, corticosteroid therapy is usually started at a high dosage (ie, topical or systemic) and then tapered as the inflammation subsides, rather than initiated at a low dose that may have to be progressively increased to control inflammation. To minimize side effects, the maintenance dose should be the lowest amount necessary to control inflammation. If systemic corticosteroids are administered for more than 2 to 3 weeks, they must be tapered gradually (ie, over days to weeks) to prevent cortisol deficiency from hypothalamic–pituitary–adrenal axis suppression.

For uveitis that is not immediately vision threatening or chronic, corticosteroids are slowly tapered, and the disease is closely monitored. If inflammation recurs before a low corticosteroid dose is reached, then additional anti-inflammatory treatment is usually required to control ocular inflammation. Systemic corticosteroids are often used as a therapeutic bridge to long-term immunosuppressive therapy. When ophthalmic surgery is performed on an eye with uveitis, the corticosteroid may need to be increased or restarted to prevent postoperative uveitis exacerbation.

Any route of corticosteroid administration can cause adverse effects, so the risk–benefit ratio of treatment should be considered carefully and discussed with the patient before initiation. Local corticosteroids convey the highest risk of ocular adverse effects, notably posterior subcapsular cataract and ocular hypertension. Compared with adults, children are more likely to have ocular adverse effects, and they can be more severe. The systemic risks of corticosteroids are discussed later in this chapter. See also BCSC Section 1, *Update on General Medicine,* and Section 2, *Fundamentals and Principles of Ophthalmology.*

CLINICAL PEARL

The following are some important points to remember when local corticosteroid treatment for noninfectious uveitis is being considered:

- Anterior and mild intermediate uveitis may be initially treated with topical corticosteroids.
- Local corticosteroid injections achieve a greater depth of penetration than topical formulations and may be used for a more posterior effect or as an adjunct to systemic treatment.
- Serial short-acting corticosteroid injections should be avoided as the sole treatment for chronic uveitis.
- Ocular hypertension and cataract formation are common adverse effects of local corticosteroid treatment and may be more frequent and severe in children than in adults.

Topical corticosteroid administration

Topical corticosteroid drops are effective primarily for anterior uveitis, although they may have beneficial effects on vitritis or macular edema in some patients. These drops are given at intervals ranging from once daily to hourly. The drugs can also be prescribed in ointment form for nighttime use. Difluprednate (0.05%), a fluorinated corticosteroid, is highly potent and penetrates tissue more deeply than other topical preparations; 4 daily doses of difluprednate are considered the equivalent of 8 or more total drops per day of prednisolone acetate (1%). Clinical studies suggest that the adverse effect profile of difluprednate is similar to that of prednisolone; however, difluprednate is associated with more frequent and severe ocular hypertension, especially in children. Of the topical preparations, loteprednol and fluorometholone produce the lowest ocular hypertensive effect; however, these drugs are not as effective as prednisolone in controlling more severe uveitis. Of note, when branded versus generic suspensions of prednisolone acetate are being considered, differences in the physical properties of the formulations can affect bioavailability, although this discrepancy may be partially overcome by vigorous agitation of the drug before instillation. See Part V, Ocular Pharmacology, in BCSC Section 2, *Fundamentals and Principles of Ophthalmology,* for additional discussion.

Slabaugh MA, Herlihy E, Ongchin S, van Gelder RN. Efficacy and potential complications of difluprednate use for pediatric uveitis. *Am J Ophthalmol.* 2012;153(5):932–938.

Local corticosteroid administration

When a more posterior effect is needed to treat uveitis or when a patient is nonadherent with or only partially responsive to topical corticosteroids, a sustained-release agent may be delivered directly into the vitreous cavity or into the periocular space—as long as an infectious cause has been sufficiently investigated. In addition, intermediate- and short-acting local corticosteroid injections may be used intermittently to treat breakthrough inflammation in otherwise well-controlled or mild uveitis. In certain clinical settings, long-acting intravitreal corticosteroids may be alternatives to long-term IMT. However, a limitation of local therapies is the variable duration of effect, with relapse being the only sign of waning corticosteroid efficacy. Relapses before reinjection or reimplantation may cause cumulative damage, creating a "saw-tooth decline," a phenomenon in which patients initially improve after injection but then worsen below the point of their previous baseline. Each subsequent spike of improvement and valley of decline are progressively lower, like the teeth of an angled saw. This type of decline is disguised by the peaks of improvement and may go unnoticed by the treating physician without careful long-term analysis. In patients with chronic uveitis, scheduled replacement or reinjection of local corticosteroid before the effect wears off may improve long-term prognosis.

Periocular corticosteroid administration Periocular corticosteroids are traditionally given as depot injections into the sub-Tenon space or orbital floor. Triamcinolone acetonide (40 mg) and methylprednisolone acetate (40–80 mg) are the most commonly used periocular drugs. Short-acting nondepot corticosteroids, such as dexamethasone or betamethasone, may be injected subconjunctivally for a limited duration of effect. Periocular injections can be performed using either a transseptal or a sub-Tenon (Nozik technique) approach (Fig 6-1).

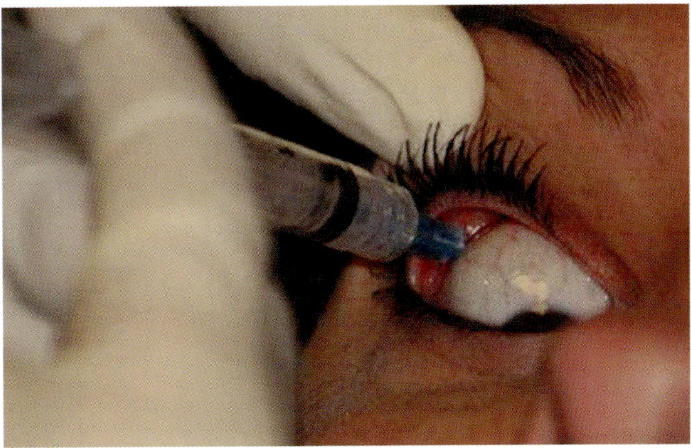

Figure 6-1 Posterior sub-Tenon injection of triamcinolone acetonide demonstrating correct position of the clinician's hands and the needle. A 25- or 27-gauge, ⅝-inch needle on a 3-mL syringe is advanced to the hub with a gentle side-to-side motion to detect any scleral engagement and directed caudad and nasally before injection of the corticosteroid. The ideal position of the tip of the needle is between the Tenon capsule and the sclera. *(Courtesy of Ramana S. Moorthy, MD.)*

For a sub-Tenon injection given in the superotemporal quadrant, the technique is as follows:

1. The upper lid is retracted and the patient instructed to look downward and nasally.
2. After proparacaine or tetracaine is applied with a cotton swab, a 25- or 27-gauge, ⅝-inch needle on a 3-mL syringe is placed bevel down against the globe and advanced through the conjunctiva and Tenon capsule using a gentle side-to-side movement, allowing the physician to determine whether the needle has entered the sclera. If the globe does not torque with the side-to-side movement of the needle, the physician can be reasonably sure that the needle has not penetrated the sclera.
3. Once the needle has been advanced to the hub, the corticosteroid is injected into the sub-Tenon space.

Complications of this superotemporal approach include upper eyelid ptosis, periorbital hemorrhage, and globe perforation. To avoid the risk of upper eyelid ptosis, an inferotemporal sub-Tenon injection, also using the Nozik technique, can be performed.

A transseptal, orbital floor approach (Fig 6-2) using a 27-gauge, ½-inch needle on a 3-mL syringe is another alternative for periocular injections, as follows:

1. The index finger is used to push the temporal lower eyelid posteriorly and to locate the equator of the globe.
2. The needle is inserted inferior to the globe through the skin of the lower eyelid and directed straight back through the orbital septum into the orbital fat.
3. The needle is advanced to the hub, and then aspirated; if there is no blood reflux, the corticosteroid is injected.

Complications of the inferior approach include periorbital and retrobulbar hemorrhage, lower eyelid retractor ptosis, orbital fat prolapse with periorbital festoon formation, orbital fat atrophy, and skin discoloration.

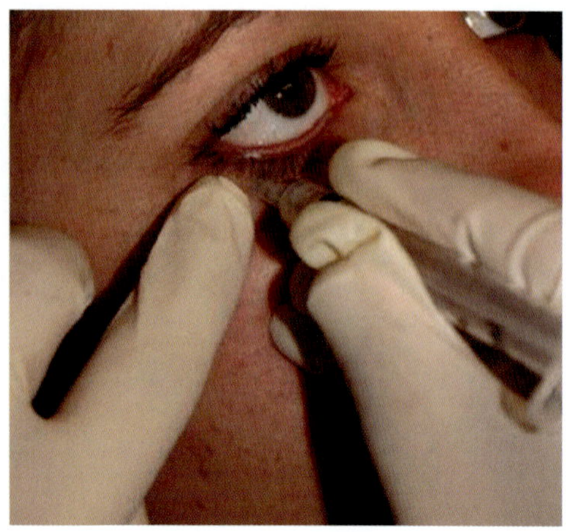

Figure 6-2 Inferior transseptal (orbital floor) injection of triamcinolone acetonide in the right eye. A 27-gauge, ½-inch needle on a 3-mL syringe is inserted through the skin of the lower eyelid and the inferior orbital septum. By using the index finger of the opposite hand, the physician can determine the location of the equator of the globe to prevent perforation and to place the depot corticosteroid as posteriorly as possible. *(Courtesy of Ramana S. Moorthy, MD.)*

Periocular injections are contraindicated in certain patients, including those with active infectious uveitis. They are also not recommended in patients with necrotizing scleritis because of cases of scleral thinning and perforation (see Chapter 7). Although systemic absorption of periocular corticosteroids is minimal, the drugs can still cause systemic adverse effects similar to those of oral corticosteroids. The physician should be aware that periocular corticosteroid injections have the potential to raise intraocular pressure (IOP) precipitously or for an extended period, particularly when longer-acting depot drugs are used. If this effect occurs, the periocular corticosteroid may be removed surgically if it is located anterior to the septum or in a subconjunctival space.

In 2021, the US Food and Drug Administration (FDA) approved a novel suprachoroidal drug delivery system to treat macular edema associated with noninfectious uveitis using a preservative-free triamcinolone suspension (CLS-TA). An integrated 30-g microinjector is used to administer 4 mg/0.1 mL of the drug. The microinjector is held perpendicular to the sclera, where it is inserted 4–5 mm posterior to the limbus. The short 900-μm or 1100-μm needle penetrates only to the level of the suprachoroidal space (SCS) between the sclera and the choroid. The drug is then slowly administered, allowing a fluid wave to propagate posteriorly and circumferentially and resulting in low levels of corticosteroid in the anterior segment and high levels in the posterior segment.

Phase 3 data from the PEACHTREE study with post hoc analysis and the MAGNOLIA extension study comparing SCS CLS-TA injection with sham injection (2 administrations 12 weeks apart) for the treatment of macular edema secondary to noninfectious uveitis revealed that 47% of patients receiving CLS-TA treatment achieved the primary endpoint of improvement of ≥15 ETDRS letters (vs 16% of patients receiving sham treatment). In addition, compared with sham treatment, SCS CLS-TA resulted in superior reduction in mean central subfield macular thickness, 152.6 μm vs 17.9 μm, CLS-TA vs sham, respectively. Approximately 50% of patients receiving SCS injection did not require additional treatment at 9 months. Percentages of patients with elevated IOP (11.5% vs 15.6%) and cataract formation (7.3% vs 6.3%) were comparable in the SCS CLS-TA and sham treatment groups, respectively.

Leder HA, Jabs DA, Galor A, Dunn JP, Thorne JE. Periocular triamcinolone acetonide injections for cystoid macular edema complicating noninfectious uveitis. *Am J Ophthalmol.* 2011;152(3):441–448.e2.

Yeh S, Khurana RN, Shah M, et al; PEACHTREE Study Investigators. Efficacy and safety of suprachoroidal CLS-TA for macular edema secondary to noninfectious uveitis: phase 3 randomized trial. *Ophthalmology*. 2020;127(7):948–955.

Intravitreal corticosteroid administration Intravitreal therapy achieves a higher, more predictable concentration of corticosteroids in the posterior segment than traditional periocular injection. In the United States, intravitreal corticosteroid administration for uveitis currently takes several forms:

- triamcinolone acetonide (4 mg/0.1 mL), preservative-free, via pars plana injection with a 30-gauge needle
- dexamethasone pellet (700 μg), biodegradable, via shelved pars plana injection with an integrated 22-gauge injector
- fluocinolone acetonide intravitreal insert (0.18 or 0.19 mg), via pars plana injection with integrated 25-gauge injector
- fluocinolone acetonide implant (0.59 mg), surgically implantable, via pars plana incision

In nonvitrectomized eyes, intravitreal injections of preservative-free triamcinolone acetonide (2–4 mg) through the pars plana have produced sustained visual acuity improvements for 3–6 months; the technique is the same as for standard intravitreal injection (see BCSC Section 12, *Retina and Vitreous*). For recalcitrant uveitic macular edema, published literature on intravitreal triamcinolone administration suggests a definite treatment benefit, although of limited duration. However, IOP may be transiently elevated in more than half of these patients, up to 25% may require topical medications to control IOP, and 1%–2% may require filtering surgery. Infectious endophthalmitis and rhegmatogenous retinal detachment may also occur, but these complications are rare when proper technique is used. Of note, this method of treatment does not cure chronic uveitic conditions and should be used judiciously because its effects are relatively short-lived.

A biodegradable injectable pellet containing 700 μg of dexamethasone has been approved in the United States and in Europe for the treatment of retinal vein occlusion and noninfectious uveitis affecting the posterior segment of the eye. With this therapy, an injector is used to create a shelved wound, and the pellet is injected through the pars plana into the vitreous cavity (Video 6-1). A prospective, randomized, controlled clinical trial demonstrated that at 8 weeks, 47% of eyes treated with the dexamethasone pellet had improved vitreous haze compared with 12% of eyes in the sham treatment group. Statistically significant improvements in visual acuity and macula thickness were also reported with the pellet, and fewer eyes required rescue medication. IOP elevation and cataracts were the most commonly reported treatment-related ocular adverse effects in this study. Several longer-term, multicenter, retrospective studies have reported relatively positive safety and efficacy results with repeated dexamethasone intravitreal pellets in patients with uveitis and refractory macular edema, with an average time to reinjection of 6 months. Relative contraindications to the dexamethasone pellet are aphakia, prior vitrectomy, and absence of lens capsule owing to the risk of implant migration into the anterior chamber.

VIDEO 6-1 Injection of dexamethasone pellet.
Courtesy of Thomas A. Albini, MD.

Sustained-release, injectable fluocinolone acetonide intravitreal inserts (0.18- or 0.19-mg inserts) are approved in the United States and Europe for the treatment of noninfectious posterior uveitis. The nonbioerodible insert is injected via a nonshelved wound through the pars plana into the vitreous cavity and releases approximately 0.2 mg/day over 36 months. A prospective, randomized, placebo-controlled clinical trial of a fluocinolone acetonide insert in noninfectious intermediate uveitis, posterior uveitis, or panuveitis demonstrated statistically significant lower uveitis recurrence rates in the insert group (87 patients) than in the placebo group (42 patients) at 6 months (27.6% vs 90.5%), 12 months (37.9% vs 97.6%), and 3 years (65.5% vs 97.6%), respectively. However, cataract surgery was required more frequently in the insert treatment group (73.8% vs 23.8%, respectively). At 3 years, IOP was similar for both study groups, and approximately half as many eyes in the fluocinolone acetonide intravitreal insert group underwent IOP-lowering surgery (5.7% vs 11.9%, respectively), possibly because of the adjunctive corticosteroid treatments administered in the sham treatment group.

In the United States, a surgically implantable, sustained-release 0.59-mg fluocinolone acetonide implant has been approved by the FDA for the treatment of chronic noninfectious uveitis affecting the posterior segment. The implant is inserted through a small pars plana incision and sutured to the sclera. The implant is effective in controlling inflammation for a median of 30 months, reducing recurrence rates and allowing discontinuation of systemic therapy and other corticosteroid injections. Visual acuity outcomes are equivalent to those associated with systemic immunosuppressive therapy for up to 4.5 years. The 7-year data strongly favor systemic treatment, presumably because of retinal damage from relapse of the uveitis before reimplantation. Postoperative complications (eg, endophthalmitis, wound leaks, hypotony, vitreous hemorrhage, and retinal detachments) have been reported with this therapy, and reimplantation or exchange may be performed. Adverse event rates are high in eyes treated with the implant, with nearly all phakic eyes developing cataract within 2 years after implantation, 75% experiencing IOP elevation requiring topical therapy, and nearly 40% requiring filtering surgery (Table 6-1).

The prospective, multicenter, randomized, controlled POINT trial compared the effectiveness of three of these local corticosteroid injections for uveitic macular edema: periocular triamcinolone acetonide, intravitreal triamcinolone acetonide, and intravitreal dexamethasone pellet. All three modalities decreased central subfoveolar thickness, but statistically significantly greater improvements were observed with the two intravitreal modalities versus periocular triamcinolone acetonide. In contrast, IOP ≥24 mm Hg or ≥10 mm Hg from baseline was more likely in the two intravitreal corticosteroid groups than in the periocular group (see Table 6-1).

Goldstein DA, Godfrey DG, Hall A, et al. Intraocular pressure in patients with uveitis treated with fluocinolone acetonide implants. *Arch Ophthalmol.* 2007;125(11):1478–1485.

Jaffe GJ, Pavesio CE; Study Investigators. Effect of a fluocinolone acetonide insert on recurrence rates in noninfectious intermediate, posterior, or panuveitis: three-year results. *Ophthalmology.* 2020;127(10):1395–1404.

Table 6-1 Selected List of Major Treatment Studies in Uveitis

Study/Year	Study Questions	Results
Local therapy		
Fluocinolone Acetonide Insert (FAi) Trial/2020 Effect of a Fluocinolone Acetonide Insert on Recurrence Rates in Noninfectious Intermediate, Posterior, or Panuveitis • Participants: 129 patients with noninfectious uveitis involving the posterior segment; 87 eyes randomly assigned to 0.2-μg/day FAi treatment, 42 eyes to sham treatment • Primary endpoint: uveitis recurrence rates at 6 months	Efficacy and safety of intravitreal injection of a slow-release (approximately 0.2 mg/day over 36 months) FAi or sham (plus reference standard) treatment	Significantly lower rates of uveitis recurrence were observed in the FAi group compared with the sham group at 6 months (27.6% vs 90.5%), 12 months (37.9% vs 97.6%), and 3 years (65.5% vs 97.6%), respectively. Cataract surgery was required significantly more frequently in the treatment group than in the sham group (73.8% vs 23.8%, respectively). IOP was similar for both study groups. Approximately half as many eyes in the FAi-treated group vs the sham-treated group underwent IOP-lowering surgery (5.7% vs 11.9%, respectively).
POINT/2019 Periocular Triamcinolone vs. Intravitreal Triamcinolone vs. Intravitreal Dexamethasone Implant for the Treatment of Uveitic Macular Edema • 192 patients (235 eyes) with uveitic macular edema (ME) • Endpoint: improvement in uveitic ME on OCT at 8 weeks	Comparative effectiveness of periocular triamcinolone (PTA), intravitreal triamcinolone (ITA), and intravitreal dexamethasone implant (IDI) for treatment of uveitic ME	At 8 weeks, eyes in all 3 treatment arms had improvements in ME on OCT. ITA and IDI groups had significantly greater reductions in ME (39% and 46%, respectively) than the PTA group (23%). Risk of having IOP ≥24 mm Hg or an increase of ≥10 mm Hg from baseline in IOP was higher in the ITA and IDI groups than in the PTA group. No significant difference was observed between the 2 intravitreal treatment groups.
Local vs systemic therapy		
MUST/2010 Multicenter Uveitis Steroid Treatment Trial • 255 patients (479 eyes) with noninfectious intermediate uveitis, posterior uveitis, or panuveitis • Endpoint: change in BCVA	Efficacy and safety of local therapy of a surgically placed 0.59-mg fluocinolone acetonide slow-release (36-month) intravitreal implant compared with systemic therapy (corticosteroid monotherapy or combination steroid-IMT therapy)	2- and 4.5-year analyses: There was no significant difference in BCVA or systemic outcomes between the two groups but more local adverse outcomes in the implant group. 7-year analysis: Systemic therapy was favored for BCVA outcome by 7.1 letters as a result of visual decline in the implant group, likely due to loss of efficacy of the implant.

(Continued)

Table 6-1 *(continued)*

Study/Year	Study Questions	Results
Systemic therapy		
SITE/2009, 2019 Systemic Immunosuppressive Therapy for Eye Diseases Cohort Study • 7957 patients expanded to 15,938 patients with noninfectious ocular inflammatory disease treated with systemic immunosuppression; analysis of 187,151 person-years • Endpoint: cancer mortality	To determine overall and cancer mortality rates in patients with uveitis receiving systemic immunosuppression for ocular inflammatory disease	Cancer mortality rates were not increased in patients treated with azathioprine, methotrexate (MTX), mycophenolate mofetil, cyclosporine, or systemic corticosteroids. Extension of follow-up study confirmed that TNF inhibitors were not associated with increased overall cancer or cancer mortality rates. Alkylating agents were associated with higher overall mortality, but not after confounding factors were excluded. Mortality was higher in patients receiving tacrolimus and etanercept, which might reflect selection factors (eg, transplantation). Further study is required.
SYCAMORE/2017 Adalimumab (ADA) plus Methotrexate (MTX) for juvenile idiopathic arthritis (JIA)–associated uveitis • 60 children and adolescents with active uveitis taking a stable MTX dosage randomly assigned (2:1) to ADA vs placebo • Endpoint: time to treatment failure	Efficacy and safety of adding ADA in active JIA-associated uveitis treated with MTX	The ADA group was less likely than the placebo group to have treatment failure (HR, 0.25; 95% CI, 0.12–0.49). Significantly greater proportions of patients in the ADA group were able to eliminate or reduce topical corticosteroids. Adverse events (AEs) and serious adverse events (SAEs) were more common in the ADA group than in the placebo group (10.07 vs 6.51 AEs and 0.29 vs 0.19 SAEs per patient-year, respectively).
VISUAL I, II, III/2016–2018 ADA for noninfectious intermediate uveitis, posterior uveitis, or panuveitis • I: 217 patients with active disease • II: 226 patients with controlled disease • III: 371 patients from I or II who completed the study or met treatment failure criteria • Endpoint: time to treatment failure	I: Efficacy and safety of ADA in controlling inflammation in active noninfectious uveitis II: Efficacy and safety of ADA in preventing flare-up in pharmacologically (prednisone and/or 1 immunomodulatory therapy) controlled noninfectious uveitis III: Long-term efficacy and safety of ADA in active or controlled noninfectious uveitis	I: The ADA group was less likely than the placebo group to have treatment failure (HR, 0.50; 95% CI, 0.36–0.70). AEs and SAEs were more common in the ADA group (1052 vs 972 AEs and 29 vs 14 SAEs, respectively, per 100-person-years). II: The ADA group was less likely than the placebo group to have treatment failure (HR, 0.57; 95% CI, 0.39–0.84). The incidences of AE and SAEs were similar between treatment groups.

Study/Year	Study Questions	Results
		III: Of 242 patients with active uveitis, 60% achieved quiescence at week 78, 66% of whom were corticosteroid free. Of 129 patients with inactive uveitis, 74% achieved quiescence at week 78, 93% of whom were corticosteroid free. AEs and SAEs were comparable to those in previous VISUAL trials.
FAST/2018 Effect of Corticosteroid-Sparing Treatment With Mycophenolate Mofetil vs Methotrexate on Inflammation in Patients With Uveitis • 194 patients with noninfectious uveitis • Endpoints: corticosteroid-sparing[a] disease control in both eyes and absence of treatment failure due to safety or intolerability at 6 months	Comparative efficacy and safety of systemic mycophenolate mofetil vs MTX for first-line treatment of noninfectious uveitis.	Treatment was successful in 66.7% of patients in the MTX group vs 57.1% in the mycophenolate mofetil group, a nonstatistically significant difference.

BCVA = best-corrected visual acuity; IMT = immunomodulatory therapy; IOP = intraocular pressure; OCT = optical coherence tomography; TNF = tumor necrosis factor.

[a] Less than or equal to 7.5 mg daily oral prednisone and ≤2 drops of prednisolone acetate 1%.

Khurana RN, Appa SN, McCannel CA, et al. Dexamethasone implant anterior chamber migration: risk factors, complications, and management strategies. *Ophthalmology.* 2014;121(1):67–71.

Lowder C, Belfort R Jr, Lightman S, et al; Ozurdex HURON Study Group. Dexamethasone intravitreal implant for noninfectious intermediate or posterior uveitis. *Arch Ophthalmol.* 2011;129(5):545–553.

Thorne JE, Sugar EA, Holbrook JT, et al; Multicenter Uveitis Steroid Treatment Trial Research Group. Periocular triamcinolone vs. intravitreal triamcinolone vs. intravitreal dexamethasone implant for the treatment of uveitic macular edema: the PeriOcular vs. INTravitreal corticosteroids for uveitic macular edema (POINT) Trial. *Ophthalmology.* 2019;126(2):283–295.

Tomkins-Netzer O, Taylor SRJ, Bar A, et al. Treatment with repeat dexamethasone implants results in long-term disease control in eyes with noninfectious uveitis. *Ophthalmology.* 2014;121(8):1649–1654.

Writing Committee for the Multicenter Uveitis Steroid Treatment (MUST) Trial and Follow-up Study Research Group; Kempen JH, Altaweel MM, Holbrook JT, et al. Association between long-lasting intravitreous fluocinolone acetonide implant vs systemic anti-inflammatory therapy and visual acuity at 7 years among patients with intermediate, posterior, or panuveitis. *JAMA.* 2017;317(19):1993–2005.

Zarranz-Ventura J, Carreño E, Johnston RL, et al. Multicenter study of intravitreal dexamethasone implant in noninfectious uveitis: indications, outcomes, and reinjection frequency. *Am J Ophthalmol.* 2014;158(6):1136–1145.e5.

CLINICAL PEARL

The following are some important points to remember when systemic corticosteroid treatment for noninfectious uveitis is being considered:

- Systemic corticosteroids are used for immediate control of severe uveitis when local corticosteroids are insufficient or contraindicated or when systemic inflammatory disease also requires treatment.
- Prescribers need to be aware of the myriad adverse effects of corticosteroids, and a team approach with specialists in rheumatology, internal medicine, or pediatrics may be used to improve patient safety.
- When systemic corticosteroids cannot be tapered to 7.5 mg/day or less, additional immunosuppression (systemic or regional) is required.
- Systemic IMT should be favored over long-term/high-dose corticosteroid use.

Systemic corticosteroid administration

Systemic corticosteroids are used for vision-threatening uveitis when local corticosteroids are insufficient or contraindicated or when systemic inflammatory disease also requires therapy. Of the many oral corticosteroid formulations available, prednisone is most commonly used. Of note, the readily available blister packages of methylprednisolone, which contain predetermined taper schedules, should not be used to treat uveitis because the dose is too low and the duration is too short. Most patients require a starting prednisone dose of 1 mg/kg/day (up to 60 mg/day), which is gradually tapered every 1–2 weeks. Doses greater than 60 mg/day are avoided because of an increased risk of avascular bone necrosis. The goal is to control ocular inflammation *and* minimize adverse effects by tapering to the lowest possible prednisone dose (preferably with prednisone tapered off completely). When prednisone cannot be tapered to 7.5 mg/day or less within 3 months, systemic IMT is typically initiated. Prednisone doses of 7.5 mg/day or less are believed to be safe in the intermediate and long term, although some data suggest increased cardiovascular risks with large cumulative doses of prednisone (eg, 5 mg/day over 20 years).

For severe cases of noninfectious uveitis or scleritis, the most aggressive immediate treatment is intravenous, high-dose, pulse methylprednisolone (1 g/day infused over 1 hour) for 3 days, followed by a gradual taper of oral prednisone starting at 1 mg/kg/day. Although this mode of therapy may control ocular inflammation, it should only be administered by a physician experienced with the approach, as multiple adverse effects have been observed, some of which may be life-threatening.

The many adverse effects associated with short-term and long-term use of systemic corticosteroids must be discussed with patients, and their general health must be closely monitored, often with the assistance of an internist. Short-term risks include ocular hypertension, hyperglycemia, systemic hypertension, gastric reflux, insomnia, emotional lability, weight gain, and fluid retention. Intermediate-term risks include cataract, osteopenia, avascular necrosis of joints, and diabetes. If possible, corticosteroids should be avoided in patients at high risk for exacerbations of existing conditions (eg, diabetes, hypertension, congestive heart failure, peptic ulcer or gastroesophageal reflux disease, psychiatric conditions, or immune compromise). Alcohol intake can also increase risk of gastrointestinal ulcer in patients taking corticosteroids, whereas diet modification to reduce carbohydrates and simple sugars may help reduce the risk of hyperglycemia. Patients taking systemic corticosteroids and NSAIDs have an elevated risk of gastric ulcers; therefore, this combination is best avoided. Patients with risk factors for gastric ulcer should take a histamine-H2 receptor antagonist or proton-pump inhibitor.

Corticosteroid use can also lead to bone loss, osteoporosis, and bone fractures; thus, partnering with an internist or a patient's primary care physician for screening and treatment of corticosteroid-induced bone loss is common. Patients receiving long-term systemic corticosteroids are encouraged to supplement their diets with calcium and vitamin D to lower the risk of osteoporosis and typically undergo formal bone density screening via dual-energy x-ray absorptiometry scan. If indicated, medication may be prescribed for the prevention and treatment of corticosteroid-induced osteoporosis in at-risk men and women receiving prednisone. For patients taking corticosteroids at doses of 20 mg/day or greater for more than 4 weeks, clinicians may also consider trimethoprim-sulfamethoxazole every other day as prophylaxis against *Pneumocystis jirovecii* infection.

The systemic adverse effects and potency of commonly used corticosteroids are discussed further in BCSC Section 1, *Update on General Medicine*. See also BCSC Section 2, *Fundamentals and Principles of Ophthalmology*.

LoPiccolo J, Mehta SA, Lipson EJ. Corticosteroid use and *Pneumocystis* pneumonia prophylaxis: a teachable moment. *JAMA Intern Med*. 2018;178(8):1106–1107.

Systemic Immunomodulatory Therapy

Introduction

Patients with chronic, severe, or corticosteroid-dependent noninfectious uveitis may benefit greatly from the use of systemic IMT, sometimes referred to as *immunosuppressive* or *disease-modifying antirheumatic drugs (DMARDS)*. Depending on the class of the medications, these drugs can modify or regulate one or more immune functions via different mechanisms (see Chapter 1, Table 1-4).

Immunomodulatory medications may be loosely divided into nonbiologic IMT agents and biologic agents. Nonbiologic IMT agents are further divided into antimetabolites, T-cell inhibitors, and alkylating agents. Biologic agents are a newer and rapidly expanding group of genetically engineered proteins that target specific immune mechanisms. They include drugs that inhibit tumor necrosis factor (TNF)-α (ie, TNF inhibitors) and other pro-inflammatory immune mediators. In clinical practice, nonbiologic alkylating agents are reserved for the most severe or recalcitrant inflammation because of risks of malignancy and infertility. Currently, all systemic IMT is used off-label to treat uveitis, except for the TNF inhibitor adalimumab, which is FDA approved for noninfectious uveitis affecting the posterior segment.

Although many case series on use of nonbiologic IMT agents in uveitis have been published, most data come primarily from the Systemic Immunosuppressive Therapy for Eye Diseases (SITE) Cohort Study, a standardized retrospective study that evaluated the adverse effect profile and efficacy of azathioprine, methotrexate, mycophenolate mofetil, cyclosporine, or systemic corticosteroids in clinical practice (see Table 6-1 and further discussion later in this section). However, data on the comparative effectiveness of systemic immunomodulatory medications for treatment of uveitis are limited. See Table 6-2 for a list of relevant IMTs and suggested monitoring schedules.

Indications Systemic IMT should be considered for treatment of noninfectious ocular inflammation in the following settings:

- vision-threatening intraocular inflammation or necrotizing scleritis
- inadequate response to corticosteroid treatment
- cases in which systemic or local corticosteroids are contraindicated or intolerable because of systemic or ocular adverse effects (eg, glaucoma, cataract)
- cases in which systemic corticosteroids cannot be tapered below 7.5 mg/day

Certain ocular inflammatory diseases warrant the early use of IMT, including mucous membrane pemphigoid (also known as *ocular cicatricial pemphigoid*), serpiginous choroiditis, macula-threatening multifocal choroiditis with panuveitis, Behçet disease, sympathetic ophthalmia, Vogt-Koyanagi-Harada (VKH) syndrome, birdshot chorioretinopathy, and necrotizing scleritis associated with systemic vasculitis. Although these disorders may initially respond well to corticosteroids, the immediate use of IMT has improved long-term prognosis and lessened visual morbidity. Several expert-panel recommendations have established a consensus on how and when to select, initiate, modify, and withdraw nonbiologic IMT or biologic agents.

Table 6-2 Selected Immunomodulatory Medications Used in Noninfectious Uveitis

Class	Name	Adult Dosing	Potential Adverse Effects	Suggested Monitoring	Obstetric Complications
Antimetabolite	Methotrexate	Subcutaneous or oral: 15–25 mg/week	Fatigue, malaise, nausea, alopecia, transaminitis or cirrhosis, anemia, leukopenia, thrombocytopenia, mouth sores	CBC, CMP every 6–12 weeks	High risk (spontaneous abortion, fetal abnormalities)
	Mycophenolate mofetil	1–1.5 g bid	Diarrhea, transaminitis, anemia, leukopenia, thrombocytopenia	CBC, CMP every 6–12 weeks	High risk (fetal abnormalities)
	Azathioprine	2–2.5 mg/kg/day	Gastrointestinal upset, transaminitis, anemia, leukopenia, thrombocytopenia	Check TPMT before initiation; CBC, CMP monthly × 3 months, then every 6–12 weeks	Minimal risk (preterm birth, IUGR)
T-cell inhibitor	Cyclosporine	2 mg/kg bid	Hypertension, nephrotoxicity, anemia, hypertrichosis, gingival hyperplasia, gastrointestinal upset, paresthesias	CBC, CMP every 6–12 weeks; blood pressure	Minimal risk (preterm birth and infants who are small for gestational age)
	Tacrolimus	1–3 mg bid	Tremor, hypertension, nephrotoxicity	CBC, CMP every 6–12 weeks; tacrolimus trough levels	Minimal risk (preterm birth and infants who are small for gestational age)
Alkylating agent	Chlorambucil	0.1–0.2 mg/kg/day	Infertility, malignancy, pancytopenia	CBC weekly	High risk (teratogenic)
	Cyclophosphamide	2 mg/kg/day	Bladder toxicity, infertility, malignancy, pancytopenia	CBC and urinalysis weekly to monthly	High risk (teratogenic)

(Continued)

Table 6-2 *(continued)*

Class	Name	Adult Dosing	Potential Adverse Effects	Suggested Monitoring	Obstetric Complications
TNF inhibitor	Adalimumab	Subcutaneous: 80 mg on day 1, 40 mg on day 8, then 40 mg every other week; may increase to weekly	Injection site reaction or infusion reactions, precipitation or unmasking of demyelinating CNS disease, congestive heart failure, opportunistic infection, possible increased lymphoma risk	Routine laboratory testing interval varies; ongoing monitoring for neurologic or cardiovascular symptoms; anti-drug antibody testing for loss of efficacy	Unknown risk; generally considered safe
	Infliximab	5–10 mg/kg intravenous induction at 0, 2, and 6 weeks followed by maintenance every 4–8 weeks May increase up to 20 mg/kg in children			Certolizumab has less third-trimester transplacental transfer than other TNF inhibitors
Anti-interleukin 6	Tocilizumab	4 mg/kg intravenously every 4 weeks or 162 mg subcutaneous every other week; uveitis dose has not been established	Injection site reaction or infusion reactions, opportunistic infection, gastric perforation, hepatotoxicity, cytopenias, lipid abnormalities	CBC, CMP every 4–8 weeks for 6 months Then every 3 months and lipid panel every 6 months	Unknown risk; generally considered safe
Glucocorticoids	Prednisone	0.5–1 mg/kg/day; individualized dosing, tapered to 7.5 mg/day or lower over 3 months	Acid reflux/gastritis, insomnia, hyperglycemia, hunger, emotional lability, weight gain Long-term use: osteopenia, hypertension, hypercholesterolemia, diabetes	Blood glucose monitoring while taking high dose; HgA_{1c} and lipid panel every 6 months while taking long-term low dose; bone density scan annually	Minimal risk (maternal diabetes, IUGR)

bid = twice a day; CBC = complete blood count; CMP = comprehensive metabolic panel; CNS = central nervous system; HgA_{1c} = glycosylated hemoglobin; IUGR = intrauterine growth restriction; TNF = tumor necrosis factor; TPMT = thiopurine S-methyltransferase.

CLINICAL PEARL

The following are some important points to remember regarding IMT for noninfectious ocular inflammation:

- Early use of IMT improves the prognosis for patients with a sight-threatening, chronic ocular inflammatory condition.
- IMT is generally well tolerated, but proper patient selection, patient education, and ongoing monitoring are mandatory.
- TNF inhibitors should be considered as first-line therapy for patients with Behçet uveitis and those with other severe ocular inflammatory disorders who have not had success with or are not candidates for conventional IMT.

Treatment IMT should be managed by a physician who is qualified to counsel, prescribe, and safely monitor such medications. Before initiation of IMT, the physician should assess patients for the following conditions:

- infection
- recent live vaccine administration
- hepatic, renal, and hematologic contraindications
- pregnancy or breastfeeding
- status of family planning and contraception
- disease activity that can be objectively and longitudinally monitored

Unlike biologic agents, which typically have a rapid onset, nonbiologic IMT takes weeks to months to develop therapeutic effectiveness. Until IMT takes effect, most patients require maintenance with a judicious amount of local and/or systemic corticosteroid. In addition, patients may need to trial more than one IMT agent to find a regimen that is effective and well tolerated; this therapeutic refinement may take 6–18 months. When ocular inflammation has been quiescent on IMT and the lowest possible dose of corticosteroids for at least 12 months (longer for pediatric patients), a slow drug taper may be considered. IMT discontinuation is tailored according to uveitis severity, the presence or absence of systemic features, and the plan for monitoring and rescue therapy.

The physician should thoroughly discuss the risks of adverse effects with the patient before initiating IMT. Although IMT is generally well tolerated, patients must be monitored regularly with laboratory testing because of the potential for serious complications. Depending on the IMT agent administered, monitoring may include complete blood count with differential and liver and renal function tests. Serious complications of nonbiologic IMT include renal and hepatic toxicity and bone marrow suppression. Alkylating agents may cause sterility and are associated with an increased risk of malignant diseases, such as leukemia or lymphoma. Certain biologic agents may cause an infusion or injection reaction; TNF inhibitors increase the risk of multiple sclerosis, congestive heart failure, and lymphoma. In addition, all IMT increases the risk of opportunistic and secondary infections.

Despite these risks, the SITE cohort study of 7957 US patients (66,802 patient-years) with noninfectious uveitis treated with IMT showed that patients who took azathioprine, methotrexate, mycophenolate mofetil, cyclosporine, or systemic corticosteroids had overall cancer mortality rates similar to those of patients who never used these IMT agents. The study was expanded to include 15,938 patients who were followed for 187,151 person-years and confirmed that most IMT agents, including TNF inhibitors, were not associated with increased overall or cancer-related mortality (see Table 6-1). Other data suggest that IMT may be associated with an increased risk of nonmelanoma skin cancer, warranting sunscreen counseling.

Other precautionary steps to avoid IMT-related adverse events include consideration of trimethoprim–sulfamethoxazole prophylaxis against *P jirovecii* infection in patients receiving alkylating agents or prolonged courses of high-dose corticosteroids and IMT. Ideally, all routine vaccines or boosters should be administered 2 weeks before the initiation of IMT (4 weeks for live vaccines). In addition to routine vaccines, pneumococcal vaccine should be given regardless of age. Additional suggested vaccinations include the inactivated zoster vaccine, an annual inactivated influenza vaccine, and the COVID-19 vaccine. Additional doses of COVID-19 immunization are typically indicated for immunosuppressed patients per evolving Centers for Disease Control and Prevention guidelines.

Finally, male and female patients require counseling regarding fertility, birth control, and family planning before initiation of IMT. Many IMT medications have absolute contraindications in pregnancy (ie, methotrexate, mycophenolate mofetil); these medications should be discontinued (in both men and women) at least 3 months before they try to conceive. See Table 6-2.

Dick AD, Rosenbaum JT, Al-Dhibi HA, et al; Fundamentals of Care for Uveitis International Consensus Group. Guidance on noncorticosteroid systemic immunomodulatory therapy in noninfectious uveitis: Fundamentals Of Care for UveitiS (FOCUS) initiative. *Ophthalmology.* 2018;125(5):757–773.

Jabs DA. Immunosuppression for the uveitides. *Ophthalmology.* 2018;125(2):193–202.

Kempen JH, Daniel E, Dunn JP, et al. Overall and cancer related mortality among patients with ocular inflammation treated with immunosuppressive drugs: retrospective cohort study. *BMJ.* 2009;339:b2480.

Kempen JH, Newcomb CW, Foster CS, et al. Risk of overall and cancer mortality after immunosuppression of patients with non-infectious ocular inflammatory diseases. *Invest Ophthalmol Vis Sci.* 2019;60(9):3854.

Leroy C, Rigot J-M, Leroy M, et al. Immunosuppressive drugs and fertility. *Orphanet J Rare Dis.* 2015;10:136.

Levy-Clarke G, Jabs DA, Read RW, Rosenbaum JT, Vitale A, Van Gelder RN. Expert panel recommendations for the use of anti-tumor necrosis factor biologic agents in patients with ocular inflammatory disorders. *Ophthalmology.* 2014;121(3):785–796e3.

Wakefield D, McCluskey P, Wildner G, et al. Inflammatory eye disease: pre-treatment assessment of patients prior to commencing immunosuppressive and biologic therapy: recommendations from an expert committee. *Autoimmun Rev.* 2017;16(3):213–222.

Yates WB, Vajdic CM, Na R, McCluskey PJ, Wakefield D. Malignancy risk in patients with inflammatory eye disease treated with systemic immunosuppressive therapy: a tertiary referral cohort study. *Ophthalmology.* 2015;122(2):265–273.

Nonbiologic immunomodulatory therapy

Antimetabolites The antimetabolites include azathioprine, methotrexate, and mycophenolate mofetil. Retrospective and prospective data support the use of antimetabolites for successful control of uveitis. In fact, antimetabolites are often the first IMTs used when corticosteroid sparing is necessary. Compared with the other antimetabolites, azathioprine has a slightly higher incidence of adverse effects, and mycophenolate mofetil has a significantly shorter time to therapeutic efficacy. A head-to-head prospective study of 216 patients with uveitis (FAST trial) randomly assigned to methotrexate or mycophenolate mofetil reported similar efficacy for the 2 medications (see Table 6-1). Antimetabolites require long-term use, as disease control may continue to improve for 6–12 months. Although antimetabolites are generally effective, ongoing low-dose systemic corticosteroid therapy is often necessary to achieve complete inflammatory control.

AZATHIOPRINE Azathioprine, a purine nucleoside analogue, interferes with DNA replication and RNA transcription. It is administered orally at a dose of up to 2–2.5 mg/kg/day in adults. On average, 25% of patients discontinue azathioprine therapy because of adverse effects, with nausea, vomiting, and upset stomach being the most common events. Bone marrow suppression is unusual at the doses used to treat uveitis; however, patients taking allopurinol and azathioprine concomitantly are at higher risk for bone marrow suppression. Azathioprine-related mild hepatic toxicity can usually be reversed by dose reduction. Complete blood count with differential and liver function tests must be closely monitored.

The variability of clinical response to azathioprine is probably related to genetic variability in the activity of thiopurine S-methyltransferase (TPMT), an enzyme responsible for the metabolism of 6-mercaptopurine. A genotypic test is available to classify a patient's TPMT activity level and to help clinicians individualize drug doses as appropriate:

- patients with low/no TPMT activity (0.3% of patients); azathioprine therapy not recommended
- patients with intermediate TPMT activity (11% of patients); azathioprine therapy at reduced dosage
- patients with normal/high TPMT activity (89% of patients); azathioprine therapy at higher doses than for intermediate TPMT activity

Azathioprine is beneficial in many types of noninfectious ocular inflammatory diseases, including Behçet disease, intermediate uveitis, VKH syndrome, sympathetic ophthalmia, and necrotizing scleritis. Overall, nearly 50% of patients treated with azathioprine achieve inflammatory control and can taper their prednisone dosage to 10 mg/day or less.

Pasadhika S, Kempen JH, Newcomb CW, et al. Azathioprine for ocular inflammatory diseases. *Am J Ophthalmol.* 2009;148(4):500–509.e2.

METHOTREXATE This agent is a folic acid analogue and inhibitor of dihydrofolate reductase; it inhibits DNA replication, but its anti-inflammatory effects result from extracellular release of adenosine. Unlike other antimetabolites, methotrexate is given as a *weekly* dose of 15–25 mg in adults. In children, the dosage is based on body surface area. Methotrexate can be given orally, subcutaneously, intramuscularly, or intravenously and is usually well tolerated. The drug has increased bioavailability when given parenterally. Methotrexate may take up to 6 months to develop a full therapeutic effect in controlling ocular inflammation.

To reduce adverse effects of methotrexate, including hair loss and mouth sores, folate is given concurrently at a dose of 1–2 mg/day. Gastrointestinal distress and anorexia also occur in 10% of patients. Reversible hepatotoxicity has been reported in up to 15% of patients, and cirrhosis develops in fewer than 0.1% of patients receiving methotrexate long term. Methotrexate is teratogenic; data on the safety of male conception while receiving methotrexate therapy are mixed. Regular alcohol consumption is contraindicated with methotrexate. Complete blood count with differential and liver function tests should be monitored regularly.

Numerous studies have shown methotrexate to be effective for various types of ocular inflammation, including juvenile idiopathic arthritis (JIA)–associated anterior uveitis, sarcoidosis, panuveitis, and scleritis. It is often the first-line IMT choice for children. In uncontrolled clinical trials of methotrexate, corticosteroid sparing was successful in two-thirds of patients with chronic ocular inflammatory disorders. Intravitreal methotrexate is used to treat vitreoretinal lymphoma; its role in treating uveitis and uveitic macular edema is under investigation.

Gangaputra S, Newcomb CW, Liesegang TL, et al; Systemic Immunosuppressive Therapy for Eye Diseases Cohort Study. Methotrexate for ocular inflammatory diseases. *Ophthalmology.* 2009;116(11):2188–2198.e1.

Malik AR, Pavesio C. The use of low dose methotrexate in children with chronic anterior and intermediate uveitis. *Br J Ophthalmol.* 2005;89(7):806–808.

MYCOPHENOLATE MOFETIL This drug inhibits both inosine monophosphate dehydrogenase and DNA replication. It is given orally at a dosage of 1–1.5 g twice daily in adults. Median time to successful control of ocular inflammation (in combination with less than 10 mg/day of prednisone) is approximately 4 months. Fewer than 20% of patients receiving mycophenolate mofetil have adverse effects (reversible gastrointestinal distress and diarrhea are common), and these are usually managed by gradual dose up-titration or dose reduction. Few patients find the drug intolerable. Regular laboratory monitoring includes complete blood count with differential; in rare cases, CD4 T-lymphocyte deficiency may develop.

Two large, retrospective studies found mycophenolate mofetil was an effective corticosteroid-sparing agent in up to 85% of patients with chronic uveitis. It has similar efficacy in children (88%) and can be a safe alternative to methotrexate in pediatric uveitis. Mycophenolate mofetil is contraindicated in pregnancy and should be discontinued in men and women before conception.

Doycheva D, Deuter C, Stuebiger N, Biester S, Zierhut M. Mycophenolate mofetil in the treatment of uveitis in children. *Br J Ophthalmol.* 2007;91(2):180–184.

Rathinam SR, Gonzales JA, Thundikandy R, et al. Effect of corticosteroid-sparing treatment with mycophenolate mofetil vs methotrexate on inflammation in patients with uveitis: a randomized clinical trial. *JAMA.* 2019;322(10):936–945.

Siepmann K, Huber M, Stübiger N, Deuter C, Zierhut M. Mycophenolate mofetil is a highly effective and safe immunosuppressive agent for the treatment of uveitis: a retrospective analysis of 106 patients. *Graefes Arch Clin Exp Ophthalmol.* 2006;244(7):788–794.

Teoh SC, Hogan AC, Dick AD, Lee RWJ. Mycophenolate mofetil for the treatment of uveitis. *Am J Ophthalmol.* 2008;146(5):752–760.e1–3.

Thorne JE, Jabs DA, Qazi FA, Nguyen QD, Kempen JH, Dunn JP. Mycophenolate mofetil therapy for inflammatory eye disease. *Ophthalmology.* 2005;112(8):1472–1477.

T-cell inhibitors Cyclosporine, a macrolide product of the fungus *Beauveria nivea,* and tacrolimus, a product of *Streptomyces tsukubaensis,* are calcineurin inhibitors that eliminate T-cell receptor signal transduction and downregulate interleukin-2 gene transcription and receptor expression of $CD4^+$ T lymphocytes.

CYCLOSPORINE This drug is available in 2 oral preparations: microemulsion and standard. The microemulsion formulation has better bioavailability than the standard preparation. It is initiated at 2 mg/kg/day, and the standard formulation is initiated at 2.5 mg/kg/day in adults. Dosing is adjusted to 1–5 mg/kg/day based on trough levels, toxicity, and clinical response. The most common adverse effects with cyclosporine are systemic hypertension and nephrotoxicity. Additional adverse effects include paresthesia, gastrointestinal upset, fatigue, hypertrichosis, and gingival hyperplasia. Blood pressure, serum creatinine levels, and complete blood counts are assessed regularly. If serum creatinine levels rise by 30%, the dose is adjusted; sustained elevation usually results in discontinuation of the medication.

In a randomized, controlled clinical trial, cyclosporine was effective for the treatment of Behçet uveitis, controlling inflammation in 50% of patients. However, the dose used in this study was 10 mg/kg/day—substantially higher than current dosing (up to 5 mg/kg/day), which led to substantial nephrotoxicity. Even at standard dosages of cyclosporine, toxicity necessitating cessation of therapy is more common in patients older than 55 years. Overall, cyclosporine is modestly effective in controlling ocular inflammation (33.4% and 51.9% of patients achieved control by 6 and 12 months, respectively in the SITE Study). As with antimetabolites, ongoing low-dose systemic corticosteroid therapy is often necessary to achieve complete inflammatory control with cyclosporine.

Kaçmaz RO, Kempen JH, Newcomb C, et al. Cyclosporine for ocular inflammatory diseases. *Ophthalmology.* 2010;117(3):576–584.

TACROLIMUS This agent is given orally at 0.10–0.15 mg/kg/day in adults. Because tacrolimus is prescribed at a lower dose than cyclosporine and has increased potency, nephrotoxicity is less common with this drug than with cyclosporine. Nevertheless, serum creatinine level, complete blood count with differential, and serum potassium level are monitored regularly in patients taking tacrolimus, with the drug dose escalated until a therapeutic trough blood level has been reached.

A prospective trial comparing cyclosporine and tacrolimus suggested the agents had equal efficacy in controlling chronic posterior and intermediate uveitis, with tacrolimus demonstrating greater safety (ie, lower risk of hypertension and hyperlipidemia). Long-term tolerability and efficacy with tacrolimus are excellent as well, with patients having an 85% chance of reducing their prednisone dosage to less than 10 mg/day. A randomized trial of tacrolimus monotherapy versus tacrolimus plus prednisone for the treatment of uveitis showed no difference in uveitis activity between groups, confirming that corticosteroid discontinuation can be achieved in many cases.

Hogan AC, McAvoy CE, Dick AD, Lee RWJ. Long-term efficacy and tolerance of tacrolimus for the treatment of uveitis. *Ophthalmology.* 2007;114(5):1000–1006.

Lee RWJ, Greenwood R, Taylor H, et al. A randomized trial of tacrolimus versus tacrolimus and prednisone for the maintenance of disease remission in noninfectious uveitis. *Ophthalmology.* 2012;119(6):1223–1230.

Murphy CC, Greiner K, Plskova J, et al. Cyclosporine vs tacrolimus therapy for posterior and intermediate uveitis. *Arch Ophthalmol.* 2005;123(5):634–641.

Alkylating agents Alkylating agents, which include cyclophosphamide and chlorambucil, are generally used for uveitis only when other IMT agents fail to control the condition. Increasingly, alkylating agents are being bypassed in favor of biologic agents because of the latter's targeted efficacy and preferred safety profile.

The most serious adverse effect of alkylating agents is an increased risk of malignancy. Cyclophosphamide treatment may confer a more than 10-fold increased risk of bladder cancer that is dependent on cumulative dose, and a two- to fourfold elevated risk of other cancers. Chlorambucil treatment may increase risk of leukemia over baseline by more than 10-fold. Despite the risks, use of alkylating agents for a limited duration may be justified for patients with severe, vision- or life-threatening, recalcitrant disease such as necrotizing scleritis associated with systemic vasculitis (eg, granulomatosis with polyangiitis or relapsing polychondritis). The alkylating agents also have shown efficacy in severe intermediate uveitis, VKH syndrome, sympathetic ophthalmia, serpiginous choroiditis, and Behçet disease. These drugs should be used with great caution and only by clinicians experienced in their dosing and potential toxicities. Before beginning treatment, patients may consider sperm or egg banking owing to a high rate of sterility if the cumulative dose exceeds certain limits. Concomitant administration of gonadotropin-releasing hormone agonists may help preserve ovarian function and fertility.

CYCLOPHOSPHAMIDE Cyclophosphamide is an agent with active metabolites that can alkylate purines in DNA and RNA, impairing DNA replication and cell death. To control ocular inflammation, oral dosing (2 mg/kg/day in adults) may be more effective than intermittent intravenous pulses. Myelosuppression and hemorrhagic cystitis are the most common adverse effects of cyclophosphamide treatment. Complete blood counts and urinalysis results are monitored weekly to monthly. Microscopic hematuria is a warning for the patient to increase hydration, and gross hematuria is an indication to discontinue therapy. Other toxicities include teratogenicity, sterility, and reversible alopecia. Opportunistic infections such as *P jirovecii* pneumonia occur more often in patients receiving cyclophosphamide than in those being treated with other systemic IMT; trimethoprim–sulfamethoxazole prophylaxis is usually utilized in patients taking cyclophosphamide. In three-fourths of patients taking the drug, inflammation is controlled within 12 months, and two-thirds of patients achieve disease remission within 2 years. However, one-third of patients discontinue therapy within 1 year because of adverse effects.

Faurschou M, Sorensen IJ, Mellemkjaer L, et al. Malignancies in Wegener's granulomatosis: incidence and relation to cyclophosphamide therapy in a cohort of 293 patients. *J Rheumatol.* 2008;35(1):100–105.

Pujari SS, Kempen JH, Newcomb CW, et al. Cyclophosphamide for ocular inflammatory diseases. *Ophthalmology.* 2010;117(2):356–365.

CHLORAMBUCIL Chlorambucil is a very long-acting alkylating agent that also interferes with DNA replication. It is absorbed well when administered orally. The drug is traditionally given as a single daily dose of 0.1–0.2 mg/kg in adults. It may also be administered as a short-term, high-dose therapy for uveitis. Because chlorambucil is myelosuppressive, complete blood count values should be monitored closely while the patient takes the drug. Like cyclophosphamide, it is associated with increased risk of hematologic malignancy. It is also teratogenic and causes sterility. Uncontrolled case series suggest that chlorambucil is effective in 66%–75% of patients with recalcitrant sympathetic ophthalmia, Behçet disease, and other vision-threatening uveitic syndromes, providing long-term, drug-free remission of disease.

Patel SS, Dodds EM, Echandi LV, et al. Long-term, drug-free remission of sympathetic ophthalmia with high-dose, short-term chlorambucil therapy. *Ophthalmology.* 2014;121(2):596–602.

Biologic agents

Inflammation is driven by a complex series of cell–cell and cell–cytokine interactions. Inhibitors of various cytokines and inflammatory mechanisms are called *biologic agents* or *biologic response modifiers.* These drugs enable targeted immunomodulation, thereby theoretically reducing the short-term, systemic adverse effects associated with the previously discussed nonbiologic IMT. However, biologic agents are more expensive and may carry higher long-term risks of serious infections or secondary malignancies than antimetabolites and T-cell inhibitors.

Tumor necrosis factor inhibitors Tumor necrosis factor α is believed to play a major role in the pathogenesis of JIA, ankylosing spondylitis, and other spondyloarthropathies. For treatment of uveitis, the best-studied TNF inhibitors are adalimumab and infliximab; their high degree of efficacy and favorable side effect profile have improved the management of many types of uveitis. According to expert consensus, TNF inhibitors should be considered first-line treatment for Behçet disease. Data on the efficacy of the TNF inhibitors certolizumab and golimumab are more limited, and etanercept is not effective for ocular inflammatory diseases.

TNF inhibitors are usually prescribed by specialists (ie, rheumatologists, uveitis specialists) experienced with their use, adverse effects, and toxicities. They are relatively contraindicated in patients with congestive heart failure. Latent tuberculosis must be ruled out or treated with the oversight of a specialist in infectious diseases before drug initiation. TNF inhibitors have been associated with central nervous system demyelination (promoting or unmasking of multiple sclerosis), hepatitis B reactivation, and deep fungal and other serious atypical infections. Because TNF inhibitors themselves are sometimes immunogenic, patients can develop antibodies against the drug that lower its efficacy. Patients taking TNF inhibitors should also avoid live vaccines. Although there are individual case reports on the *intravitreal* administration of TNF inhibitors, this form of delivery has not been fully investigated and may be retinotoxic; further study is needed.

Sfikakis PP, Markomichelakis N, Alpsoy E, et al. Anti-TNF therapy in the management of Behçet's disease—review and basis for recommendations. *Rheumatology (Oxford).* 2007;46(5):736–741.

ADALIMUMAB Adalimumab, a fully human monoclonal immunoglobulin G1 antibody directed against TNF-α, is the first FDA-approved systemic medication for noninfectious uveitis. Self-administered via subcutaneous injection, the initial dosage is usually 80 mg, followed by a maintenance dose of 40 mg/0.8 mL every other week starting 1 week after the initial injection. Because adalimumab is a fully human antibody, risk of antidrug–antibody formation is lower than with infliximab, a mouse/human chimeric antibody. Injection site reactions may occur but are usually mild. When the drug is administered in conjunction with methotrexate, serum levels of adalimumab are higher, and rates of antidrug-antibody formation are reduced.

In an industry-sponsored, randomized, double-masked, controlled trial in adults with noninfectious uveitis (VISUAL I/II) that included an open-label extension arm (VISUAL III), adalimumab was associated with significant reductions in treatment failure compared with placebo for both active and controlled uveitis. Significantly higher rates of quiescence and corticosteroid-free quiescence were also achieved and maintained through 52 weeks, regardless of disease status at entry. However, adverse events and serious adverse events were reported more frequently among patients who took adalimumab than among those taking placebo (see Table 6-1).

Adalimumab has been as effective as infliximab in controlling inflammation, with success rates of up to 88% in pediatric patients with uveitis and at least 90% in adult patients with Behçet uveitis, posterior uveitis, and panuveitis. However, uveitis relapses requiring local corticosteroid injections may occur. Adalimumab has also reduced the rate of anterior uveitis flares and recurrences in HLA-B27–associated uveitis. In SYCAMORE, a randomized placebo-controlled trial involving pediatric patients with JIA-associated uveitis who were assigned to methotrexate alone versus methotrexate plus adalimumab, the addition of adalimumab delayed time to treatment failure and increased the likelihood of reducing topical corticosteroid use. Adverse events were seen in 5% of the adalimumab group, with 22% of these reports considered serious adverse events (see Table 6-1).

Ramanan AV, Dick AD, Jones AP, et al; SYCAMORE Study Group. Adalimumab plus methotrexate for uveitis in juvenile idiopathic arthritis. *N Engl J Med.* 2017;376(17):1637–1646.

Suhler EB, Adán A, Brézin AP, et al. Safety and efficacy of adalimumab in patients with noninfectious uveitis in an ongoing open-label study: VISUAL III. *Ophthalmology.* 2018;125(7):1075–1087.

INFLIXIMAB This agent is a mouse/human-chimeric immunoglobulin G1 kappa monoclonal antibody directed against TNF-α. It is administered through intravenous infusions of 5–10 mg/kg at weeks 0, 2, and 6 and then every 4–8 weeks thereafter for maintenance. Infliximab has been effective in controlling active inflammation and decreasing the likelihood of future attacks in more than 75% of patients, including those with Behçet uveitis, undifferentiated uveitis, sarcoidosis, VKH disease, and human leukocyte antigen (HLA)-B27–associated anterior uveitis. However, one study showed that despite treatment success, nearly one-half of patients could not complete 50 weeks of therapy because of adverse events, including drug-induced lupus, systemic vascular thrombosis, congestive heart failure, new malignancy, demyelinating disease, and vitreous hemorrhage. As many as 75% of patients receiving more than 3 infusions developed antinuclear antibodies.

To reduce the risk of infliximab-induced lupus syndrome and loss of efficacy due to the formation of anti-drug antibodies, low-dose methotrexate (5–7.5 mg/week) may be administered concurrently. Although increasing the dose and frequency of infliximab may achieve control in patients with the most severe ocular inflammatory diseases, antibody formation is more likely to occur.

Giganti M, Beer PM, Lemanski N, Hartman C, Schartman J, Falk N. Adverse events after intravitreal infliximab (Remicade). *Retina.* 2010;30(1):71–80.

Tugal-Tutkun I, Mudun A, Urgancioglu M, et al. Efficacy of infliximab in the treatment of uveitis that is resistant to treatment with the combination of azathioprine, cyclosporine, and corticosteroids in Behçet's disease: an open-label trial. *Arthritis Rheum.* 2005;52(8):2478–2484.

Other biologic agents *Tocilizumab,* an anti–interleukin-6 agent, may have efficacy in treating noninfectious uveitis in some patients. In the phase 1/2 STOP-Uveitis randomized clinical trial (n = 37), patients with noninfectious uveitis who received 4 or 8 mg/kg intravenous tocilizumab for 6 months showed improvements in visual acuity and a reduction in vitreous haze. In the APTITUDE study, a multicenter trial of subcutaneous tocilizumab in children with active JIA-associated uveitis recalcitrant to a TNF-inhibitor, 7 of 21 patients had decreased uveitis activity at 12 weeks and macular edema resolved in 3 of 4 patients. However, the primary outcome was not met, and a phase 3 trial was not justified. Nonetheless, several retrospective cohort studies have shown tocilizumab can effectively treat refractory uveitic macular edema.

Rituximab, a chimeric monoclonal antibody directed against $CD20^{+}$ cells (mainly B lymphocytes) is given as a set of intravenous infusions every 6 months. It may be useful in the treatment of Behçet retinal vasculitis, scleritis associated with granulomatosis with polyangiitis or rheumatoid arthritis, and mucous membrane pemphigoid. Case series have also reported success in treating refractory JIA-associated uveitis.

Interferon alfa-2a/2b, administered subcutaneously, has been beneficial in some patients with uveitis. Reports in the European literature indicate that interferon alfa-2a, which has antiviral, immunomodulatory, and antiangiogenic effects, is efficacious and well tolerated in patients with Behçet uveitis, controlling inflammation in almost 90%; it is somewhat less effective in non-Behçet uveitis, with inflammation control in 60% of patients. There are also reports of interferon alfa-2b successfully treating patients with uveitic macular edema.

Before initiation of interferon alfa-2a therapy, patients should discontinue any other immunomodulatory drugs, as a flulike syndrome has been observed, most frequently during the first weeks of therapy. However, symptoms may be reduced through prophylactic administration of acetaminophen. Despite the use of low interferon doses, leukopenia or thrombocytopenia may occur with the drug. Depression is another important adverse effect of interferon therapy.

Abatacept, a T-cell costimulation inhibitor given as a subcutaneous injection or an intravenous infusion, has been used with mixed results in patients with JIA-associated uveitis, including one small study suggesting that only 14% experienced sustained inflammation control. Another study showed a 49% success rate at 1 year.

Gueudry J, Wechsler B, Terrada C, et al. Long-term efficacy and safety of low-dose interferon alpha2a therapy in severe uveitis associated with Behçet disease. *Am J Ophthalmol.* 2008;146(6):837–844.e1.

Kötter I, Zierhut M, Eckstein AK, et al. Human recombinant interferon alfa-2a for the treatment of Behçet's disease with sight threatening posterior or panuveitis. *Br J Ophthalmol.* 2003;87(4):423–431.

Ramanan AV, Dick AD, Guly C, et al; APTITUDE Trial Management Group. Tocilizumab in patients with anti-TNF refractory juvenile idiopathic arthritis-associated uveitis (APTITUDE): a multicentre, single-arm, phase 2 trial. *Lancet Rheumatol.* 2020;2(3): e135–e141.

Sepah YJ, Sadiq MA, Chu DS, et al. Primary (month-6) outcomes of the STOP-Uveitis Study: evaluating the safety, tolerability, and efficacy of tocilizumab in patients with noninfectious uveitis. *Am J Ophthalmol.* 2017;183:71–80.

Other Therapeutic Agents

Topical mydriatic and cycloplegic drugs are beneficial for breaking or preventing the formation of posterior synechiae and for relieving photophobia secondary to ciliary spasm. Short-acting cycloplegics, such as tropicamide and cyclopentolate hydrochloride (1%) or phenylephrine (2.5%), allow the pupil to remain mobile and permit rapid recovery when discontinued.

Oral NSAIDs are used in the treatment of mild to moderate nonnecrotizing anterior scleritis (see Chapter 7). Potential complications of prolonged systemic NSAID use include cardiovascular, gastrointestinal, renal, and hepatic toxicity. (See also BCSC Section 1, *Update on General Medicine,* for more information.) Topical NSAIDs may be used in mild cases of diffuse episcleritis, as well as for macular edema. However, in rare instances, topical NSAIDs can cause severe corneal complications such as keratitis and corneal perforations. (See also BCSC Section 8, *External Disease and Cornea.*)

The use of oral *carbonic anhydrase inhibitors* as an adjunct in the treatment of uveitic macular edema is supported by a small but notable body of literature spanning several decades. These agents may be particularly useful in ameliorating diffuse leakage from the retinal pigment epithelium, rather than treating leakage from retinal vessels.

Intravenous immunoglobulin has been effective in some patients with uveitis that is otherwise refractory to IMT, as well as in patients with mucous membrane pemphigoid.

Intracameral *fibrinolytic agents* such as recombinant tissue plasminogen activator have been used to treat severe fibrinous reactions in the anterior segment after cataract surgery and in the setting of acute fibrinous HLA-B27–associated anterior uveitis.

Surgical Management of Uveitis

Drug delivery to the eye for treatment of uveitis may require a procedure involving ocular injection or surgical implantation, as discussed elsewhere in this chapter. For patients with uveitis, surgery in the operating room may be scheduled for diagnostic and/or therapeutic reasons. These additional therapeutic surgical procedures for uveitis and uveitic complications are discussed in Chapter 16.

CHAPTER 7

Scleritis

Highlights

- Scleritis is a primary inflammation of the sclera, typically manifesting with marked ocular pain and congestion of the deep episcleral plexus.
- Systemic inflammatory conditions are frequently associated with scleritis. It is important to properly investigate and treat these conditions.
- Treatment of scleritis requires systemic anti-inflammatory and/or immunomodulatory drugs.
- Patients with infectious, posterior, or necrotizing scleral inflammation have a high risk of permanent vision loss.

Introduction

Scleritis, inflammation of the sclera, is typically a painful, destructive condition that carries a potential risk of permanent ocular structural damage and visual compromise. Scleritis often manifests with an acute episode of marked ocular pain, swelling, and redness. It can progress to decreased vision when there is necrotizing disease or inflammation of the posterior sclera that affects the choroid and retina. Scleritis can be immune mediated, or it can be associated with infection, trauma, surgery, or medications. Approximately 40% of scleritis cases are associated with a systemic disease (eg, rheumatoid arthritis). Necrotizing scleritis is associated with a systemic process even more frequently, in 50%–60% of cases. Early and accurate diagnosis is critical, as scleral inflammation may be the first sign of a treatable sight-threatening or life-threatening disease.

Classification of Scleritis

Scleritis is classified based on the site (anterior vs posterior), severity (necrotizing vs nonnecrotizing), and pattern of scleral inflammation (diffuse vs nodular). This classification system can help the clinician predict the clinical course, uncover associated systemic disease, plan treatment, and make a prognosis (Table 7-1).

Similar to uveitis, scleritis can also be classified as *noninfectious* or *infectious.* The latter is frequently associated with surgery or trauma. Distinguishing between noninfectious and infectious scleritis is critical because aggressive use of systemic corticosteroids or immunomodulatory therapy in cases with an unidentified underlying infectious etiology can lead to devastating visual consequences.

Table 7-1 Classification of Scleritis

Type	Subtype
Anterior scleritis	Diffuse scleritis
	Nodular scleritis
	Necrotizing scleritis
	With inflammation (granulomatous, vaso-occlusive, postsurgical [surgically induced necrotizing scleritis])
	Scleromalacia perforans (without overt inflammation)
Posterior scleritis	

Pathophysiology

Noninfectious scleritis is an immune-mediated condition that frequently involves the small blood vessels of the sclera. Pathophysiologic mechanisms vary according to the type of scleritis and the associated systemic disease, if any.

The onset is usually characterized by inflammatory cell infiltration of the sclera and episclera that is mediated by proinflammatory cytokines and intercellular adhesion molecules. The diffuse anterior subtype of scleritis is associated with a nongranulomatous response involving macrophages, lymphocytes, and plasma cells that often assumes a perivascular distribution.

In nodular scleritis and particularly in necrotizing scleritis, the inflammatory response is more substantial and specific, involving direct antibody-mediated damage, deposition of immune complexes, or a delayed hypersensitivity response mainly characterized by granulomatous inflammation of the sclera. Inflammation may progress to an essentially vasculitic response, culminating in fibrinoid necrosis of the vessel walls and, eventually, necrosis of the sclera, episclera, conjunctiva, and cornea. Proinflammatory cytokines and activated metalloproteinases may play a role in local scleral and corneal damage.

Fong LP, Sainz de la Maza M, Rice BA, Kupferman AE, Foster CS. Immunopathology of scleritis. *Ophthalmology.* 1991;98(4):472–479.

Usui Y, Parikh J, Goto H, Rao NA. Immunopathology of necrotising scleritis. *Br J Ophthalmol.* 2008;92(3):417–419.

Epidemiology

Scleritis is a relatively uncommon ocular disease. In the United States, the incidence of scleritis is estimated at 3.4–4.1 per 100,000 persons; the prevalence, at 5.2 per 100,000 persons. There are no geographic or racial differences in scleritis incidence and prevalence, but most epidemiologic studies show that the disease is more common in females. In tertiary centers, scleritis makes up 0.1%–2.6% of newly referred cases. Diffuse anterior scleritis is the most common form of the disease. Although noninfectious scleritis is more common in the United States, it is important to consider infectious causes of scleritis (ie, herpetic, nocardial, mycobacterial, and fungal) in patients who have risk factors related to their medical or surgical history or geographic origin.

Homayounfar G, Nardone N, Borkar DS, et al. Incidence of scleritis and episcleritis: results from the Pacific Ocular Inflammation Study. *Am J Ophthalmol.* 2013;156(4):752–758.

Honik G, Wong IG, Gritz DC. Incidence and prevalence of episcleritis and scleritis in Northern California. *Cornea.* 2013;32(12):1562–1566.

Williamson J. Incidence of eye disease in cases of connective tissue disease. *Trans Ophthalmol Soc UK.* 1974;94(3):742–752.

Clinical Presentation

Anterior scleritis is defined as scleral inflammation anterior to the recti muscles. Individuals with anterior scleritis usually present with tenderness and severe pain in the affected eye and periocular area. The pain may worsen with eye movement and radiate to the face and jaw. When cornea or posterior sclera is involved, vision may be affected. Anterior chamber reaction may occasionally be seen.

Sometimes the clinician will find it easier to appreciate the severity of scleritis activity by looking at the eye externally, lifting the upper eyelid, and using daylight or full-room lights rather than the slit lamp. The eye with scleritis typically shows scleral edema and intense hyperemia (Fig 7-1), leading to a characteristic violaceous hue on external examination. Slit-lamp examination characteristically discloses marked dilatation of the deep episcleral plexus, which is displaced outward because of scleral edema/inflammatory cell infiltration. This is an important distinction from episcleritis, in which no scleral edema is found and only the superficial episcleral plexus is affected. Careful utilization of a topical vasoconstrictor (eg, phenylephrine drops) can also help distinguish episcleritis, in which the vessels blanch, from scleritis, in which there is partial or no blanching. However, nonblanching conjunctival injection can occur in other forms of ocular inflammation, such as acute anterior uveitis and endophthalmitis, so the phenylephrine test does not solely indicate the presence of scleritis. (The presence of high-grade intraocular inflammation distinguishes these forms of ocular inflammation from scleritis.) Close biomicroscopic inspection is also important to assess for the presence of signs of necrotizing disease (Fig 7-2).

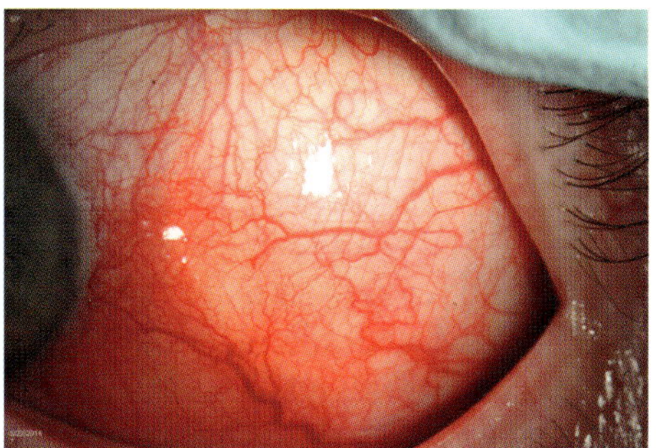
A

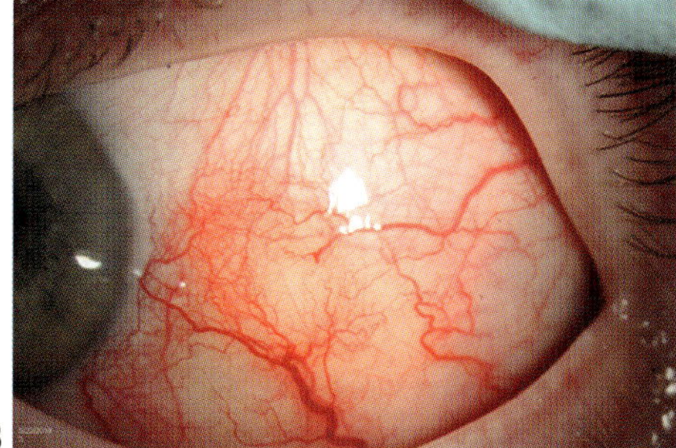
B

Figure 7-1 Diffuse anterior scleritis. Dilation of deep episcleral vessels before **(A)** and after **(B)** instillation of phenylephrine is demonstrated. *(Courtesy of H. Nida Sen, MD/National Eye Institute.)*

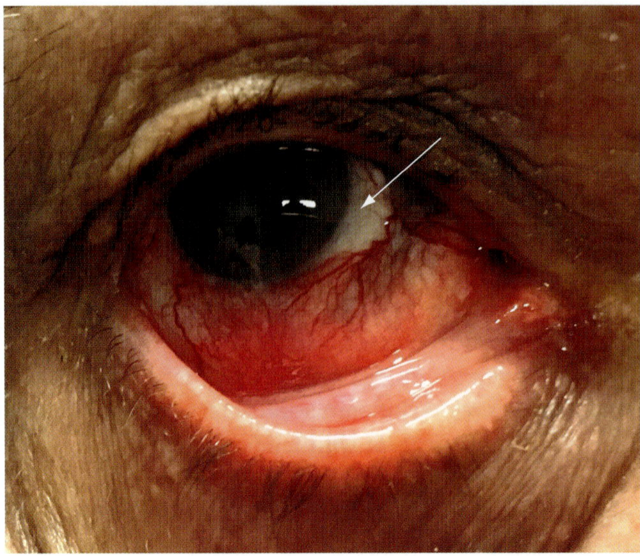

Figure 7-2 Anterior necrotizing scleritis. The eye shows active scleral inflammation associated with an avascular area *(arrow)* close to the limbus, adjacent to an area of scleral thinning. *(Courtesy of Daniel V. Vasconcelos-Santos, MD, PhD.)*

Sainz de la Maza M, Molina N, Gonzalez-Gonzalez LA, Doctor PP, Tauber J, Foster CS. Clinical characteristics of a large cohort of patients with scleritis and episcleritis. *Ophthalmology*. 2012;119(1):43–50.

Sainz de la Maza M, Vitale AT. Scleritis and episcleritis. *Focal Points: Clinical Modules for Ophthalmologists*. American Academy of Ophthalmology; 2009, module 4.

Diffuse Anterior Scleritis

The diffuse form of anterior scleritis is the most common and least severe type of scleritis; in most affected individuals, the risk of complications is less than 10%. Onset is frequently insidious, beginning slowly and building up to severe pain with deep episcleral vascular congestion. Scleral swelling/infiltration is more diffuse (see Fig 7-1), so no nodule is formed. Recurrences are very common. The main systemic associations include rheumatoid arthritis, systemic lupus erythematosus, and relapsing polychondritis. Inflammatory bowel disease, reactive arthritis, and less frequently, ankylosing spondylitis can also be implicated.

Nodular Anterior Scleritis

Features of nodular anterior scleritis include a tender and typically immobile scleral nodule, in addition to the local or diffuse violaceous hue associated with markedly engorged deep episcleral vessels. In up to 10% of patients who present with nodular anterior scleritis, the condition progresses to necrotizing disease, particularly when there is an underlying systemic inflammatory condition. It is important to rule out infectious etiologies of nodular anterior scleritis, especially in the presence of necrosis (Fig 7-3). Necrotic change often manifests as an avascular area in the center of the nodule (eventually with superficial ulceration) or as a new, discrete lesion that extends circumferentially. After scleral inflammation resolves, increased scleral translucency may be seen, eventually with thinning that reveals the bluish hue of underlying uveal tissue (Fig 7-4).

Necrotizing Scleritis

Necrotizing scleritis is the most severe and destructive type of scleritis, and therefore, it is more likely to lead to vision loss. It is frequently associated with systemic disease (approximately 50%–60% of cases), including life-threatening vasculitic diseases, and more commonly affects older individuals. Mortality rates of patients with necrotizing scleritis associated with systemic inflammatory disease had been as high as 30% but improved significantly with the development of biologic therapies.

Necrotizing scleritis can be divided into 2 groups: necrotizing scleritis with inflammation and scleromalacia perforans (necrotizing scleritis without overt inflammation). These are discussed in the following subsections.

Doshi RR, Harocopos GJ, Schwab IR, Cunningham ET Jr. The spectrum of postoperative scleral necrosis. *Surv Ophthalmol.* 2013;58(6):620–633.

Lin CP, Su CY. Infectious scleritis and surgical induced necrotizing scleritis. *Eye (Lond).* 2010;24(4):740.

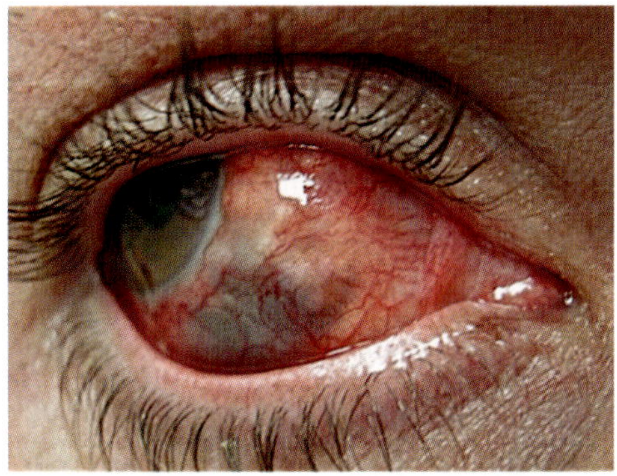

Figure 7-3 Infectious scleritis due to actinomycetes. A nodule is visible superotemporally, and a large area of scleral thinning can be seen inferiorly. *(Courtesy of Daniel V. Vasconcelos-Santos, MD, PhD.)*

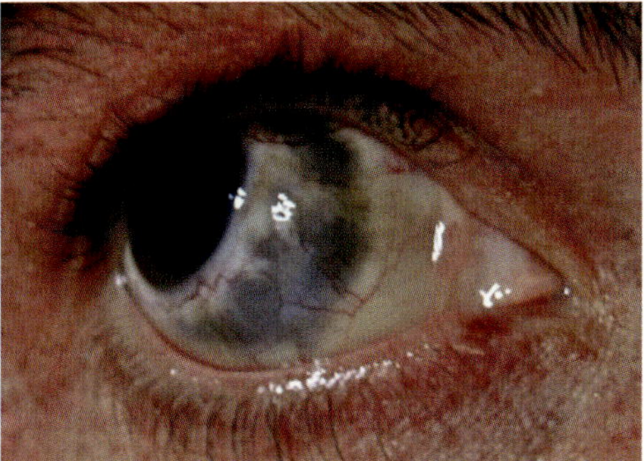

Figure 7-4 Infectious scleritis due to actinomycetes (same patient as in Fig 7-3). The inflammation resolved after antibiotic treatment, but an arch of scleral thinning remained. *(Courtesy of Daniel V. Vasconcelos-Santos, MD, PhD.)*

Necrotizing scleritis with inflammation

Necrotizing scleritis with inflammation is characterized by overt signs and symptoms of scleral inflammation. It can be subdivided into 3 forms: vaso-occlusive, granulomatous, and postsurgical (surgically induced necrotizing scleritis).

In the *vaso-occlusive form,* inflammation causes destruction of the vessel walls, leading to ischemia and nonperfusion, associated with scleral edema/infiltration (Fig 7-5). The limbal area and peripheral cornea are often spared. The vaso-occlusive form is usually associated with infection or an underlying systemic inflammatory disease.

The *granulomatous* form typically starts with necrotizing inflammation of the limbal area, subsequently extending anteriorly to the cornea and posteriorly to the sclera. The inflamed area assumes a "lumpy" aspect, associated with inflammatory cell infiltration and edema. Eventually, necrosis and ulceration of the affected tissues (cornea, conjunctiva, episclera, and sclera) develop. The granulomatous form is frequently associated with systemic vasculitides, particularly granulomatosis with polyangiitis (formerly, Wegener granulomatosis) (Fig 7-6) and polyarteritis nodosa. It is important to note that other forms of necrotizing scleritis may also display granulomatous inflammation on histologic examination.

When necrotizing scleritis arises after surgical trauma to the sclera, it is termed *surgically induced necrotizing scleritis (SINS).* This rare condition may arise a few months to several years after the surgery. It is important to exclude infection in these cases to distinguish SINS from postoperative infectious scleritis. Procedures associated with postsurgical scleritis include cataract, strabismus, or retinal surgery; trabeculectomy; cryotherapy; and pterygium excision with use of mitomycin C or beta radiation. Recalcitrant inflammation, with progressive necrosis of the sclera, develops commonly at the site of the surgical insult (Fig 7-7), or sometimes more distant from the surgical incision. Many patients with SINS have an underlying autoimmune disease; surgical injury of the sclera is the possible trigger for the local inflammatory process.

Watson PG, Hazleman BL, McCluskey P, Pavésio CE. *The Sclera and Systemic Disorders.* 3rd ed. JP Medical; 2012.

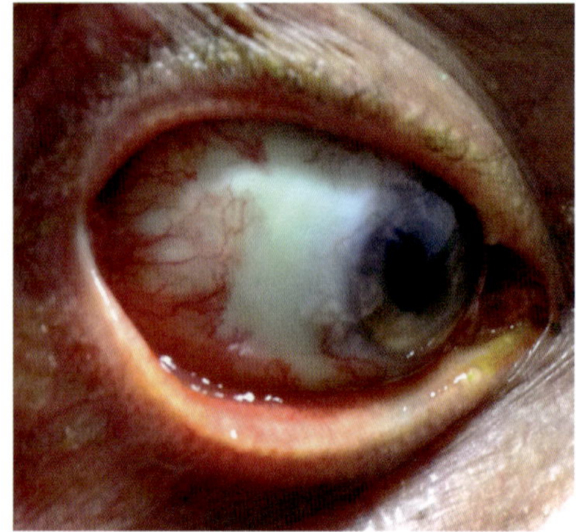

Figure 7-5 Vaso-occlusive form of necrotizing scleritis. A large avascular area adjacent to the limbus is evident. *(Courtesy of Daniel V. Vasconcelos-Santos, MD, PhD.)*

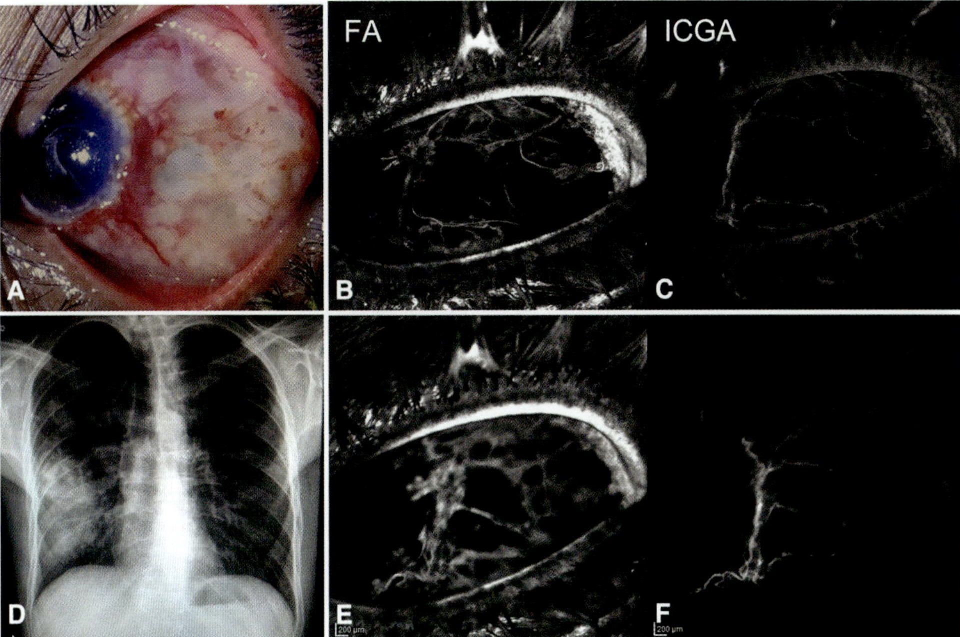

Figure 7-6 Granulomatous form of necrotizing scleritis in a patient who had granulomatosis with polyangiitis with concomitant lung and kidney disease. Infiltration of the sclera and peripheral cornea is seen, with formation of multiple necrotic and avascular areas **(A).** Simultaneous fluorescein angiography **(B, E)** and indocyanine green angiography **(C, F)** delineate areas of necrosis (with absence of episcleral and conjunctival vessels) and peripheral corneal neovascularization. Chest radiograph **(D)** shows infiltrates in the right lung *(bottom left)*. *(Courtesy of Daniel V. Vasconcelos-Santos, MD, PhD.)*

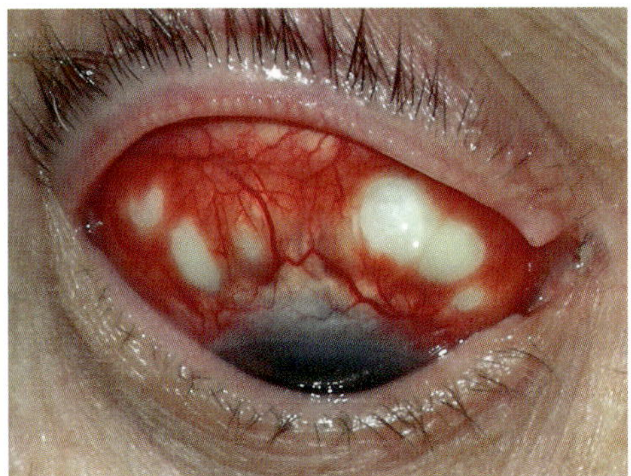

Figure 7-7 Surgically induced necrotizing scleritis. Multiple foci of scleral necrosis are present after extracapsular cataract surgery. *(Courtesy of Daniel V. Vasconcelos-Santos, MD, PhD.)*

Scleromalacia perforans (necrotizing scleritis without overt inflammation)

Scleromalacia perforans is characterized by a lack of significant symptoms and signs of clinical scleral inflammation. On histologic examination, there is inflammatory cell infiltration in the sclera. (Historically, this entity has been called *scleritis without inflammation,* which is a misnomer.) The necrotizing granulomatous response leads to progressive (and "silent") destruction of the scleral tissue, which may extend circumferentially, eventually

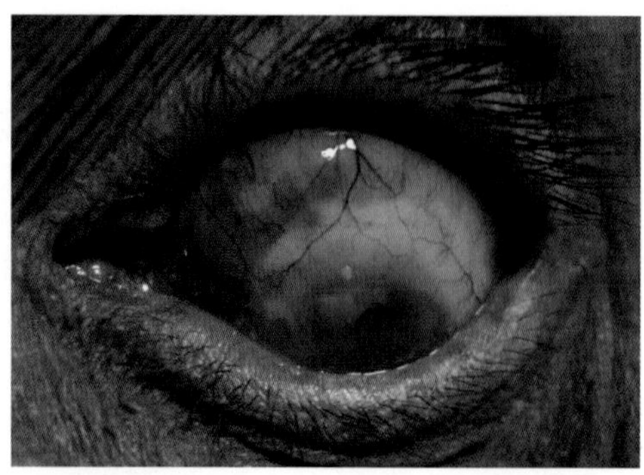

Figure 7-8 Scleromalacia perforans. The eye has profuse loss of scleral tissue with protrusion of underlying uveal tissue, which is covered by conjunctiva. There are no overt inflammatory signs. *(Courtesy of Daniel V. Vasconcelos-Santos, MD, PhD.)*

leaving a staphyloma. Patients with scleromalacia perforans are often older adult women with long-standing rheumatoid arthritis. They typically present with yellowish or white necrotic plaques involving the sclera and episclera (sequestrum) of both eyes. These plaques are surrounded by mildly dilated episcleral vessels. Associated staphylomata are covered by conjunctiva and a thin, translucent layer of fibrous tissue (Fig 7-8). Despite the term *perforans,* these lesions do not usually perforate spontaneously.

Posterior Scleritis

Posterior scleritis is a sight-threatening entity that is defined as scleral inflammation posterior to the ora serrata. Unless it is concomitant with anterior scleritis, posterior scleritis may be difficult to recognize because of the lack of inflammatory signs in the anterior part of the sclera. The rate of association with systemic inflammatory conditions is comparable to that of anterior scleritis. Patients often report severe deep, boring eye pain and tenderness on palpation, but in 30%–40% of patients, these symptoms are mild or absent. Decreased vision is often reported; the location of the inflammation and the involvement of underlying structures determine whether vision is affected. Possible signs include choroidal detachment and folds, subretinal fluid, and optic disc edema (Fig 7-9). Anterior rotation of the pars plicata (ciliary body) can displace the lens–iris diaphragm anteriorly, leading to angle closure and acute elevation of intraocular pressure. Involvement of extraocular muscles (myositis) occasionally leads to diplopia.

McCluskey PJ, Watson PG, Lightman S, Haybittle J, Restori M, Branley M. Posterior scleritis: clinical features, systemic associations, and outcome in a large series of patients. *Ophthalmology.* 1999;106(12):2380–2386.

Infectious Scleritis

A wide variety of agents can infect the sclera, including *Pseudomonas* organisms (most common after pterygium excision), *Actinomyces* and *Nocardia* species, mycobacteria, fungi such as *Fusarium* and *Aspergillus* species, and gram-positive cocci (*Staphylococcus pneumoniae* and *Streptococcus* species). In addition, infection with herpes simplex virus or varicella-zoster virus can cause chronic scleritis. Infectious scleritis can occur after any ocular surgery, including pterygium surgery (especially when beta radiation or mitomycin C

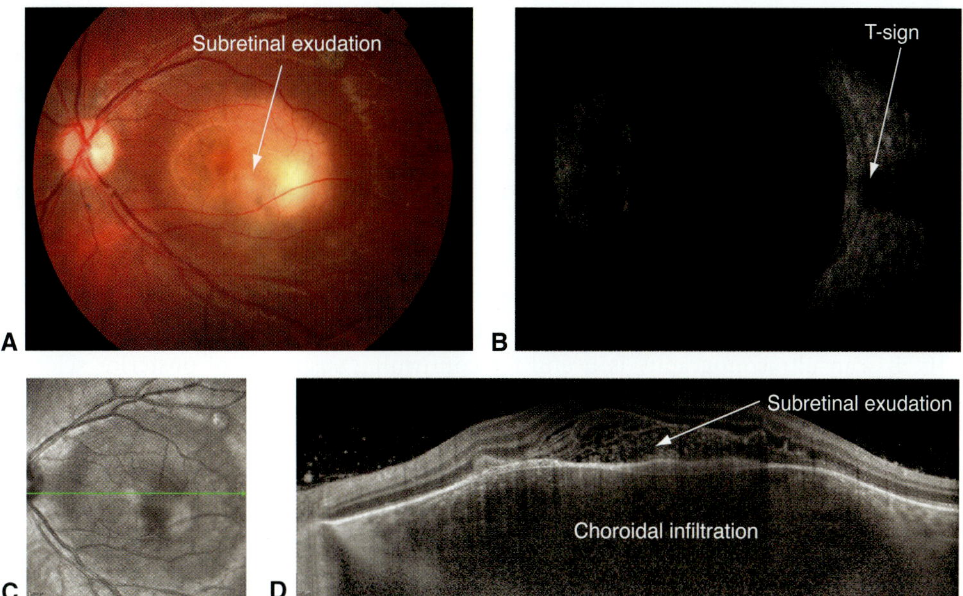

Figure 7-9 Posterior scleritis. **A,** Subretinal exudation is seen on fundus photography. **B,** B-scan reveals accumulation of sub-Tenon fluid contiguous to the optic nerve shadow (T-sign). **C, D,** Spectral-domain optical coherence tomography shows marked choroidal infiltration leading to serous detachment of the neurosensory retina and the underlying retinal pigment epithelium. *(Courtesy of Daniel V. Vasconcelos-Santos, MD, PhD.)*

is used), scleral buckling, cataract surgery, and pars plana vitrectomy. The precipitating surgery may have occurred recently, several months earlier, or in rare cases, many years before. Infectious scleritis can also develop if a penetrating ocular injury site is contaminated by vegetable or organic matter.

Similar to noninfectious scleritis, infectious scleritis can manifest with eye pain, redness, and decreased vision. Nodular and necrotizing scleral disease are more common in infectious versus noninfectious scleritis, and if there is associated intraocular inflammation (sclerouveitis), it can be disproportionately more substantial in infectious scleritis. The sclera appears necrotic, thin, and avascular, with inflammation at the edges (see Fig 7-3), usually at the site of a surgical or traumatic wound. A mucopurulent discharge may be present, depending on the infectious agent.

Raiji VR, Palestine AG, Parver DL. Scleritis and systemic disease association in a community-based referral practice. *Am J Ophthalmol.* 2009;148(6):946–950.

Riono WP, Hidayat AA, Rao NA. Scleritis: a clinicopathologic study of 55 cases. *Ophthalmology.* 1999;106(7):1328–1333.

Diagnosis

Diagnosis of scleritis is based on a detailed clinical history, careful external eye inspection, and findings from slit-lamp and fundus examinations; these findings are discussed in the section Clinical Presentation. Complementary B-scan ultrasonography, fundus angiography, and optical coherence tomography (OCT) can help better delineate scleral involvement. An appropriate laboratory workup is warranted to rule out underlying systemic inflammatory diseases (Table 7-2), which are often associated with scleritis and may be life-threatening, especially those diseases associated with necrotizing scleritis. Referral to a rheumatologist may be required for confirmatory diagnosis of systemic diseases.

Anterior segment spectral-domain OCT provides noninvasive imaging that may document local changes at the level of the sclera, episclera, Tenon capsule, conjunctiva, cornea, and angle structures; however, its clinical utility is unclear at this time. Ultrasound biomicroscopy may be used to image the anterior segment and ciliary body, but this technique is often technically cumbersome and painful in tender eyes with scleritis. B-scan ultrasonography is useful for confirming suspicion of posterior scleritis

Table 7-2 Investigations for Noninfectious Inflammatory Conditions Associated With Scleritis

Disease	Potentially Useful Investigations
Rheumatoid arthritis	RF, anti-CCP, ESR, CRP, joint radiography, C3, C4
Systemic lupus erythematosus	ANA, CBC, urine sediment, C3, C4
Juvenile idiopathic arthritis	ANA, HLA-B27, RF, anti-CCP, joint radiography
Ankylosing spondylitis	HLA-B27, ESR, CRP, lumbosacral radiography
Reactive arthritis	HLA-B27, ESR, CRP, joint radiography, cultures (urogenital tract, throat, stool, synovial fluid)
Enteropathic arthritis	HLA-B27, lumbosacral radiography
Psoriatic arthritis	HLA-B27, ESR, CRP
Granulomatosis with polyangiitis	c-ANCA-specific antibodies (anti-PR3), tissue biopsy, radiography (chest/sinuses), urine sediment, C3, C4
Polyarteritis nodosa	p-ANCA-specific antibodies (anti-MPO), tissue biopsy, urine sediment
Microscopic polyangiitis	p-ANCA-specific antibodies (anti-MPO)
Relapsing polychondritis	ESR, CRP, cartilage biopsy
Churg-Strauss syndrome (allergic granulomatous angiitis)	CBC (eosinophilia), p-ANCA-specific antibodies (anti-MPO), tissue biopsy, urine sediment, C3, C4
Leukocytoclastic vasculitis	Anti-HCV, RF, ESR, CRP
Cogan syndrome	Hearing test
Giant cell arteritis	ESR, CRP, CBC, temporal artery biopsy
Takayasu arteritis	Cardiac catheterization
Sarcoidosis	ACE (lysozyme for patients using ACE inhibitors), chest x-ray or CT, tuberculin skin test or interferon-gamma release assay, tissue biopsy

ACE = angiotensin-converting enzyme; ANA = antinuclear antibodies; c-ANCA = cytoplasmic pattern of antineutrophil cytoplasmic antibodies; CBC = complete blood count; CCP = cyclic citrullinated peptide; CRP = C-reactive protein; CT = computed tomography; ESR = erythrocyte sedimentation rate; HCV = hepatitis C virus; HLA = human leukocyte antigen; MPO = myeloperoxidase; p-ANCA = perinuclear antineutrophil cytoplasmic antibodies; PR3 = serine proteinase 3; RF = rheumatoid factor.

or assessing concomitant posterior scleral involvement in eyes with anterior scleritis; imaging typically reveals thickening of the sclera, associated with accumulation of fluid in the sub-Tenon space. When adjacent to the optic nerve shadow, this accumulation may lead to the classic "T-sign" (see Fig 7-9). Ultrasonography may also be helpful to assess the involvement of adjacent structures, including the choroid, ciliary body, retina, extraocular muscles, and orbit. Concern about an orbital process requires further workup with computed tomography and magnetic resonance imaging with and without gadolinium.

In cases of posterior scleritis, fundus fluorescein or indocyanine green angiography can delineate the extent of disease and may be helpful in differential diagnosis. Fluorescein can show optic nerve staining, multiple pinpoint leakages, and pooling of dye within subretinal fluid in the late phase of the angiogram.

If there is high clinical suspicion for infectious scleritis, microbiological examination of scleral scrapings and incisional biopsy of the sclera can be very helpful. Biopsy is also valuable when there is a possibility of neoplastic conditions, such as conjunctival carcinomas and lymphomas. These can masquerade as or be associated with a variable degree of scleral inflammation. Intraocular tumors, particularly large uveal melanomas, occasionally lead to engorgement of overlying episcleral *(sentinel)* vessels.

Levison AL, Lowder CY, Baynes KM, Kaiser PK, Srivastava SK. Anterior segment spectral domain optical coherence tomography imaging of patients with anterior scleritis. *Int Ophthalmol.* 2016;36(4):499–508.

Liu Z, Zhao W, Tao Q, Lin S, Li X, Zhang X. Comparison of the clinical features between posterior scleritis with exudative retinal detachment and Vogt-Koyanagi-Harada disease. *Int Ophthalmol.* 2021;42(2):479–488.

Nieuwenhuizen J, Watson PG, Emmanouilidis-van der Spek K, Keunen JE, Jager MJ. The value of combining anterior segment fluorescein angiography with indocyanine green angiography in scleral inflammation. *Ophthalmology.* 2003;110(8):1653–1666.

Okhravi N, Odufuwa B, McCluskey P, Lightman S. Scleritis. *Surv Ophthalmol.* 2005;50(4): 351–363.

Treatment

Treatment of scleritis depends on the type and extent of scleral inflammation and the results of diagnostic investigations (see Table 7-2). When an underlying systemic disease is present, particularly when it is associated with necrotizing scleritis, aggressive control of the disease is essential, as it may be a major determinant of mortality. It is also important to manage infectious and neoplastic etiologies accordingly. Although it is an infrequent occurrence (up to 15% of cases), if necrotizing scleritis develops in a patient who initially had nonnecrotizing disease, further investigation for associated causes and escalation of therapy are warranted.

Topical corticosteroids may be used to control associated iridocyclitis, present in nearly one-third of individuals with severe scleritis. This measure may prevent complications such as anterior/posterior synechiae, uveitic glaucoma, and cataract.

Systemic Treatment

Topical therapy is usually ineffective to treat scleritis; therefore, treatment is systemic, ranging from oral nonsteroidal anti-inflammatory drugs (NSAIDs) to immunomodulatory agents.

In individuals with mild to moderate noninfectious anterior scleritis, either diffuse or nodular, primary management consists of oral NSAIDs for no more than 2 weeks, in the absence of specific contraindications (Table 7-3). Caution is advised because of the risk of gastroduodenal ulceration, which may be decreased by concomitant use of histamine H_2 receptor antagonists or proton pump inhibitors. Also, it is important to monitor renal function closely.

Severe noninfectious anterior scleritis, refractory to NSAIDs or with posterior or necrotizing disease, is managed with systemic corticosteroids, typically with an initial dosage of 1 mg/kg/day of prednisone (up to 60–80 mg/day) or equivalent, followed by a slow tapering regimen. Careful monitoring for adverse effects is critical. It is important to distinguish noninfectious scleritis from infectious scleritis because high-dose corticosteroids or immunosuppressive agents can worsen scleritis in the presence of active, untreated infection. Systemic corticosteroids should not be given until infection has been ruled out or treated.

When scleral inflammation recurs or is refractory to systemic corticosteroids, especially in necrotizing scleritis, immunomodulatory drugs (mainly antimetabolites, such as methotrexate, mycophenolate mofetil, or azathioprine) are indicated either as corticosteroid-sparing agents or as adjuvants. Biologic immunomodulatory agents, such as tumor necrosis factor inhibitors (eg, infliximab, adalimumab), and anti-CD20 agents (rituximab), have also been successfully employed for refractory cases.

In the setting of severe necrotizing or nonnecrotizing scleritis, intravenous pulse therapy with methylprednisolone (1 g daily for 3 days) can be used initially, followed by high-dose oral prednisone (up to 60–80 mg per day). Alkylating agents, such as cyclophosphamide, are reserved for severe necrotizing involvement of the sclera and cornea, especially if there is impending risk of perforation. Scleritis associated with granulomatosis with polyangiitis and polyarteritis nodosa typically requires more aggressive therapy with rituximab or cyclophosphamide.

Infectious scleritis can be treated with systemic (and topical) antimicrobials plus surgical debridement as needed. Microorganisms may be difficult to eradicate from the

Table 7-3 NSAID Dosage for Management of Mild to Moderate Noninfectious Anterior Scleritis[a]

Drug	Dosage
Flurbiprofen	50–100 mg 3 times daily
Ibuprofen	600 mg 3–4 times daily
Indomethacin	25–50 mg 3 times daily
Naproxen	500 mg 2 times daily

NSAID = nonsteroidal anti-inflammatory drug.
[a] NSAIDs should not be used for long-term management of scleritis.

sclera, and long-term antimicrobial treatment may be necessary. If there is severe scleral thinning, scleral grafting may be utilized.

Individuals with nonnecrotizing, noninfectious scleritis who cannot tolerate systemic therapy or who have residual scleral inflammation after treatment may be candidates for subconjunctival injection of triamcinolone (40 mg/mL, 0.2 mL in each active quadrant). Before administering a local corticosteroid injection, it is paramount to rule out infectious etiologies. Associated systemic inflammatory diseases should also be under control. In each case, it is important to weigh the risks of the injection—cataract and secondary ocular hypertension/glaucoma and, less likely, of scleral melting and infection—against the possible benefits.

Cao JH, Oray M, Cocho L, Foster CS. Rituximab in the treatment of refractory noninfectious scleritis. *Am J Ophthalmol.* 2016;164:22–28.

Daniel Diaz J, Sobol EK, Gritz DC. Treatment and management of scleral disorders. *Surv Ophthalmol.* 2016;61(6):702–717.

Jabs DA, Mudun A, Dunn JP, Marsh MJ. Episcleritis and scleritis: clinical features and treatment results. *Am J Ophthalmol.* 2000;130(4):469–476.

Sobrin L, Christen W, Foster CS. Mycophenolate mofetil after methotrexate failure or intolerance in treatment of scleritis and uveitis. *Ophthalmology.* 2008;115(8):1416–1421.

Sohn EH, Wang R, Read R, et al. Long-term, multicenter evaluation of subconjunctival injection of triamcinolone for non-necrotizing, noninfectious anterior scleritis. *Ophthalmology.* 2011;118(10):1932–1937.

Surgical Treatment

For eyes with severe refractory necrotizing scleritis, surgical treatment may be considered to reinforce the scleral wall in the setting of an impending perforation or to close a spontaneous or traumatic corneal and/or scleral defect (tectonic grafting). Figure 7-10 shows the postoperative appearance of an eye after scleral grafting. Cadaveric donor sclera may be used for grafting, but it can melt. Consequently, some authors recommend the use of autogenous periosteum or donor cornea. For patients with infectious scleritis, antimicrobial agents are used, sometimes accompanied by debridement of necrotic scleral tissue to reduce the load of microorganisms and improve penetration of the medication.

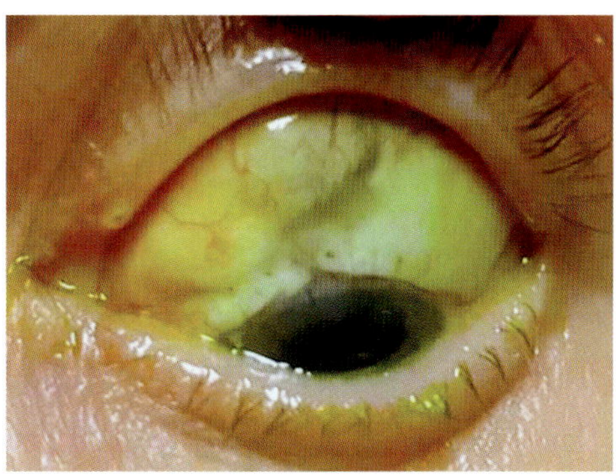

Figure 7-10 Postoperative appearance of a scleral graft. *(Courtesy of Humeyra Karacal, MD.)*

Prognosis

The prognosis of scleritis depends on the severity and extent of ocular structure involvement and the presence of underlying systemic diseases. Nonnecrotizing noninfectious anterior (diffuse or nodular) scleritis has a good prognosis with treatment; most eyes maintain good visual function over time. However, patients with posterior scleritis, necrotizing scleritis, or infectious scleritis have a high risk of permanent vision loss. Individuals with necrotizing scleritis also have higher mortality rates because of the frequent association with life-threatening vasculitic disorders. Proper and timely management of these disorders is thus very important.

CHAPTER 8

Noninfectious Anterior and Intermediate Uveitis

Highlights

- Anterior uveitis, the most common form of uveitis, is usually treated with topical corticosteroids.
- The first episode of mild, nongranulomatous, unilateral anterior uveitis may not require further systemic workup.
- Intermediate uveitis can be associated with systemic diseases, including sarcoidosis and multiple sclerosis.
- Pars planitis, a subtype of idiopathic or undifferentiated intermediate uveitis, is characterized by the presence of snowballs (aggregates of inflammatory cells in the vitreous) and snowbanks (inflammatory exudates on the pars plana).

Anterior Uveitis

Anterior uveitis is the most common type of uveitis, accounting for more than 90% of cases in a community-based practice. Incidence in the United States varies by age, from approximately 7 cases per 100,000 person-years in individuals aged 14 years and younger to approximately 220 cases per 100,000 person-years in adults aged 65 years and older.

Because uveitis may occur secondary to inflammation of the cornea and/or sclera, it is important for the physician to evaluate these structures carefully to rule out primary keratitis or scleritis. Inflammation of the sclera and the cornea is covered in depth in BCSC Section 8, *External Disease and Cornea*. See Chapter 7 in this volume for discussion of scleritis.

Gritz DC, Wong IG. Incidence and prevalence of uveitis in Northern California; the Northern California Epidemiology of Uveitis Study. *Ophthalmology.* 2004;111(3): 491–500.

Reeves SW, Sloan FA, Lee PP, Jaffe GJ. Uveitis in the elderly: epidemiological data from the National Long-term Care Survey Medicare Cohort. *Ophthalmology.* 2006;113(2):307–321.

Acute Anterior Uveitis

The classic presentation of acute anterior uveitis is the sudden onset of eye pain, redness, and photophobia that can be associated with decreased vision. In nongranulomatous anterior uveitis, the inflammatory infiltrate is typically composed of lymphocytic and plasma cells; clinically, fine keratic precipitates (KPs) can dust the corneal endothelium. The clinical description of granulomatous anterior uveitis is related to the appearance of the KPs (large, yellow, and "greasy," with inferior cornea distribution). See Chapter 5 for further discussion about KPs and other findings associated with anterior uveitis.

Active anterior uveitis is characterized by inflammatory cells and flare in the anterior chamber, which distinguishes anterior uveitis from non-uveitic entities such as dry eye and conjunctivitis. Severe cases may show a protein coagulum in the aqueous (fibrin) or, less commonly, a hypopyon (Fig 8-1). Occasionally, a fibrin net forms across the pupillary margin (Fig 8-2), potentially producing a seclusion membrane and iris bombé. Iris vessels may be dilated, and on rare occasions, a spontaneous hyphema occurs. Cells may also be present in the anterior vitreous. Fundus lesions are not characteristic, although uveitic macular edema and optic disc edema may occur with high-grade inflammation. Intraocular pressure (IOP) is often low due to increased uveoscleral outflow or decreased aqueous production secondary to ciliary body inflammation. Occasionally, IOP is elevated due to trabeculitis, obstruction of the trabecular meshwork by debris and cells, or pupillary block.

The inflammation usually lasts several days to weeks, up to 3 months. There are 2 patterns of inflammation: One is acute and bilateral. The other is an acute and unilateral attack, with recurrences alternating between the 2 eyes, although the disease is usually not active in both eyes simultaneously. This pattern is typical for *human leukocyte antigen (HLA)-B27–associated anterior uveitis.* Other features of HLA-B27–associated anterior uveitis include high-grade inflammation (ie, significant number of anterior chamber cells [see Chapter 5, Table 5-7]) at presentation, hypopyon, fibrin, and posterior synechiae. The age at onset of HLA-B27–associated anterior uveitis ranges from 20 to 40 years, and men are more likely to be affected than women.

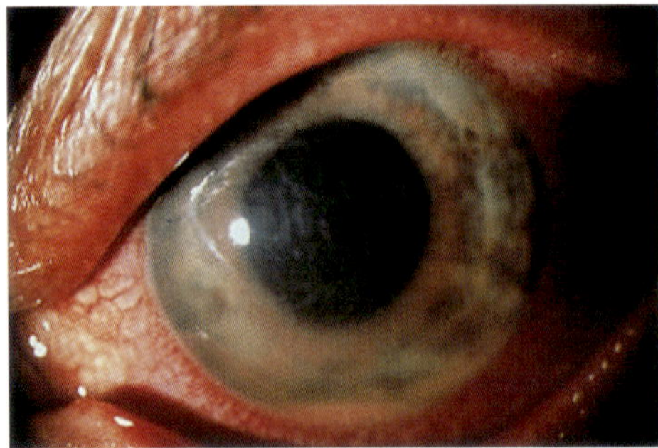

Figure 8-1 Acute HLA-B27–positive anterior uveitis accompanied by marked conjunctival injection, fixed pupil, loss of iris detail from corneal edema, and hypopyon. The patient had eye pain and photophobia. *(Courtesy of David Meisler, MD.)*

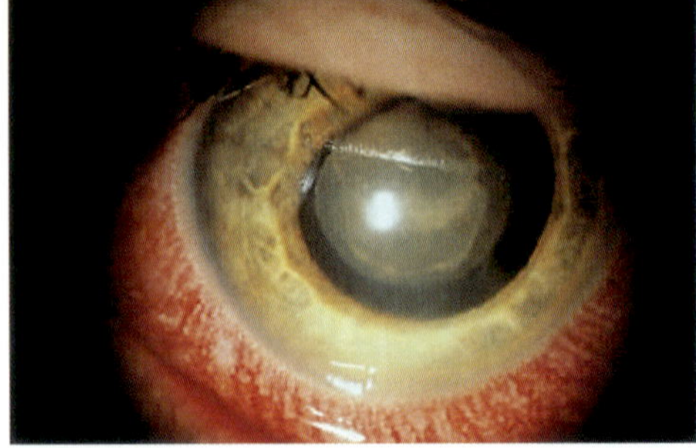

Figure 8-2 Ankylosing spondylitis. Acute unilateral anterior uveitis with severe anterior chamber reaction, central fibrinous exudate contracting anterior to the lens capsule, and posterior synechiae from the 10 o'clock to 12 o'clock position. *(Courtesy of David Meisler, MD.)*

Unilateral anterior uveitis should also raise suspicion for an infectious etiology, especially herpetic anterior uveitis. Sarcoidosis can present as an acute, bilateral or unilateral, granulomatous anterior uveitis. In most cases, the first episode of acute anterior uveitis does not require a systemic workup, although high-grade or bilateral uveitis might warrant targeted testing. See Chapter 5 for further discussion about indications for testing.

For all forms of acute nongranulomatous anterior uveitis, ocular morbidity can be reduced by timely diagnosis, aggressive initial therapy, and patient adherence. Topical corticosteroids are first-line treatment, and administration every 1–2 hours may be necessary. Very severe inflammation may require periocular and/or oral corticosteroids in addition to topical treatment. Periocular corticosteroids should not be used unless infectious etiologies have been thoroughly investigated or infection has been treated before corticosteroid use. Topical cycloplegic agents can relieve pain due to ciliary body spasm, as well as lyse or prevent formation of posterior synechiae. Mydriasis may also be attained with conjunctival cotton pledgets soaked in tropicamide, cyclopentolate, or phenylephrine hydrochloride (Fig 8-3).

Although a protracted course of treatment is typically not required for acute nongranulomatous anterior uveitis, systemic corticosteroid-sparing immunomodulatory therapy (IMT) may be necessary for long-term therapy if the inflammation recurs frequently or becomes chronic, or if complications arise from long-term use of topical or periocular corticosteroids. Antimetabolites are usually the first-line treatment for anterior uveitis without associated systemic inflammatory disease. A tumor necrosis factor (TNF) inhibitor may be considered for second-line treatment of anterior uveitis, particularly in patients who are HLA-B27 positive. Of note, *none* of the TNF inhibitors are approved by the US Food and Drug Administration (FDA) to treat undifferentiated or isolated anterior uveitis; the FDA indications for adalimumab are for noninfectious intermediate, posterior, and panuveitis.

Rosenbaum JT. Evolving "diagnostic" criteria for axial spondyloarthritis in the context of anterior uveitis. *Ocul Immunol Inflamm.* 2016;24(4):445–449.

Van Gelder RN. Diagnostic testing in uveitis. *Focal Points: Clinical Modules for Ophthalmologists.* American Academy of Ophthalmology; 2013, module 4.

HLA-B27–related diseases

HLA-B27 is a major histocompatibility complex (MHC) class I antigen present in approximately 8% of the general population in the United States. In some populations, approximately 40%–50% of patients with acute anterior uveitis are HLA-B27 positive. Although

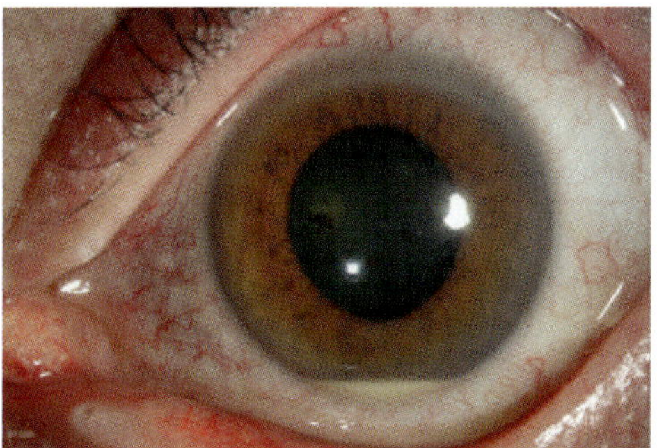

Figure 8-3 Acute nongranulomatous anterior uveitis. Hypopyon and anterior capsule ring of pigment after lysis of posterior synechiae by treatment with dilating agents. *(Courtesy of H. Nida Sen, MD/National Eye Institute.)*

patients with recurrent acute nongranulomatous anterior uveitis should be tested for HLA-B27, the presence of HLA-B27 does not necessarily indicate that the uveitis is HLA-B27 associated. The clinical characteristics of the uveitis should be consistent with those of HLA-B27–associated uveitis. Thus, for example, a patient with multifocal choroidal lesions who is HLA-B27 positive does *not* have HLA-B27–associated uveitis, because choroidal lesions are not a characteristic of this entity. See Chapter 4 for additional discussion of HLA–disease associations.

Several autoimmune diseases known collectively as the *seronegative spondyloarthropathies* are strongly associated with both acute nongranulomatous anterior uveitis and HLA-B27. Patients with these diseases, by definition, do not test positive for rheumatoid factor (RF). The seronegative spondyloarthropathies include

- ankylosing spondylitis (AS)
- reactive arthritis
- inflammatory bowel disease–related arthropathy
- psoriatic arthritis

These entities are sometimes clinically indistinguishable, and all may be associated with spondylitis and sacroiliitis. Women are more likely than men to experience atypical spondyloarthropathies.

Up to 90% of patients with AS test positive for HLA-B27, although most HLA-B27–positive individuals do not develop the disease. The chance that an HLA-B27–positive patient will develop spondyloarthritis or eye disease is 1 in 4. Family members may also have AS or anterior uveitis.

Ankylosing spondylitis AS ranges in severity from asymptomatic to crippling. Symptoms of this disorder include lower back pain and morning stiffness that improves with movement. AS typically affects young men between 20 and 40 years of age. Patients with anterior uveitis may lack symptoms of inflammatory arthritis, or they may not report lower back pain and stiffness unless specifically asked about these symptoms. Sacroiliac imaging studies can be used to screen for evidence of joint inflammation. Patients with anterior uveitis who have possible symptoms of inflammatory arthritis or enthesitis may be referred to a rheumatologist for further evaluation. Pulmonary apical fibrosis and cardiovascular disease (aortic valvular insufficiency) can also occur in AS.

Early diagnosis of AS is important because nonpharmacologic interventions such as exercise, physical therapy, and smoking cessation may help slow disease progression. Nonsteroidal anti-inflammatory drugs (NSAIDs) are the first-line systemic treatment for AS. Sulfasalazine may be used for joint disease not controlled with NSAIDs and may reduce the frequency of uveitis recurrences. However, TNF inhibitors are gaining favor as second-line treatment because of their rapid therapeutic effect, overall efficacy, and side effect profile.

Ahn SM, Kim M, Kim YJ, Lee Y, Kim YG. Risk of Acute Anterior Uveitis in Ankylosing Spondylitis According to the Type of Tumor Necrosis Factor-Alpha Inhibitor and History of Uveitis: A Nationwide Population-Based Study. *J Clin Med.* 2022;11(3):631. doi:10.3390/jcm11030631

Chung YM, Liao HT, Lin KC, et al. Prevalence of spondyloarthritis in 504 Chinese patients with HLA-B27-associated acute anterior uveitis. *Scand J Rheumatol.* 2009;38(2):84–90.

Haroon M, O'Rourke M, Ramasamy P, Murphy CC, FitzGerald O. A novel evidence-based detection of undiagnosed spondyloarthritis in patients presenting with acute anterior uveitis: the DUET (Dublin Uveitis Evaluation Tool). *Ann Rheum Dis.* 2015;74(11):1990–1995.

Reactive arthritis Reactive arthritis (formerly, Reiter syndrome) consists of the classic diagnostic triad of nonspecific urethritis, polyarthritis, and conjunctival inflammation, sometimes accompanied by nongranulomatous anterior uveitis. The HLA-B27 allele is found in approximately 50%–75% of patients with reactive arthritis. The condition constitutes less than 2% of all spondyloarthropathies and occurs most frequently in young adult men, although 10% of patients are female.

Episodes of diarrhea or dysentery without urethritis can trigger reactive arthritis. *Ureaplasma urealyticum,* as well as *Chlamydia, Shigella, Salmonella,* and *Yersinia* species have all been implicated as triggering infections, although pathogens cannot be isolated from affected joints. Arthritis begins within 30 days of infection in 80% of patients. The knees, ankles, feet, and wrists are affected asymmetrically and in an oligoarticular (4 or fewer joints) distribution. Sacroiliitis is present in as many as 70% of patients.

In addition to the classic triad, 2 other conditions are considered major diagnostic criteria:

- keratoderma blennorrhagicum: a scaly, erythematous, irritating disorder of the palms and soles of the feet (Fig 8-4)
- circinate balanitis: a persistent, scaly, erythematous, circumferential rash of the distal penis

Extraarticular findings such as nail bed pitting, oral ulcers, conjunctivitis, uveitis, and constitutional symptoms help establish a diagnosis of reactive arthritis. Most cases resolve after a short episode. Occasionally, the disease becomes chronic.

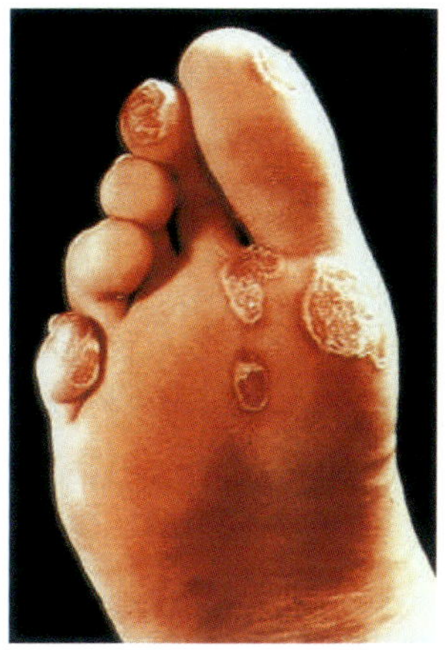

Figure 8-4 Reactive arthritis with pedal discoid keratoderma blennorrhagicum. *(Courtesy of John D. Sheppard Jr, MD.)*

Eye involvement occurs in approximately 20% of cases. Conjunctivitis, the most common ocular finding associated with this disease, is usually mucopurulent and papillary. Punctate and subepithelial keratitis may also occur, occasionally leaving permanent corneal scars. Acute nongranulomatous anterior uveitis occurs in up to 10% of affected patients and may become bilateral and chronic.

Inflammatory bowel disease–related arthropathy Acute nongranulomatous anterior uveitis develops in up to 12% of patients with ulcerative colitis and 2.4% of patients with Crohn disease. Occasionally, bowel disease is asymptomatic and follows the onset of uveitis. Twenty percent of patients with inflammatory bowel disease (IBD) have sacroiliitis; of these, 60% are HLA-B27 positive. Patients with both acute anterior uveitis and IBD are more likely to be HLA-B27 positive and have sacroiliitis. Patients with IBD may also develop sclerouveitis, but they are usually HLA-B27 negative and do not develop sacroiliitis, although they can have rheumatoid arthritis–like symptoms. HLA-B27–negative patients with IBD are also more likely to develop intermediate uveitis.

Psoriatic arthritis The diagnosis of psoriatic arthritis is based on the presence of typical cutaneous changes (Fig 8-5), distal interphalangeal joint inflammation (Fig 8-6), and ungual involvement. Twenty percent of patients have sacroiliitis, and IBD occurs more frequently than would be expected by chance. Up to 25% of patients develop anterior uveitis, which tends to be insidious and bilateral; it is also more likely to be chronic compared with the uveitis associated with other spondyloarthropathies, and the risk is highest in patients with psoriatic spondylitis. Uveitis may be more severe in HLA-B27–positive patients. Treatment consists of cycloplegic and mydriatic agents and corticosteroids, which are usually given topically. In severe cases, periocular or systemic corticosteroids may be required, and chronic cases may need systemic IMT.

Anterior uveitis in patients with psoriasis without arthritis has distinct clinical features. The mean age at onset is older than in idiopathic or HLA-B27–associated uveitis,

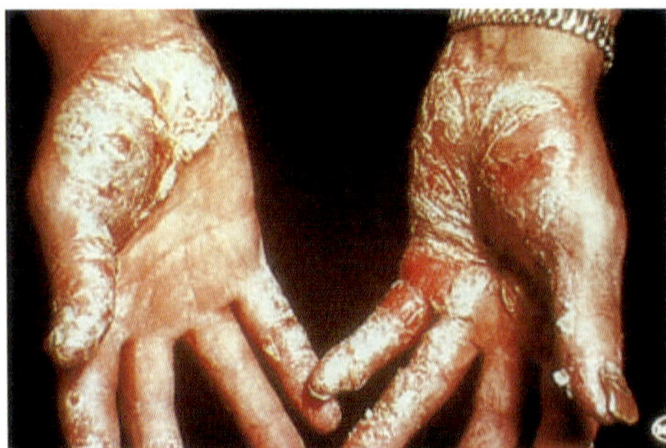

Figure 8-5 Psoriatic arthritis with classic erythematous, hyperkeratotic rash. *(Courtesy of John D. Sheppard Jr, MD.)*

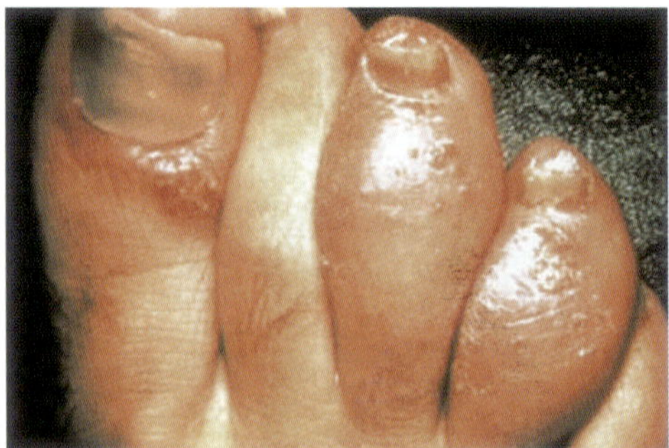

Figure 8-6 Psoriatic arthritis. The patient has "sausage" digits resulting from tissue swelling and distal interphalangeal joint inflammation. *(Courtesy of John D. Sheppard Jr, MD.)*

and the uveitis may be bilateral and of longer duration. Posterior segment involvement can be present.

Egeberg A, Khalid U, Gislason GH, Mallbris L, Skov L, Hansen PR. Association of psoriatic disease with uveitis: a Danish nationwide cohort study. *JAMA Dermatol.* 2015;151(11): 1200–1205.

Köse B, Uzlu D, Erdöl H. Psoriasis and uveitis. *Int Ophthalmol.* 2022;42(7):2303–2310. doi:10.1007/s10792-022-02225-5

Sampaio-Barros PD, Pereira IA, Hernández-Cuevas C, et al; RESPONDIA Group. An analysis of 372 patients with anterior uveitis in a large Ibero-American cohort of spondyloarthritis: the RESPONDIA Group. *Clin Exp Rheumatol.* 2013;31(4):484–489.

Tubulointerstitial nephritis and uveitis syndrome

Tubulointerstitial nephritis and uveitis (TINU) syndrome was originally described as anterior uveitis and renal inflammation occurring predominantly in adolescent girls and women up to their early 30s. It is now recognized that TINU has a variety of ophthalmic manifestations and occurs across a wide age range, with a median age at onset of 15 years. The associated anterior uveitis is typically acute, bilateral and nongranulomatous; it may be recurrent. Ocular symptoms and findings are more severe in patients with recurrent disease, with development of fibrin, posterior synechiae, larger KPs, and in rare cases, hypopyon. Posterior segment involvement may include vitritis, multifocal chorioretinal lesions or scars (Fig 8-7), and retinal vascular leakage, as well as optic disc and macular edema.

In many cases, systemic symptoms precede the development of uveitis. However, patients may be asymptomatic or develop systemic symptoms and tubulointerstitial nephritis

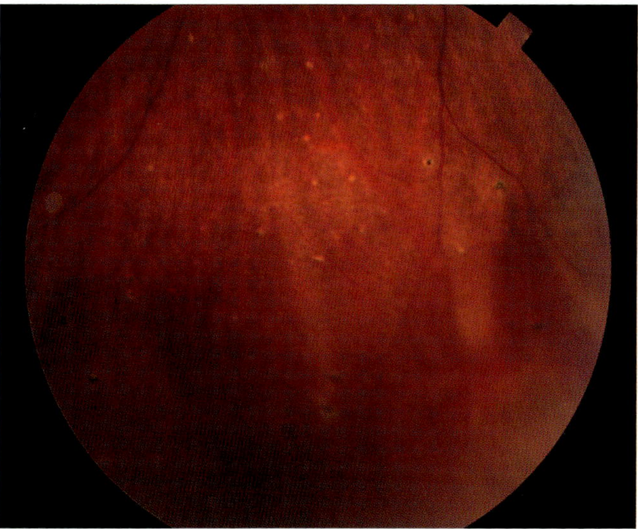

Figure 8-7 Tubulointerstitial nephritis–associated uveitis with chorioretinal scars in the peripheral retina. *(Courtesy of Debra A. Goldstein, MD.)*

after the onset of uveitis. The following findings are required for a clinical diagnosis of TINU syndrome:

- abnormal serum creatinine level or decreased creatinine clearance
- abnormal urinalysis findings, with increased β_2-microglobulin level, proteinuria, presence of eosinophils, pyuria or hematuria, urinary white cell casts, and normoglycemic glycosuria
- associated systemic illness, consisting of fever, weight loss, anorexia, fatigue, arthralgias, and myalgias; there may also be abnormal liver function, eosinophilia, and an elevated erythrocyte sedimentation rate

The etiology remains unclear. The syndrome has been reported to be strongly associated with HLA-DRB1*01:02. The predominance of activated $CD4^+$ (helper) T lymphocytes in the kidney interstitium suggests a role for cellular immunity. Renal biopsies have shown severe interstitial fibrosis. Seroreactivity against retinal and renal antigens has been demonstrated. Infection and drug reaction are among the potential triggers. Flares of renal disease do not occur simultaneously with ocular flares.

Initially, TINU syndrome is very responsive to treatment with high-dose oral corticosteroids. The renal disease tends to resolve over time, but ocular inflammation can be chronic and require systemic IMT.

Ali A, Rosenbaum JT. TINU (tubulointerstitial nephritis uveitis) can be associated with chorioretinal scars. *Ocul Immunol Inflamm.* 2014;22(3):213–217.

Koreishi AF, Zhou M, Goldstein DA. Tubulointerstitial nephritis and uveitis syndrome: characterization of clinical features. *Ocul Immunol Inflamm.* 2021;29(7–8):1312–1317.

Okafor LO, Hewins P, Murray PI, Denniston AK. Tubulointerstitial nephritis and uveitis (TINU) syndrome: a systematic review of its epidemiology, demographics, and risk factors. *Orphanet J Rare Dis.* 2017;12(1):128.

Pakzad-Vaezi K, Pepple KL. Tubulointerstitial nephritis and uveitis. *Curr Opin Ophthalmol.* 2017;28(6):629–635.

Glaucomatocyclitic crisis

Glaucomatocyclitic crisis (also known as *Posner-Schlossman syndrome*) usually manifests as a recurrent unilateral, acute, mild nongranulomatous anterior uveitis associated with markedly elevated IOP. Symptoms are vague: discomfort, blurred vision, and halos. In addition to elevated IOP, signs include corneal edema, small KPs, low-grade anterior chamber inflammation, and a slightly dilated pupil. Episodes last from several hours to several days, and recurrences are common over many years. An increase in KPs is often noted with recurrences.

Recent studies suggest ocular cytomegalovirus (CMV) infection as a possible cause of glaucomatocyclitic crisis, with specific genotypes of CMV associated with anterior uveitis versus retinitis. Corneal endotheliitis, linear KPs, and male preponderance are more common in CMV-associated glaucomatocyclitic crisis. Polymerase chain reaction testing can be performed on aqueous humor to confirm the presence of CMV DNA; there may be a role for antiviral therapy in such cases. See BCSC Section 10, *Glaucoma,* for additional discussion.

Traditionally, treatment for acute inflammation has been topical corticosteroids and antiglaucoma medications, including systemic carbonic anhydrase inhibitors, if necessary. Long-term surveillance may be required in addition to careful IOP monitoring.

Chee SP, Jap A. Presumed Fuchs heterochromic iridocyclitis and Posner-Schlossman syndrome: comparison of cytomegalovirus-positive and negative eyes. *Am J Ophthalmol.* 2008;146(6):883–889.

Oka N, Suzuki T, Inoue T, Kobayashi T, Ohashi Y. Polymorphisms in cytomegalovirus genotype in immunocompetent patients with corneal endotheliitis or iridocyclitis. *J Med Virol.* 2015;87(8):1441–1445.

Lens-associated uveitis

Although the exact mechanism is unknown, an immune reaction to lens material may result in ocular inflammatory disease, including acute nongranulomatous anterior uveitis (Table 8-1).

Phacoantigenic uveitis Phacoantigenic uveitis (also called *phacoantigenic glaucoma*) was previously termed *phacoanaphylactic uveitis,* which was a misnomer because none of the mediators of anaphylaxis (ie, immunoglobulin E, mast cells, and basophils) are present in the eye. Phacoantigenic uveitis is an ocular inflammation that occurs after disruption of the lens capsule (traumatic or surgical) in patients previously sensitized to lens protein, for example, as a result of cataract extraction in the fellow eye; this inflammation may occur within 24 hours of capsular rupture.

Clinically, patients exhibit an anterior uveitis that may be granulomatous or nongranulomatous (Fig 8-8). Small or large KPs are usually present. Anterior chamber reaction varies from mild (eg, postoperative inflammation involving a small amount of retained lens cortex) to severe (eg, traumatic lens capsule disruption); hypopyon may be present. Posterior synechiae are common, and IOP is often elevated. Inflammation in the anterior vitreous cavity is common, but fundus lesions do not occur.

Histologically, a zonal granulomatous inflammation is present at the site of lens injury. Neutrophils are clustered around the lens material with surrounding lymphocytes, plasma cells, epithelioid cells, and occasional giant cells.

Table 8-1 Lens-Induced Uveitis

	Etiology	Clinical Features	Treatment
Phacoantigenic uveitis	Disrupted lens capsule (as a result of surgery, trauma)	Red eye, anterior chamber cells and flare, keratic precipitates, posterior synechiae, elevated IOP	Topical or systemic corticosteroids Removal of lens material
Phacolytic uveitis	Leakage of lens protein through intact capsule	Elevated IOP, anterior chamber cell and flare, refractile bodies, mature/hypermature cataract	Reduction of IOP Cataract surgery

IOP = intraocular pressure.

Treatment consists of topical and in severe cases, systemic corticosteroids, as well as cycloplegic and mydriatic agents. Surgical removal of all lens material is usually curative. When small amounts of lens material remain, corticosteroid therapy alone may be sufficient to allow resorption of the inciting material. It is important to differentiate this inflammatory process from postoperative infectious endophthalmitis. Visual outcomes can deteriorate rapidly in patients with infectious endophthalmitis if the infection is not treated quickly and aggressively.

Phacolytic uveitis Phacolytic uveitis (or *phacolytic glaucoma*) is due to leakage of lens protein through microscopic openings in the intact lens capsule of a mature or hypermature cataract (Fig 8-9). Macrophages engorged with lens proteins clog the trabecular meshwork and cause an acute increase in IOP. Refractile bodies (lipid-laden macrophages) can be seen in the aqueous, but KPs and synechiae are often absent. Therapy includes IOP reduction, often through use of osmotic agents and topical medications, followed quickly by cataract extraction. See BCSC Section 10, *Glaucoma*, for additional discussion and images of phacolytic glaucoma.

Nche EN, Amer R. Lens-induced uveitis: an update. *Graefes Arch Clin Exp Ophthalmol.* 2020;258(7):1359–1365.

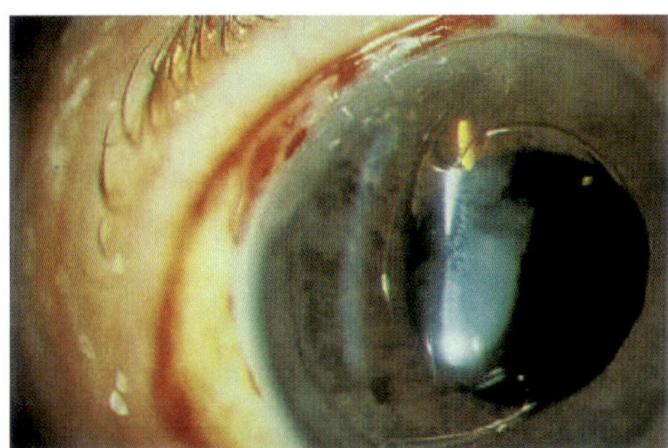

Figure 8-8 Low-grade postoperative uveitis in this patient could be secondary to retained lens cortex or to the anterior chamber intraocular lens (IOL). *(Courtesy of John D. Sheppard Jr, MD.)*

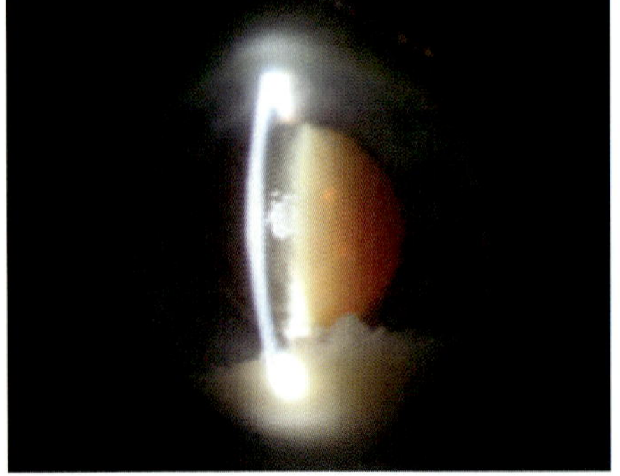

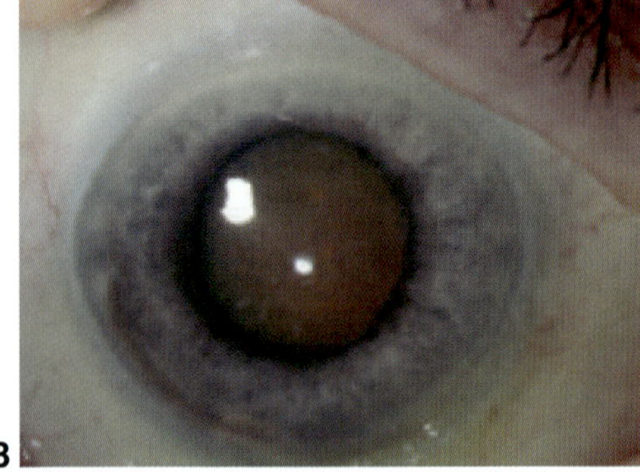

Figure 8-9 Phacolytic uveitis. **A,** Phacolytic uveitis with glaucoma, corneal edema, anterior uveitis, and pseudohypopyon in a patient with hypermature cataract. **B,** Resolution of anterior chamber inflammation with intense topical corticosteroid use; the patient eventually required cataract surgery. *(Courtesy of H. Nida Sen, MD/National Eye Institute.)*

Postoperative inflammation: infectious endophthalmitis

Infectious endophthalmitis must be included in the differential diagnosis of postoperative inflammation, especially in the presence of hypopyon. Delayed or late-onset endophthalmitis may be caused by infection with low-virulence organisms such as *Cutibacterium acnes* (formerly, *Propionibacterium acnes*) and *Staphylococcus epidermidis,* as well as with fungal species. Chronic postoperative endophthalmitis is discussed in more detail in Chapter 14. See BCSC Section 12, *Retina and Vitreous,* for information about acute postoperative endophthalmitis.

Postoperative inflammation: intraocular lens–associated uveitis

All forms of surgical manipulation result in a breakdown of the blood–aqueous barrier, leading to vulnerability in the early postoperative period. Intraocular lens (IOL) implantation can activate complement cascades and promote neutrophil chemotaxis. This leads to cellular deposits on the IOL, synechiae formation, capsular opacification, and anterior capsule phimosis. Residual lens material can exacerbate the typically transient postoperative inflammation.

In general, the more biocompatible the IOL material, the less likely it is to incite an inflammatory response. Irregular or damaged IOL surfaces and polypropylene haptics have been associated with enhanced bacterial and leukocyte binding and should be avoided in patients with a preoperative diagnosis of uveitis. Acrylic IOLs appear to have excellent biocompatibility, with low rates of cellular deposits and capsular opacification.

IOL-associated uveitis can occur when chafing of the anterior or posterior surface of the iris by the edges or loops of an IOL causes mechanical irritation and inflammation. This uveitis ranges from mild inflammation to the uveitis-glaucoma-hyphema (UGH) syndrome.

The motion of an iris-supported IOL or anterior chamber IOL (ACIOL) can cause intermittent corneal touch and lead to corneal edema due to endothelial damage. Other ocular complications from IOL contact with anterior chamber structures include low-grade anterior uveitis, peripheral anterior synechiae, recurrent microhyphema, recalcitrant glaucoma, and macular edema (Fig 8-10). UGH syndrome and corneal decompensation are more likely to develop with older rigid ACIOLs versus newer ACIOLs and scleral-fixated IOLs. ACIOLs should be removed and exchanged when penetrating keratoplasty is performed.

Because ACIOL use is rare, UGH syndrome is encountered most commonly with unintentional sulcus placement of a single-piece hydrophobic acrylic IOL. UGH or IOL-associated uveitis can occur even with appropriate IOL placement; the IOL-capsule complex may be mobile, as for example in eyes with pseudoexfoliation syndrome. In cases of chronic pseudophakic uveitis, ultrasound biomicroscopy or anterior segment optical coherence tomography (OCT) can be used to evaluate the IOL position (Fig 8-11). Many cases can be managed with topical corticosteroids and/or cycloplegia, although some may require IOL repositioning or explantation. UGH syndrome and chronic uveitis are also discussed in BCSC Section 11, *Lens and Cataract.*

Ozdal PC, Mansour M, Deschênes J. Ultrasound biomicroscopy of pseudophakic eyes with chronic postoperative inflammation. *J Cataract Refract Surg.* 2003;29(6):1185–1191.

Patel C, Kim SJ, Chomsky A, Saboori M. Incidence and risk factors for chronic uveitis following cataract surgery. *Ocul Immunol Inflamm.* 2013;21(2):130–134.

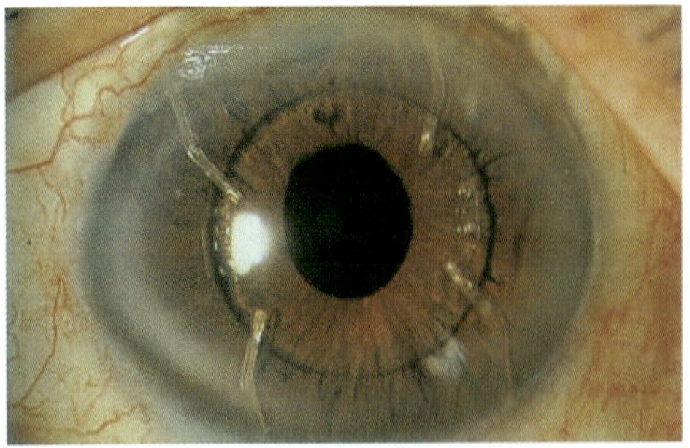

Figure 8-10 Fixed-haptic anterior chamber IOL associated with peripheral and superior corneal edema, chronic low-grade anterior uveitis, peripheral anterior synechiae, and intermittent microhyphema. *(Courtesy of John D. Sheppard Jr, MD.)*

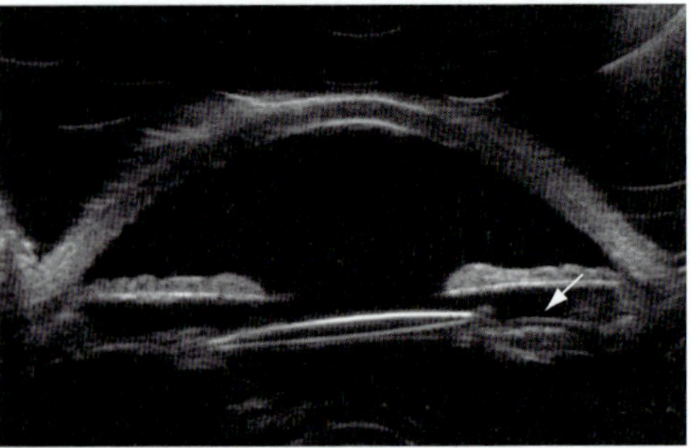

Figure 8-11 Evaluation of a patient who developed chronic anterior uveitis and macular edema after cataract surgery with IOL implantation. Ultrasound biomicroscopy shows a 1-piece posterior chamber IOL that is tilted with 1 haptic *(arrow)* in the sulcus. Clinically, an iris transillumination defect was observed overlying the haptic in the sulcus (not shown in the image). *(Courtesy of Wendy M. Smith, MD.)*

Roesel M, Heinz C, Heimes B, Koch JM, Heiligenhaus A. Uveal and capsular biocompatibility of two foldable acrylic intraocular lenses in patients with endogenous uveitis—a prospective randomized study. *Graefes Arch Clin Exp Ophthalmol.* 2008;246(11):1609–1615.

Taravati P, Lam DL, Leveque T, Van Gelder RN. Postcataract surgical inflammation. *Curr Opin Ophthalmol.* 2012;23(1):12–18.

Zhang L, Hood CT, Vrabec JP, Cullen AL, Parrish EA, Moroi SE. Mechanisms for in-the-bag uveitis-glaucoma-hyphema syndrome. *J Cataract Refract Surg.* 2014;40(3):490–492.

CLINICAL PEARL

For patients with persistent anterior uveitis following cataract surgery and IOL implantation:

- Assess for retained lens fragments.
- Evaluate for iris chafing even if the IOL is in the capsule.
- Investigate infectious causes, including *C acnes.*
- Use topical corticosteroids, tapered very slowly, to try to control the inflammation.
- Employ systemic IMT if necessary (only after infectious causes have been sufficiently investigated).

Drug-induced ocular inflammation

It is important to identify cases of drug-induced ocular inflammation, which is rare, because discontinuation of the offending agent may be curative. The causal relationship between a medication and an adverse reaction (eg, ocular inflammation) can be graded by using the Naranjo Algorithm, or Adverse Drug Reaction Probability Scale, which consists of 10 questions inquiring about the frequency of the patient's reaction and whether the reaction resolved with discontinuation of medication, worsened with dose increase, and recurred with medication rechallenge. Point values are given to each response, and the total score indicates whether the reaction is definite, probable, possible, or doubtful. Medications associated with ocular inflammation include systemic, intravitreal, and topical formulations, as well as vaccines.

The systemic medications most strongly associated with ocular inflammation, including anterior uveitis, are the antiviral cidofovir and the antibiotic rifabutin (used in the treatment of *Mycobacterium avium* complex [*M avium-Mycobacterium intracellulare* infection]). Bisphosphonates (eg, pamidronate, alendronate) are highly associated with scleritis and uveitis. Systemic medications that are moderately associated with uveitis include systemic fluoroquinolones (especially moxifloxacin, which may induce iris depigmentation and uveitis), sulfonamides, and diethylcarbamazine (an antifilarial drug). Paradoxically, some TNF inhibitors (eg, etanercept, adalimumab) have also been associated with new-onset uveitis, psoriasis-like rash (Fig 8-12), and a systemic sarcoid-like syndrome. Vaccines such as BCG vaccine and influenza vaccines, as well as the purified protein derivative used in the tuberculin skin test, have been implicated in the development of uveitis. Intravesical BCG vaccine (sometimes used in the treatment of bladder cancer) can result in uveitis that may be immune mediated or infectious. More recently, cancer immunotherapy, particularly with immune checkpoint inhibitors (Fig 8-13), has been associated with a spectrum of intraocular inflammation—ranging from mild anterior uveitis to retinal vasculitis, choroiditis, and Vogt-Koyanagi-Harada syndrome–like panuveitis.

Numerous topical ocular hypotensive medications have been associated with uveitis, including brimonidine (α_2-adrenergic agonist), pilocarpine, and prostaglandin $F_{2\alpha}$ analogues.

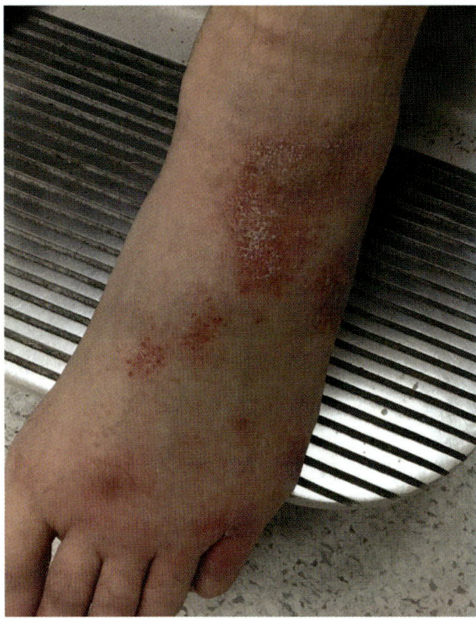

Figure 8-12 Adalimumab-induced psoriasis-like rash on the dorsal surface of the left foot of a young patient with chronic pars planitis. The rash resolved after discontinuation of the drug.

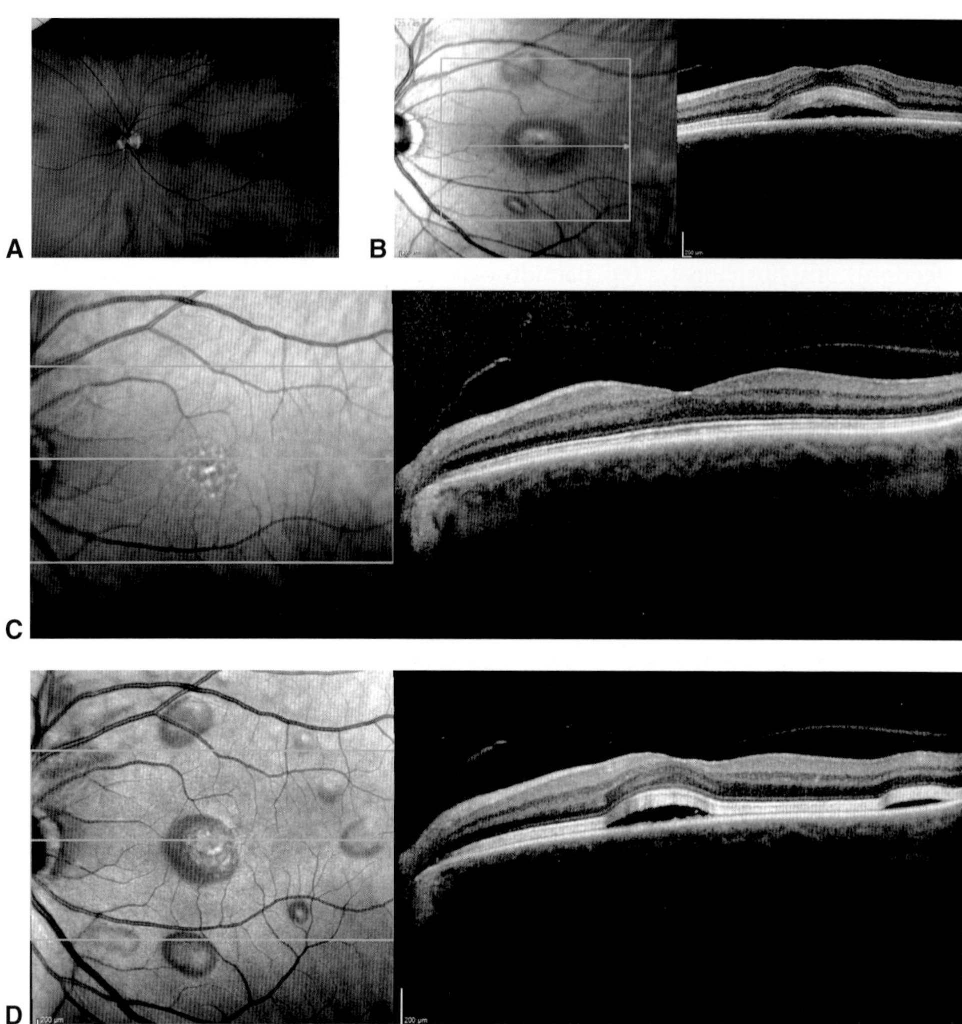

Figure 8-13 Immune checkpoint inhibitor (nivolumab)–induced Vogt-Koyanagi-Harada syndrome–like panuveitis in a patient with metastatic melanoma. **A, B,** Subretinal fluid noted on optical coherence tomography, despite relatively unremarkable fundus findings. **C,** Fluid resolved with periocular corticosteroids, but residual retinal pigment epithelium changes were noted on infrared imaging *(left)*. **D,** There was recurrence when the next cycle of anticancer treatment was started. *(Courtesy of Bryn M. Burkholder, MD, and H. Nida Sen, MD.)*

A common presentation of brimonidine-associated uveitis is a red and irritated eye with extensive (often granulomatous) KPs and low-grade anterior uveitis in a patient receiving long-term brimonidine therapy. Corneal edema and vitreous inflammation may also be present. While prostaglandin analogues have been reported to induce or worsen macular edema, this adverse effect is rare; therefore, these glaucoma drops can be used in patients with uveitis when other medications are not sufficient to lower IOP.

Intravitreal medications associated with uveitis include antibiotics, urokinase (a plasminogen activator), cidofovir (a cytosine analogue effective against CMV), and vascular endothelial growth factor (VEGF) inhibitors (brolucizumab, aflibercept).

Treatment of drug-induced ocular inflammation often includes temporarily discontinuing the offending agent. If the inflammation is primarily anterior uveitis, topical corticosteroids can be effective. Scleritis and higher-grade uveitis or inflammation involving the posterior segment may require oral corticosteroids. If inflammation is vision threatening or recurs with medication rechallenge, the causative medication may need to be discontinued.

Conrady CD, Larochelle M, Pecen P, Palestine A, Shakoor A, Singh A. Checkpoint inhibitor-induced uveitis: a case series. *Graefes Arch Clin Exp Ophthalmol.* 2018;256(1):187–191.

Cunningham ET Jr, Pasadhika S, Suhler EB, Zierhut M. Drug-induced inflammation in patients on TNF-α inhibitors. *Ocul Immunol Inflamm.* 2012;20(1):2–5.

Horsley MB, Chen TC. The use of prostaglandin analogs in the uveitic patient. *Semin Ophthalmol.* 2011;26(4–5):285–289.

Moorthy RS, London NJ, Garg SJ, Cunningham ET Jr. Drug-induced uveitis. *Curr Opin Ophthalmol.* 2013;24(6):589–597.

Naranjo CA, Busto U, Sellers EM, et al. A method for estimating the probability of adverse drug reactions. *Clin Pharmacol Ther.* 1981;30(2):239–245.

Chronic Anterior Uveitis

Inflammation of the anterior segment that is persistent and relapses less than 3 months after discontinuation of therapy is termed *chronic anterior uveitis;* it may persist for years. This type of inflammation usually starts insidiously, with variable amounts of redness, discomfort, and photophobia. Some patients have no symptoms. The disease can be unilateral or bilateral, and the amount of inflammatory activity is variable. Uveitic macular edema, cataract progression, and secondary glaucoma are common complications. Common causes of chronic anterior uveitis include juvenile idiopathic arthritis–associated uveitis in children and sarcoidosis in adults. See Chapter 10 for further discussion of sarcoidosis.

Juvenile idiopathic arthritis

Juvenile idiopathic arthritis (JIA; formerly called *juvenile chronic arthritis* and *juvenile rheumatoid arthritis*) is the most common systemic disease associated with anterior uveitis in the pediatric age group. It is characterized by arthritis beginning before age 16 years and lasting for at least 6 weeks.

JIA subtypes and ocular involvement According to International League of Associations for Rheumatology guidelines, JIA can be classified into 7 subtypes on the basis of number of joints involved, extra-articular manifestations, and laboratory markers of antinuclear antibody (ANA) and HLA-B27 seropositivity:

- *Oligoarticular arthritis.* This subtype, previously called *pauciarticular onset,* accounts for 50%–60% of all cases of JIA and 60% of cases of JIA-associated uveitis. Four or fewer joints may be involved during the first 6 months of disease, and patients may have no joint symptoms. In 25%–35% of these patients, uveitis develops, with most cases occurring in the first 4 years after JIA diagnosis. Girls younger than 5 years who are positive for ANA are at increased risk of developing chronic anterior uveitis.

- *RF-negative, polyarticular arthritis.* This subtype represents 10%–30% of JIA cases and approximately 20% of cases of JIA-associated chronic anterior uveitis. Patients show involvement of more than 4 joints in the first 6 months of the disease.
- *RF-positive, polyarticular arthritis.* This subtype accounts for 2%–7% of JIA cases. Patients show involvement of more than 4 joints in the first 6 months of the disease. Individuals who are positive for RF may not develop uveitis.
- *Psoriatic arthritis* (or *psoriatic JIA*). This subtype accounts for approximately 2%–15% of JIA cases and 7% of JIA-associated chronic anterior uveitis.
- *Enthesitis-related arthritis (ERA).* ERA represents 1%–7% of JIA cases and approximately 8% of JIA-associated acute anterior uveitis. Enthesitis, axial disease, and HLA-B27 positivity are common. Compared with the course of uveitis in other JIA subtypes, uveitis in these patients is more likely to be acute and recurrent, with pain, redness, and photophobia.
- *Systemic arthritis (Still disease).* This subtype, usually found in children younger than 5 years, accounts for approximately 10%–20% of all JIA cases. It is characterized by fever, evanescent rash, lymphadenopathy, and hepatosplenomegaly. Joint involvement may be minimal or absent initially. Uveitis is rare.
- Undifferentiated. Cases are categorized as undifferentiated when they do not meet criteria for one of the categories listed here or when they meet criteria for more than one category.

See also BCSC Section 6, *Pediatric Ophthalmology and Strabismus,* Chapter 25 for additional information.

Children with JIA, especially those who are ANA positive or who have oligoarticular disease, should undergo regular slit-lamp examinations. Table 8-2 outlines the schedule for screening eye examinations in patients with JIA as recommended by the American College of Rheumatology/Arthritis Foundation in 2019.

The average age at onset of uveitis in patients with JIA is 6 years. Uveitis generally develops within 5–7 years of the onset of joint disease but may occur as long as 28 years after the development of arthritis. There is usually little or no correlation between severity or timing of ocular and joint inflammation. Most patients test negative for RF. HLA-DRB1*11 and *13 may be associated with increased risk of uveitis among patients with JIA.

Table 8-2 Uveitis Screening Schedule for Patients With JIA

Eye examination every 3 months for patients with the following characteristics:

- oligoarthritis or undifferentiated
- ANA positive
- JIA onset before age 7 years
- JIA diagnosis for 4 years or less

Eye examination every 6–12 months for patients without the characteristics listed above.

ANA = antinuclear antibody; JIA = juvenile idiopathic arthritis.

Adapted from Angeles-Han ST, Ringold S, Beukelman T, et al. 2019 American College of Rheumatology/Arthritis Foundation Guideline for the Screening, Monitoring, and Treatment of Juvenile Idiopathic Arthritis-Associated Uveitis. *Arthritis Care Res (Hoboken).* 2019;71(6):703–716.

In JIA-associated uveitis, the eyes are frequently white and asymptomatic. The eye disease may be found incidentally on routine examination. When they occur, symptoms may include mild to moderate pain, photophobia, and blurred vision. Signs of inflammation include fine KPs, band keratopathy, anterior chamber cells and flare, posterior synechiae, and cataract (Fig 8-14). When JIA is suspected, ANA, RF, and HLA-B27 testing can be performed in addition to evaluation by a pediatric rheumatologist, as the joint disease may be minimal or absent at the time of uveitis diagnosis. The differential diagnosis includes TINU, Fuchs uveitis syndrome, sarcoidosis, Blau syndrome, Behçet disease, the seronegative spondyloarthropathies, and herpetic uveitis.

Angeles-Han ST, Pelajo CF, Vogler LB, et al; and the CARRA Registry Investigators. Risk markers of juvenile idiopathic arthritis-associated uveitis in the Childhood Arthritis and Rheumatology Research Alliance (CARRA) Registry. *J Rheumatol.* 2013;40(12):2088–2096.

Weiss JE, Ilowite NT. Juvenile idiopathic arthritis. *Rheum Dis Clin North Am.* 2007;33(3): 441–470, vi.

Prognosis Because the uveitis is frequently asymptomatic, profound ocular damage can occur. The long-term prognosis often depends on the extent of structural complications at the time of diagnosis. Sequelae of inflammation are frequent and often severe; they include band keratopathy, cataract, glaucoma, macular edema, chronic hypotony, and phthisis bulbi.

Treatment of JIA-associated uveitis The American College of Rheumatology and the Arthritis Foundation expert panels developed evidence-based recommendations for the screening, treatment, and monitoring of JIA-associated anterior uveitis. As mentioned previously, Table 8-2 summarizes screening recommendations. In general, the goal of treatment is to eliminate active inflammation and prevent the development of new complications. Although topical corticosteroids may be used initially, long-term use of topical treatment increases the risk of complications such as corticosteroid-induced glaucoma and cataract formation. There is evidence that even low-grade inflammation, when present for a prolonged period, can result in unacceptable ocular morbidity and vision loss. Therefore, if topical corticosteroids cannot be tapered to a frequency of 2 times daily or less, if steroid-induced ocular hypertension develops, or if the ocular inflammation is severe, there is a low threshold to begin systemic treatment. Systemic corticosteroids may be used in the

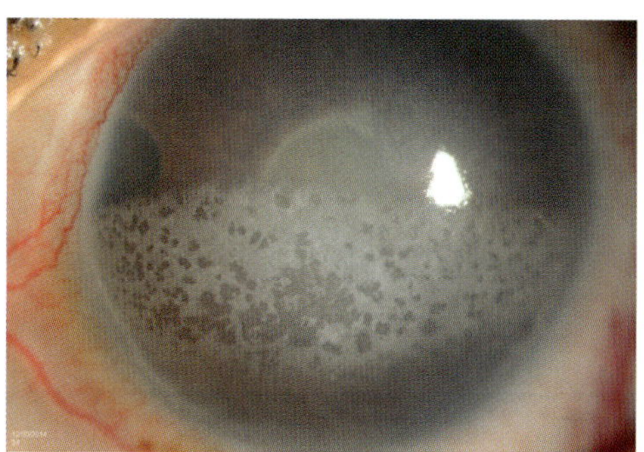

Figure 8-14 JIA-associated uveitis with complicated chronic calcific band keratopathy, cataract, and glaucoma in a patient with peripheral iridectomy superonasally. *(Courtesy of H. Nida Sen, MD/National Eye Institute.)*

short term; however, children are uniquely at risk for growth retardation from premature closure of the epiphyses, so corticosteroid-sparing systemic IMT is usually necessary.

To reduce the risk of complications of treatment and inflammation, the clinician should maintain a low threshold for beginning an antimetabolite such as methotrexate (MTX) in children with JIA-associated chronic anterior uveitis. Numerous studies have shown that this treatment approach can effectively control the uveitis, is generally well tolerated, and can spare patients the complications of long-term corticosteroid use. If uveitis is not adequately controlled with MTX, the TNF inhibitor adalimumab is often prescribed in addition to the antimetabolite. See Chapter 6 for discussion of the SYCAMORE trial, which demonstrated that there was significant improvement in the control of JIA-associated uveitis with the addition of adalimumab to MTX. Although etanercept can effectively treat the joint inflammation associated with JIA, it is usually not effective for JIA-associated uveitis.

In patients with chronic anterior chamber flare, short-acting mydriatic drugs may be useful to keep the pupil mobile and to prevent posterior synechiae formation. Use of systemic NSAIDs may permit a lower dose of corticosteroids. Treatment of JIA-associated uveitis is usually prolonged (ie, years) due to the chronic nature of the inflammatory disease. Patients with inactive uveitis (or <1+ anterior chamber cells) should be monitored every 3 months, unless tapering or discontinuing treatment. Patients should be seen at least 1 month after each change in topical medication, and within 2 months of changing systemic treatment.

Angeles-Han ST, Ringold S, Beukelman T, et al. 2019 American College of Rheumatology/Arthritis Foundation Guideline for the Screening, Monitoring, and Treatment of Juvenile Idiopathic Arthritis-Associated Uveitis. *Arthritis Care Res (Hoboken).* 2019;71(6):703–716.

Gregory AC 2nd, Kempen JH, Daniel E, et al; Systemic Immunosuppressive Therapy for Eye Diseases Cohort Study Research Group. Risk factors for loss of visual acuity among patients with uveitis associated with juvenile idiopathic arthritis: the Systemic Immunosuppressive Therapy for Eye Diseases Study. *Ophthalmology.* 2013;120(1):186–192.

Horton S, Jones AP, Guly CM, et al. Adalimumab in juvenile idiopathic arthritis-associated uveitis: 5-year follow-up of the Bristol participants of the SYCAMORE trial. *Am J Ophthalmol.* 2019;207:170–174.

Mehta PJ, Alexander JL, Sen HN. Pediatric uveitis: new and future treatments. *Curr Opin Ophthalmol.* 2013;24(5):453–462.

Thorne JE, Woreta FA, Dunn JP, Jabs DA. Risk of cataract development among children with juvenile idiopathic arthritis–related uveitis treated with topical corticosteroids. *Ophthalmology.* 2020;127(4S):S21–S26.

Zannin ME, Birolo C, Gerloni VM, et al. Safety and efficacy of infliximab and adalimumab for refractory uveitis in juvenile idiopathic arthritis: 1-year followup data from the Italian Registry. *J Rheumatol.* 2013;40(1):74–79.

Management of cataract Cataract surgery in patients with JIA remains a challenge. There is a high risk of complications due to the difficulty controlling the more aggressive inflammatory response present in these children. However, good visual outcomes can be attained if uveitis is meticulously controlled before cataract surgery as well as during the postoperative period. Band keratopathy should be treated using chelation with sodium

EDTA, and the cornea should be well healed before cataract surgery is attempted. Pars plana lensectomy with removal of the lens complex and anterior vitreous has been advocated to avoid posterior capsule opacification.

Because children who are left aphakic may develop amblyopia, it may be appropriate to place an IOL in some cases. For patients with JIA-associated uveitis who receive an IOL implant at the time of cataract surgery, it is important for the clinician to do the following:

- Ensure that uveitis is well controlled for at least 3 months before surgery without the need for frequent topical corticosteroids or high-dose systemic corticosteroids.
- Use systemic IMT preoperatively and postoperatively, not just perioperatively.
- Place an acrylic lens in the capsular bag whenever possible.
- Monitor patients frequently after cataract surgery and treat postoperative inflammation aggressively.
- Maintain a low threshold for IOL explantation in patients with chronic postoperative inflammation and recurrent cyclitic membranes.
- Strongly advise patients about the need for lifelong follow-up to detect late complications.

Grajewski RS, Zurek-Imhoff B, Roesel M, Heinz C, Heiligenhaus A. Favourable outcome after cataract surgery with IOL implantation in uveitis associated with juvenile idiopathic arthritis. *Acta Ophthalmol.* 2012;90(7):657–662.

Management of glaucoma Glaucoma should be treated with medical therapy initially, although surgical intervention is often necessary in severe cases. Standard filtering procedures are usually unsuccessful, and the use of antifibrotic drugs or aqueous drainage devices is usually required for successful IOP control. See Chapter 16 in this volume and BCSC Section 6, *Pediatric Ophthalmology and Strabismus,* for further discussion of treatment of band keratopathy, pediatric cataract, and glaucoma.

Fuchs uveitis syndrome

Fuchs uveitis syndrome (sometimes called *Fuchs heterochromic iridocyclitis* or *Fuchs heterochromic uveitis*) accounts for 2%–3% of patient referrals to uveitis clinics. Studies have shown an association between Fuchs uveitis syndrome and several infectious agents, including rubella virus, CMV, and *Toxoplasma*. Fuchs uveitis syndrome is usually unilateral, and symptoms vary from none to mild blurred vision and ocular discomfort. Signs include

- heterochromia
- diffuse iris stromal atrophy with variable pigment epithelial layer atrophy (Fig 8-15)
- small, white, stellate KPs scattered diffusely over the entire endothelium (Fig 8-16A)
- iris nodules (Fig 8-16B)
- cells in the anterior chamber and anterior vitreous
- late staining of the optic nerve on fluorescein angiography (FA)
- glaucoma and cataract, which occur frequently

Posterior synechiae, chorioretinal scars, and retinal periphlebitis are rare or absent; likewise, macular edema is seldom present. Occasionally, patients may develop extensive vitreous opacification.

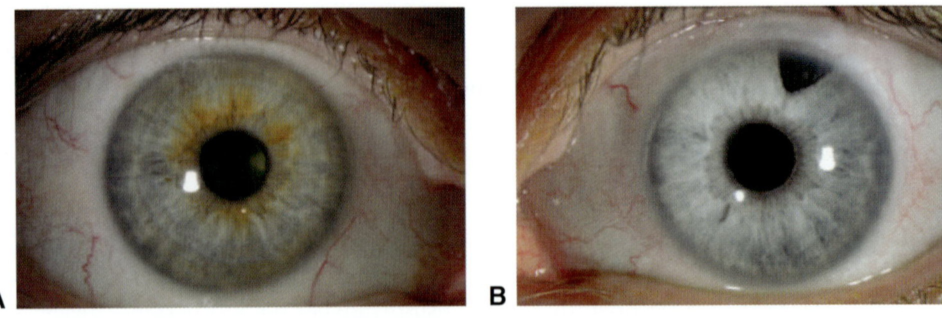

Figure 8-15 Heterochromia in Fuchs uveitis syndrome. **A,** Right (unaffected) eye. **B,** Left (affected) eye in the same patient. Note the lighter iris color and stromal atrophy ("moth-eaten appearance") in the affected eye, which underwent iridectomy at the same time as cataract surgery. *(Courtesy of H. Nida Sen, MD/National Eye Institute.)*

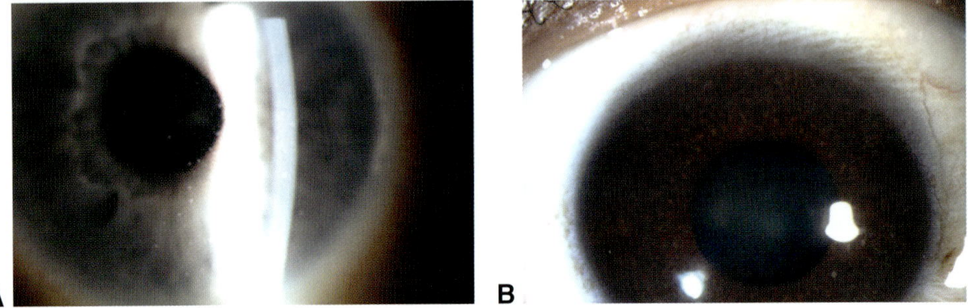

Figure 8-16 Fuchs uveitis syndrome. **A,** Diffusely distributed stellate keratic precipitates. **B,** Iris nodules have a "pasted on" appearance. *(Part A courtesy of H. Nida Sen, MD/National Eye Institute; part B courtesy of Wendy M. Smith, MD.)*

The diagnosis is made according to the distribution of KPs, presence of heterochromia, lack of synechiae, and minimal or no symptoms. The heterochromia may be subtle in brown eyes, and the clinician must look carefully for signs of iris stromal atrophy. Often, the inflammation is discovered during a routine examination, such as when a unilateral cataract develops. Usually, but not invariably, a lighter-colored iris indicates the involved eye. In patients with blue eyes, however, the affected eye may become darker as the stromal atrophy progresses and the darker iris pigment epithelium shows through.

Although topical corticosteroids can lessen the inflammation, they typically do not resolve it; thus, aggressive treatment to eradicate the cellular reaction is not indicated. Cycloplegia is usually unnecessary. Patients can have symptomatic exacerbations of uveitis that may be treated by restarting or increasing topical corticosteroids. Topical corticosteroids may also be used long-term to decrease the accumulation of KPs and inflammatory deposits on IOLs after cataract surgery. Glaucoma may be difficult to control, but otherwise the prognosis is good in most cases, even when the inflammation persists for decades.

Since the anterior chamber cellular reaction may not completely subside with treatment, cataract surgery and IOL implantation may be performed even if the eye has not been quiet for at least 3 months. Abnormal vessels bridging the angle may bleed during surgery, resulting in postoperative hyphema. In general, however, outcomes are usually good after cataract surgery. Some patients may still experience substantial visual disability after surgery, because of diffuse KPs or extensive vitreous opacification; pars plana vitrectomy may be carefully considered for such patients. See BCSC Section 10, *Glaucoma,* for further discussion of Fuchs uveitis syndrome.

Accorinti M, Spinucci G, Pirraglia MP, Bruschi S, Pesci FR, Iannetti L. Fuchs' heterochromic iridocyclitis in an Italian tertiary referral centre: epidemiology, clinical features, and prognosis. *J Ophthalmol.* 2016;2016:1458624. doi:10.1155/2016/1458624

Birnbaum AD, Tessler HH, Schultz KL, et al. Epidemiologic relationship between Fuchs heterochromic iridocyclitis and the United States rubella vaccination program. *Am J Ophthalmol.* 2007;144(3):424–428.

de Groot-Mijnes JD, de Visser L, Rothova A, Schuller M, van Loon AM, Weersink AJ. Rubella virus is associated with Fuchs heterochromic iridocyclitis. *Am J Ophthalmol.* 2006;141(1):212–214.

Undifferentiated anterior uveitis

In many cases of chronic anterior uveitis, it may not be possible to identify a cause. As long as infectious etiologies have been appropriately investigated, the uveitis should be treated with topical corticosteroids and/or cycloplegics, as well as systemic corticosteroids or IMT or both as needed. If the clinical picture evolves or new systemic signs or symptoms arise, additional diagnostic testing may be warranted. However, if the result of initial HLA-B27 testing was negative, this test does not need to be repeated.

Intermediate Uveitis

Intermediate uveitis accounts for up to 15% of all cases of uveitis. It is characterized by inflammatory cells and haze in the vitreous (see Chapter 5, Fig 5-7). Inflammation may also occur in the vitreous base overlying the ciliary body and peripheral retina–pars plana complex. Other signs may include *snowballs* (aggregates of inflammatory cells in the vitreous) and *snowbanks* (inflammatory exudative accumulation on the inferior pars plana). Snowbanks seem to correlate with a more severe disease process. Retinal phlebitis is often present peripherally or diffusely. Anterior chamber reaction of varying severity may also occur.

Intermediate uveitis can be associated with various conditions, including sarcoidosis, multiple sclerosis (MS), peripheral toxocariasis, syphilis, tuberculosis, TINU, primary Sjögren syndrome, and human T-cell lymphotropic virus type 1 infection. The most common form of intermediate uveitis is idiopathic or undifferentiated.

Pars Planitis

The term *pars planitis* refers to a form of idiopathic intermediate uveitis with snowballs as well as inflammatory membranes on the pars plana and snowbanks. It is the most common form of intermediate uveitis, constituting approximately 85%–90% of such cases. The condition most commonly affects persons aged 5–40 years in a bimodal distribution, concentrating in younger (5–15 years) and older (20–40 years) age groups. No overall sex predilection is apparent.

Approximately 80% of cases of pars planitis are bilateral, but disease activity may be asymmetric with 1 eye more affected. The initial presentation in children may include eye redness, photophobia, and discomfort with considerable anterior chamber inflammation as well as vitreous cells. The onset in teenagers and young adults may be more insidious, and the presenting symptom is often just floaters.

In addition to snowballs (Fig 8-17A), pars plana inflammatory membranes, and snowbanks (Fig 8-17B), ocular manifestations can include anterior chamber inflammation and vitreous cells and haze. Inferior peripheral retinal phlebitis with retinal venous sheathing is common. With long-standing inflammation, macular edema often develops; this condition becomes chronic and refractory in approximately 10% of patients and is the major cause of vision loss. Ischemia from retinal phlebitis, combined with angiogenic stimuli from intraocular inflammation, can lead to neovascularization along the inferior snowbank in up to 10% of cases. These neovascular complexes can result in vitreous hemorrhages, which are more common in children than in adults; the complexes also may contract, leading to peripheral tractional retinal schisis and rhegmatogenous retinal detachments. In rare cases, the complexes evolve into secondary peripheral retinal vasoproliferative tumors—vascular masses with exudative retinopathy and minimally dilated vessels—years after the initial diagnosis. Rhegmatogenous retinal detachments are rare, but localized peripheral detachments (exudative [also called *serous*] or tractional) occur in 4%–10% of patients with pars planitis. With chronic inflammation, posterior synechiae and band keratopathy may also develop. Other possible causes of vision loss include cataract, epiretinal membrane, and vitreous opacification.

Histologic examination of eyes with pars planitis shows vitreous condensation and cellular infiltration in the vitreous base. The inflammatory cells consist mostly of macrophages, lymphocytes, and a few plasma cells. Pars planitis is also characterized by peripheral lymphocytic cuffing of venules and a loose fibrovascular membrane over the pars plana.

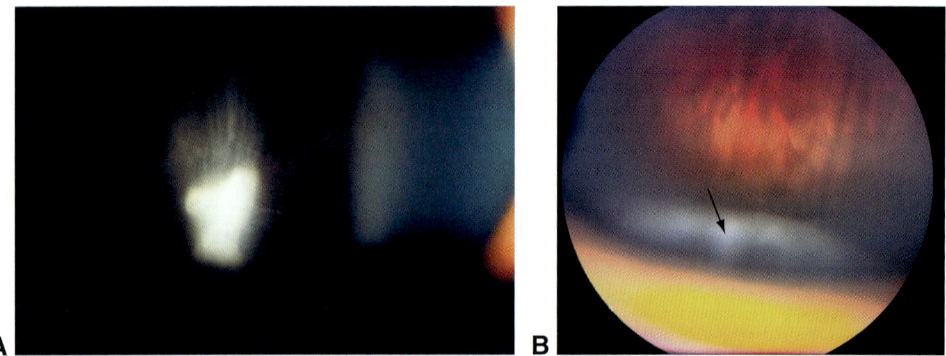

Figure 8-17 Pars planitis. **A,** Snowball opacity in the retrolental vitreous. **B,** Inferior pars plana snowbank *(arrow)*. *(Part A courtesy of Ramana S. Moorthy, MD/National Eye Institute; part B courtesy of H. Nida Sen, MD/National Eye Institute.)*

Workup and ancillary tests

The diagnosis of intermediate uveitis is based on the clinical findings, and the subtype pars planitis is established by ruling out specific etiologies. The workup should investigate any pertinent positive responses on a comprehensive review of systems and may include evaluations for sarcoidosis and MS. Sarcoidosis-associated uveitis presents as an intermediate uveitis in 7% of cases. Up to 15% of patients with pars planitis eventually develop MS. Anterior uveitis and intermediate uveitis occur in up to 20% of patients with MS; if the patient has current neurologic symptoms or a previous episode of an unexplained symptom like footdrop, magnetic resonance imaging (MRI) of the brain may be obtained to assess for evidence of demyelinating disease. Syphilis testing should be performed in all patients with new-onset uveitis, including those with intermediate uveitis. Although Lyme-associated uveitis is very rare, Lyme enzyme-linked immunosorbent assay (ELISA) screening may be appropriate in a patient who has erythema chronicum migrans ("bull's eye" rash), new-onset arthritis, and a history of tick bite in a Lyme-endemic region. A child with toxocariasis may have a peripheral or posterior pole retinal granuloma that resembles a snowbank. The complete absence of inflammation in the contralateral eye and a positive *Toxocara* antibody test result may help confirm the diagnosis of ocular toxocariasis.

The new onset of vitreous cells in an older patient should raise suspicion for vitreoretinal lymphoma. These patients are often older than the typical pars planitis patient, usually 50–60 years of age or older. Visual acuity may be better than expected despite substantial sheets of dense vitreous cells, and macular edema is usually absent. See Chapter 15 for additional discussion of vitreoretinal lymphoma.

Macular OCT may show macular thickening with or without frank intraretinal edema. The pattern of thickening can be diffuse or focal over macular vessels. Epiretinal membrane may also be present. FA should be obtained in all patients with substantial clinical signs of inflammation, such as higher-grade vitreous cell and haze and pars plana membranes or snowbanks. Reliance on clinical findings and OCT may result in underassessment of uveitis activity. FA may show peripheral or diffuse leakage of venules and capillaries as well as optic disc and macular leakage (Fig 8-18). Ultrasound biomicroscopy can demonstrate peripheral exudates or membranes on the pars plana.

Prognosis

The clinical course of pars planitis varies. Approximately 10% of cases have a self-limited, benign course; 30% have a smoldering course with remissions and exacerbations; and 60% have a chronic course without exacerbations. Chronic forms of pars planitis can remain active for many years. As mentioned previously, macular edema is the foremost vision-threatening complication. If macular edema is resolved, the long-term visual prognosis can be good, with nearly 75% of patients maintaining visual acuity of 20/40 or better after 10 years.

Treatment

Occasionally, pars planitis is very low grade and can be observed without treatment, but a substantial proportion of patients will need either long-acting regional corticosteroid injections or systemic IMT. Indications for treatment may include substantial vitritis and macular thickening with or without intraretinal fluid. Although patients may have

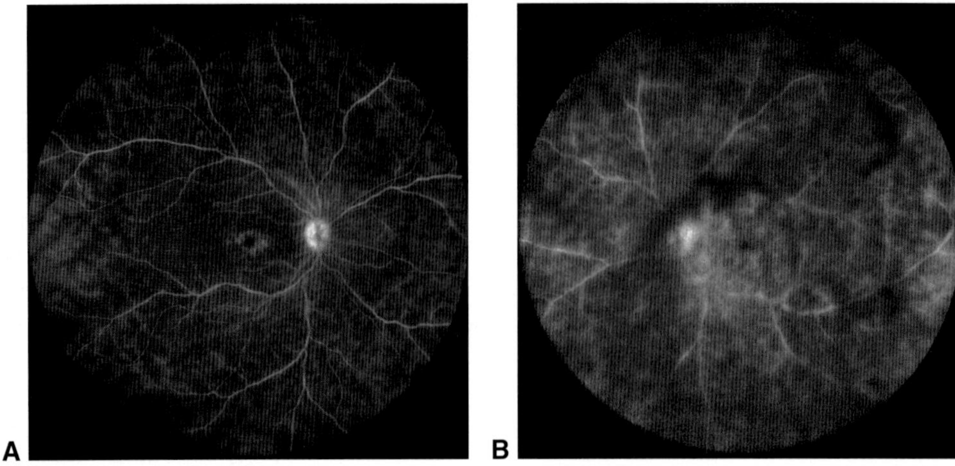

Figure 8-18 Pars planitis. **A,** Wide-angle fluorescein angiography shows diffuse venular and small-vessel leakage in the right eye. **B,** Imaging of the left eye shows a similar pattern of leakage, as well as shadowing from vitreous inflammatory debris. *(Courtesy of Wendy M. Smith, MD.)*

objectively good visual acuity, floaters and glare can be debilitating and may warrant treatment. FA may show more inflammation than is clinically apparent and should be used to monitor response to treatment.

Corticosteroids are first-line therapy. In unilateral cases, local treatment with corticosteroid injections is a particularly appealing approach as long as infectious causes of uveitis have been sufficiently investigated. Triamcinolone acetonide or methylprednisolone acetate may be given as depot injections into the posterior sub-Tenon space or orbital floor (see Chapter 6). In many cases, the inflammation resolves, and the macular edema improves; however, both conditions may persist, or they may recur within 2–3 months. Patients must be carefully monitored for corticosteroid-induced IOP elevation, which can develop weeks to years after corticosteroid injections. Cataract formation can occur with any form of corticosteroid therapy.

Intravitreal corticosteroids may also be utilized in pars planitis. The POINT (PeriOcular vs. INTravitreal corticosteroids for uveitic macular edema) Trial showed that intravitreal corticosteroids were more effective than periocular corticosteroid injections as treatment for uveitic macular edema. (See Chapter 6 for further discussion of POINT.) IOP elevation and cataract progression can also occur with intravitreal corticosteroids. Additional risks include retinal tear and detachment, vitreous hemorrhage, and endophthalmitis. Injections should be administered away from areas of snowbanking or other peripheral retinal pathology. Longer-acting forms of intravitreal corticosteroids, such as dexamethasone or fluocinolone acetonide implants, are FDA approved for the treatment of noninfectious intermediate uveitis.

In severe or bilateral cases, systemic corticosteroid therapy is required. Patients are treated with an initial dosage of 1 mg/kg/day (up to a maximum of 60–80 mg/day), with gradual tapering every 1–2 weeks to dosages of less than 7.5 mg/day after 8–10 weeks of treatment. As with all cases of noninfectious uveitis, if corticosteroid therapy fails or high doses of corticosteroids are needed to control the inflammation, systemic corticosteroid-sparing agents are added. Systemic IMT options include antimetabolites, T-cell inhibitors, and biologic agents. Several reports from the SITE (Systemic Immunosuppressive Therapy for Eye Diseases) Cohort Study and the FAST (First-line Antimetabolites as Steroid-sparing Treatment) uveitis trial indicated that methotrexate, azathioprine, mycophenolate mofetil, and cyclosporine were effective in achieving sustained control of inflammation in 70%–80% of patients with intermediate uveitis. (See Chapter 6 for more details on these studies.) The TNF inhibitor adalimumab is approved by the FDA for the treatment of noninfectious uveitis, including intermediate uveitis. Because TNF inhibitors can exacerbate MS, it is important to consider a workup for demyelinating disease, including brain MRI, before initiating this therapy. See Table 6-1 in Chapter 6 for more detailed information on IMT in uveitis.

Some practitioners utilize supplementary therapies for pars planitis, including peripheral ablation of snowbanks with cryotherapy and/or laser photocoagulation to the peripheral retina. In patients receiving systemic IMT who have persistent inflammation or retinal neovascularization, gentle, limited cryotherapy might be applied; however, there is a risk of inducing further inflammation. Peripheral laser photocoagulation to ischemic retina may prevent or involute retinal neovascularization and prevent vitreous hemorrhage; laser does not seem to increase the risk of rhegmatogenous retinal detachment. Intravitreal anti-VEGF agents can also be used for retinal or choroidal neovascularization in otherwise quiet eyes.

Pars plana vitrectomy (PPV) may be necessary to treat non-resolving vitreous hemorrhage or tractional adhesions, retinal detachment, or epiretinal membrane. In cases involving epiretinal membrane or vitreomacular traction, separation of the posterior hyaloid membrane during PPV may have a beneficial effect in reducing macular edema. PPV may also be considered for patients with substantial vitreous opacities despite adequate IMT. Potential complications of PPV include retinal detachment, endophthalmitis, and cataract formation. A perioperative increase in systemic immunosuppression and/or corticosteroids should be considered.

Mackensen F, Jakob E, Springer C, et al. Interferon versus methotrexate in intermediate uveitis with macular edema: results of a randomized controlled clinical trial. *Am J Ophthalmol.* 2013;156(3):478–486.

Rathinam SR, Gonzales JA, Thundikandy R, et al; FAST Research Group. Effect of corticosteroid-sparing treatment with mycophenolate mofetil vs methotrexate on inflammation in patients with uveitis: a randomized clinical trial. *JAMA.* 2019;322(10):936–945.

Shin YU, Shin JY, Ma DJ, Cho H, Yu HG. Preoperative inflammatory control and surgical outcome of vitrectomy in intermediate uveitis. *J Ophthalmol.* 2017;2017:5946240. doi:10.1155/2017/5946240

Sohn EH, Chaon BC, Jabs DA, Folk JC. Peripheral cryoablation for treatment of active pars planitis: long-term outcomes of a retrospective study. *Am J Ophthalmol.* 2016;162:35–42.

Thorne JE, Sugar EA, Holbrook JT, et al; Multicenter Uveitis Steroid Treatment Trial Research Group. Periocular Triamcinolone vs. Intravitreal Triamcinolone vs. Intravitreal Dexamethasone Implant for the Treatment of Uveitic Macular Edema: The PeriOcular vs. INTravitreal corticosteroids for uveitic macular edema (POINT) Trial. *Ophthalmology.* 2019;126(2):283–295.

Complications

Complications of pars planitis include cataract, glaucoma, macular edema, macular or foveal atrophy, retinal neovascularization, vitreous hemorrhage, retinoschisis, and tractional or rhegmatogenous retinal detachment. Cataract occurs in up to 60% of cases. Cataract surgery with IOL implantation may be complicated by smoldering low-grade inflammation, recurrent posterior capsule opacification, and chronic macular edema. Combining PPV with cataract extraction and IOL implantation may reduce the risk of these complications. Glaucoma—both angle-closure and open-angle—occurs in approximately 10% of patients with pars planitis. Macular edema is a hallmark of pars planitis and occurs in 50% of patients. Neovascularization of the retina, optic disc, and peripheral snowbank can develop. Occasionally, vitreous hemorrhage is the presenting sign of pars planitis, especially in children. Tractional and rhegmatogenous retinal detachments occur rarely and may require scleral buckling, sometimes combined with vitrectomy. Risk factors for rhegmatogenous retinal detachment include severe inflammation, use of cryotherapy at the time of a vitrectomy, and neovascularization of the snowbank.

Donaldson MJ, Pulido JS, Herman DC, Diehl N, Hodge D. Pars planitis: a 20-year study of incidence, clinical features, and outcomes. *Am J Ophthalmol.* 2007;144(6):812–817.

Lauer AK, Smith JR, Robertson JE, Rosenbaum JT. Vitreous hemorrhage is a common complication of pediatric pars planitis. *Ophthalmology.* 2002;109(1):95–98.

Multiple Sclerosis

Uveitis is 10 times more common in patients with MS than in the general population. The frequency of uveitis in patients with MS is reported to be as high as 30%, and the onset of uveitis may precede the diagnosis of MS by 5–10 years. MS usually affects White women 20–50 years of age; however, patients with intermediate uveitis who are in this demographic do not warrant an MRI or neurologic workup unless they have neurologic signs and symptoms of MS. An MRI might also be considered before treatment with a TNF inhibitor is initiated.

The immunopathogenesis of MS is not well understood but appears to involve humoral, cellular, and immunogenetic components directed against myelin. Studies have shown some cross-reactivity between myelin-associated glycoprotein and Müller cells. HLA-DR15 has been associated with the combination of MS and uveitis.

Intermediate uveitis is the most common manifestation of MS-associated uveitis. It is bilateral in 95% of cases, and most patients have mild vitritis with periphlebitis (Fig 8-19). In contrast to idiopathic intermediate uveitis, MS-associated intermediate uveitis is milder, and macular edema is less common. Periphlebitis in MS-associated uveitis is not clearly related to optic neuritis, systemic exacerbations, or disease severity. As in all types of intermediate uveitis, FA may show more inflammation than might be appreciated clinically.

Some of the medications used as disease-modifying therapy for MS may also treat MS-associated uveitis and associated macular edema. Interferon has been shown to be effective for macular edema in MS-associated uveitis. Ocrelizumab is a humanized anti-CD20 monoclonal antibody with a mechanism of action similar to that of rituximab, a biologic that has been used to treat other forms of noninfectious uveitis and scleritis. Of

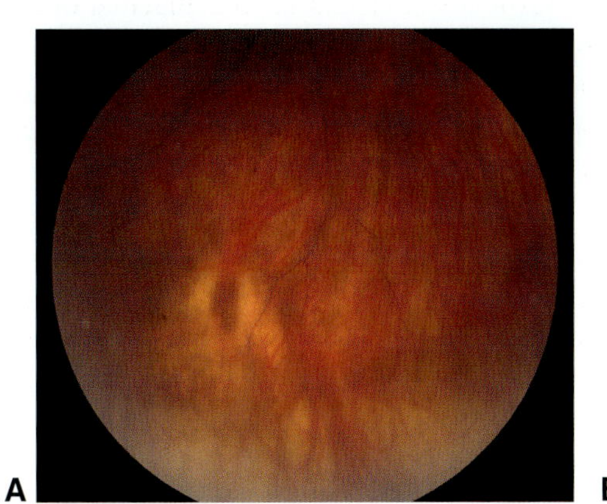

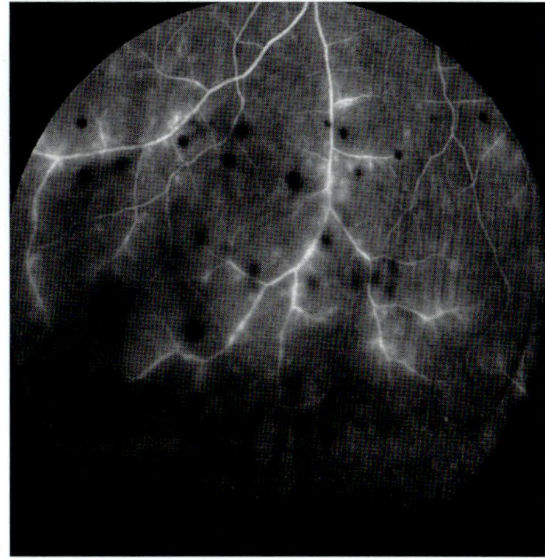

Figure 8-19 Multiple sclerosis–associated intermediate uveitis. **A,** Color fundus photograph demonstrates subtle vascular sheathing and vitreous snowballs. **B,** Corresponding fluorescein angiogram shows venular leakage and shadowing from vitreous snowballs. *(Courtesy of Wendy M. Smith, MD.)*

note, one disease-modifying therapy for MS, fingolimod, can cause macular edema, although this is a rare complication.

TNF inhibitors, a class of biologic medications that is FDA approved to treat noninfectious uveitis, are contraindicated with demyelinating disease. Therefore, before these agents are started in patients with suspected idiopathic intermediate uveitis, a brain MRI should be obtained to rule out demyelinating disease.

Abraham A, Nicholson L, Dick A, Rice C, Atan D. Intermediate uveitis associated with MS: diagnosis, clinical features, pathogenic mechanisms, and recommendations for management. *Neurol Neuroimmunol Neuroinflamm.* 2020;8(1):e909.

Becker MD, Heiligenhaus A, Hudde T, et al. Interferon as a treatment for uveitis associated with multiple sclerosis. *Br J Ophthalmol.* 2005;89(10):1254–1257.

Chen L, Gordon LK. Ocular manifestations of multiple sclerosis. *Curr Opin Ophthalmol.* 2005;16(5):315–320.

Chirpaz N, Kerever S, Gavoille A, et al. Relevance of brain MRI in patients with uveitis: retrospective cohort on 402 patients. *Ocul Immunol Inflamm.* 2021;1–7. doi:10.1080/09273948.2020.1870145

Zein G, Berta A, Foster CS. Multiple sclerosis–associated uveitis. *Ocul Immunol Inflamm.* 2004;12(2):137–142.

CHAPTER 9

Posterior Uveitis: The White Dot Syndromes

Highlights

- White dot syndromes are noninfectious inflammatory chorioretinopathies that usually have no associated systemic inflammatory disease.
- A patient with a suspected white dot syndrome should be evaluated for tuberculosis and syphilis.
- Diagnosis of a white dot syndrome is based primarily on clinical characteristics observed on ophthalmic examination and imaging; there are no confirmatory diagnostic tests.
- Many white dot syndromes require treatment with systemic immunomodulatory therapy.
- Diagnosis and management of autoimmune retinopathy can be challenging because the presence of most serum antiretinal antibodies has unclear significance and the disease may have a poor response to therapies used for other types of ocular inflammation.

Definitions

Posterior uveitis is defined as intraocular inflammation that involves mainly the retina and/or choroid. Although inflammatory cells may be observed in the vitreous, the main site of inflammation must be retinal or choroidal to be defined as posterior uveitis. Retinal vasculitis *with vascular occlusion* is also classified as posterior uveitis. Posterior segment findings such as macular edema, *peripheral* retinal vasculitis, and optic disc edema are not indicators of posterior or panuveitis unless retinal or choroidal inflammatory lesions are also present. For example, if an eye with human leukocyte antigen (HLA)-B27–associated anterior uveitis develops macular edema, the inflammation is not reclassified as posterior uveitis.

This chapter discusses the *white dot syndromes,* a group of posterior uveitic entities that usually have no associated systemic inflammatory disease:

- birdshot chorioretinopathy
- acute posterior multifocal placoid pigment epitheliopathy

- serpiginous choroiditis
- multifocal choroiditis and panuveitis
- punctate inner choroiditis
- subretinal fibrosis and uveitis syndrome
- multiple evanescent white dot syndrome
- acute retinal pigment epitheliitis
- acute zonal occult outer retinopathy
- acute idiopathic maculopathy

Although autoimmune retinopathy is not a white dot syndrome, it is also included in this chapter because it is a presumably immune-mediated retinal degeneration that shares symptoms (eg, decreased vision, scotomas, photopsias) with the white dot syndromes. Posterior uveitis and panuveitis with systemic manifestations are covered in Chapter 10.

Overview of the White Dot Syndromes

The white dot syndromes are a group of inflammatory chorioretinopathies characterized by multiple, discrete yellow-white lesions at the level of the retina, outer retina, retinal pigment epithelium (RPE), choriocapillaris, and/or choroid. The morphology of the lesions varies from syndrome to syndrome, although there is some overlap. Symptoms include photopsias, blurred vision, nyctalopia, floaters, an enlarged blind spot, and visual field loss. A viral prodrome may also be described. Although bilateral or asymmetric presentation is typical with these disorders, unilateral involvement also occurs. See Table 9-1 for a summary of patient demographics and clinical findings associated with white dot syndromes.

The etiology of the white dot syndromes is unknown. Some investigators have postulated an infectious cause; others have proposed an autoimmune/inflammatory origin. The increased prevalence of systemic autoimmune disease in patients and their family members suggests that immune dysregulation does play a role in the pathogenesis of these syndromes.

The differential diagnosis of the white dot syndromes includes both infectious (eg, syphilis, tuberculosis [TB], diffuse unilateral subacute neuroretinitis [DUSN], and ocular histoplasmosis syndrome [OHS]) and noninfectious diseases (ie, sarcoidosis, sympathetic ophthalmia, Vogt-Koyanagi-Harada syndrome, and intraocular lymphoma). Although the diagnosis of a white dot syndrome is based primarily on clinical characteristics observed on ophthalmic examination and imaging, a careful history and review of systems as well as targeted laboratory testing are indicated to investigate the differential diagnoses in the workup of patients with a suspected white dot syndrome. Of note, there are no confirmatory diagnostic tests for the majority of the white dot syndromes.

Abu-Yaghi NE, Hartono SP, Hodge DO, Pulido JS, Bakri SJ. White dot syndromes: a 20-year study of incidence, clinical features, and outcomes. *Ocul Immunol Inflamm.* 2011;19(6):426–430.

Gass JD. Are acute zonal occult outer retinopathy and the white spot syndromes (AZOOR complex) specific autoimmune diseases? *Am J Ophthalmol.* 2003;135(3):380–381.

Quillen DA, Davis JB, Gottlieb JL, et al. The white dot syndromes. *Am J Ophthalmol.* 2004;137(3):538–550.

Birdshot Chorioretinopathy

Birdshot chorioretinopathy (BCR; also known as *birdshot uveitis, birdshot retinochoroidopathy,* and *vitiliginous chorioretinitis*) is most common in women and in individuals of northern European descent. Age at onset of BCR was traditionally 50–60 years; however, owing to improvements in diagnostic testing, diagnosis is increasingly common in patients younger than 45 years. No systemic disease is consistently associated with BCR, although the disorder is highly correlated with the HLA-A29 allele, with a sensitivity of 96% and a specificity of 93%. However, given that the HLA-A29 haplotype is common (eg, occurring in approximately 7% of the US population) whereas BCR is relatively rare, identification of the allele alone does not confirm a diagnosis. Uveitis with clinical features consistent with BCR must also be present.

Manifestations

Presenting symptoms may be bilateral or asymmetric and include blurred vision, floaters, nyctalopia, and color vision disturbances. Patient-reported symptoms may be out of proportion to visual acuity measurements, reflecting diffuse retinal dysfunction. In addition, unusual visual phenomena such as pinwheels, sparkles, or flickering lights may be indicators of subtle disease activity. Anterior segment inflammation is typically minimal or absent. Although patients usually have some inflammatory cells in the vitreous, they often lack substantial vitreous haze.

Ophthalmoscopy reveals characteristic multifocal, hypopigmented, cream-colored ovoid lesions (50–1500 μm) at the level of the choroid and RPE in the posterior and midzones of the fundus. These lesions often (but not exclusively) have a nasal and radial distribution that emanates from the optic nerve and frequently follows the underlying choroidal vessels (Fig 9-1). At initial presentation, the lesions may be prominent, or they may be quite subtle. Retinal vasculitis (best seen angiographically), uveitic macular edema, and optic disc inflammation are prominent features of active disease. Late complications of BCR include optic atrophy, macular thinning, loss of peripheral visual field, and choroidal neovascularization (CNV).

Key metrics for monitoring BCR disease progression and response to therapy include fluorescein angiography (FA), indocyanine green angiography (ICGA) (as accessible), optical coherence tomography (OCT), and visual field evaluations. Serial full-field electroretinogram (ERG), with attention to the 30-Hz flicker implicit time and scotopic b-wave amplitudes, may also be used. On FA, findings vary and can be subtle or nonspecific. For example, early lesions may show initial hypofluorescence with subtle late staining, whereas retinal vasculitis of the large arcade vessels or diffuse small vessel leakage, macular edema, and optic disc leakage represent more obvious active disease (Fig 9-2). ICGA may disclose multiple hypocyanescent (hypofluorescent) spots, typically in greater numbers than observed on clinical examination or FA (Fig 9-3). Although fundus autofluorescence (FAF) imaging is less useful than other techniques in detecting active BCR, it may reveal *hypo*autofluorescent areas of RPE atrophy, suggestive of long-standing disease. Visual field evaluation, meanwhile, may show substantial field loss despite good vision and minimal or no macular edema (Fig 9-4).

OCT may show signs of disease activity such as cystoid or noncystoid macular thickening (ie, inflammatory thickening without frank intraretinal fluid). Changes in macular thickening are best appreciated on OCT change maps collected over sequential visits

Table 9-1 Selected White Dot Syndromes

	BCR	APMPPE	Serpiginous Choroiditis	MFCPU
Age, years	30–70	20–50	20–60	10–70
Sex	F>M	M=F	M=F	F>M (3:1 ratio)
Laterality	Bilateral, may be asymmetric	Bilateral, may be asymmetric	Usually bilateral, may be asymmetric	Usually bilateral, may be asymmetric
Systemic associations	80%–98% HLA-A29 allele	Viral prodrome, cerebrovasculitis, CSF abnormalities	Rule out TB-associated disease	None
Onset	Insidious	Acute	Variable	Insidious
Course	Chronic, progressive	Self-limited	Chronic, recurrent	Chronic, recurrent
Symptoms	Blurred vision, floaters, photopsias, disturbed night and color vision	Photopsias, central and/or peripheral vision loss	Blurred vision, scotomas	Blurred vision, floaters, photopsias, metamorphopsia, scotomas, blind-spot enlargement
Examination findings	Vitritis; ovoid, creamy, white-yellow, posterior and midzone lesions, 50–1500 μm; do not pigment	Multifocal, flat, yellow-white lesions, 1–2 disc areas; outer retina/RPE with evolving pigmentation	Geographic, gray-white or creamy yellow, peripapillary, macular chorioretinal lesions with centrifugal extension; activity at leading peripheral edge with RPE/choriocapillaris atrophy in its wake	Myopia, anterior uveitis (50%), vitritis (100%); active white-yellow chorioretinal lesions, 50–200 μm; evolving to punched-out scars
Structural complications	Retinal vasculitis, disc edema, ME, CNV (6%)	Disc edema, pigment alterations	CNV (25%), RPE mottling, scarring, loss of choriocapillaris	Optic disc edema, peripapillary pigment changes, ME (14%–44%), macular subretinal fibrosis, CNV
FA findings	Early hypofluorescence vs silence, subtle late stain; leakage from disc, vessels, ME; delayed retinal circulation time	Acute lesions: early blockage, late staining; late window defects	Early hypofluorescence; late staining/leakage of active border; leakage in presence of CNV	Early blockage, late staining of lesions; leakage from ME; CNV
ICGA findings	Corresponding hypocyanescent lesions more numerous than on examination, FA	Hypocyanescent spots corresponding to those seen on examination, FA	Early hypocyanescence; late staining more widespread than seen on examination, FA	Multiple hypocyanescent lesions, confluence around optic nerve more numerous than seen on examination, FA
FAF findings	HypoAF spots more numerous than clinically apparent lesions; macular hypoAF	HyperAF areas correspond to FA blockage; hypoAF areas correspond to areas of staining; FAF findings lag FA findings	HyperAF active lesions; hypoAF scarred lesions	Acute lesions variably hyper- to hypoAF; may be more numerous with FAF than clinically

PIC	SFU	MEWDS	AZOOR	AIM
20–40	20–40	10–50	15–65	20–40
F (90%)	F (>95%)	F>M (3:1 ratio)	F>M (3:1 ratio)	M=F
Usually bilateral, often asymmetric	Bilateral, asymmetric	Usually unilateral	Bilateral (76%)	Usually unilateral
None	None	Viral prodrome (50%)	Systemic autoimmune disease (28%)	Viral prodrome, coxsackievirus, and hand-foot-and-mouth disease
Acute	Insidious	Acute	Insidious	Acute
Self-limited	Chronic, recurrent	Self-limited	Chronic, recurrent (31%)	Self-limited
Paracentral scotomas, photopsias, metamorphopsia	Blurred vision	Blurred vision, paracentral scotomas, photopsias	Photopsias, scotomas	Blurred vision, central scotoma
Myopia, vitritis absent; yellow-white chorio-retinal lesions, 100–300 µm; may develop pigment	Mild to moderate vitritis; 50–500 µm white-yellow lesions posterior pole to midperiphery; RPE; hypertrophy; atrophy; large stellate zones of subretinal fibrosis	Myopia; mild anterior uveitis; vitritis; small white-orange, evanescent, perifoveal dots, 100–200 µm; outer retina/RPE; macular granularity	Initially normal to subtle RPE changes; late pigment migration; focal perivenous sheathing	Minimal to no cells; white/gray/yellow RPE discoloration and thickening; sparse intraretinal hemorrhages
CNV (17%–40%), serous detachment over confluent lesions	Neurosensory retinal detachment, ME, CNV	Disc edema, venous sheathing	RPE mottling, occasional ME	RPE granularity, rarely CNV
Early blockage or hyperfluorescence; variable late leakage/staining of acute lesions; leakage in presence of ME; CNV	Multiple areas of alternating hypo- and hyperfluorescence; late staining	Early punctate hyperfluorescence, wreathlike configuration; late staining of lesions, optic nerve	In acute stage: normal with increased retinal circulation time; in late stage: diffuse hyperfluorescence; RPE atrophy	Early hypo- or hyperfluorescence followed by late stippled hyperfluorescent staining of the RPE and pooling of dye
Multiple hypocyanescent, peripapillary, posterior pole lesions, corresponding to those seen on examination, FA	Hypocyanescent lesions	Multiple hypocyanescent spots, larger and more numerous than on examination, FA	Hypocyanescence in atrophic areas with late leakage in subacute areas	Hypocyanescence
Similar to MFCPU	No information	HyperAF spots corresponding to lesions on clinical examination	Lesions may have central hypoAF with peripheral hyperAF border	HypoAF

(Continued)

Table 9-1 *(continued)*

	BCR	APMPPE	Serpiginous Choroiditis	MFCPU
OCT findings	ME; loss of inner/outer segment line (ellipsoid zone); diffuse choroidal thickening; suprachoroidal fluid	Outer retinal hyperreflectivity with intra- and subretinal fluid	Outer retinal hyperreflectivity and thickening of underlying choroid in active lesions; retinal and RPE atrophy in scarred lesions	Sub-RPE deposits with overlying outer retinal disruption, thickening of underlying choroid (when active); CNV
Electrophysiology, VF findings	ERG: abnormal rod and cone responses; diminished b-wave; prolonged 30-Hz flicker implicit times VF: SITA 24-2 can show extensive loss even if central VA is preserved; MD may correlate with subjective vision changes	EOG: variably abnormal	ERG: normal	ERG: abnormal, extinguished responses
Visual prognosis	Guarded without treatment	Variable	Guarded	Guarded
Treatment	Systemic or local corticosteroids; IMT	Observation; systemic corticosteroids, especially with CNS involvement	Systemic and/or local corticosteroids; IMT; intravitreal anti-VEGF therapy for CNV	Systemic or local corticosteroids; IMT; intravitreal anti-VEGF therapy for inflammatory CNV

AIM = acute idiopathic maculopathy; APMPPE = acute posterior multifocal placoid pigment epitheliopathy; AZOOR = acute zonal occult outer retinopathy; BCR = birdshot chorioretinopathy; CNS = central nervous system; CNV = choroidal neovascularization; CSF = cerebrospinal fluid; EOG = electro-oculogram; ERG = electroretinogram; F = female; FA = fluorescein angiography; FAF = fundus autofluorescence; HLA = human leukocyte antigen; hyperAF = hyperautofluorescence/hyperautofluorescent; hypoAF = hypoautofluorescence/hypoautofluorescent; ICGA = indocyanine green

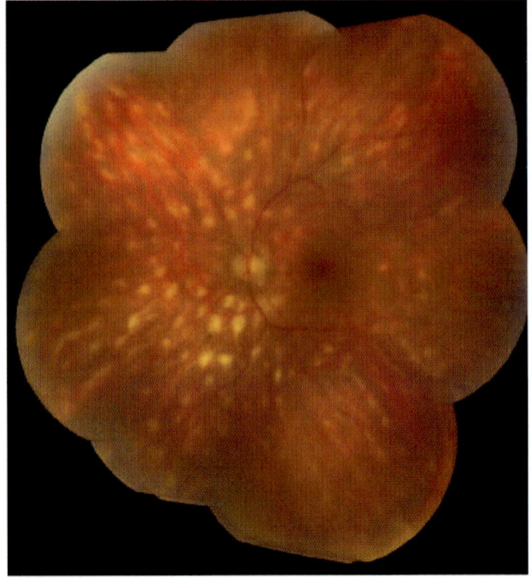

Figure 9-1 Birdshot chorioretinopathy. Fundus photograph showing multiple cream-colored ovoid lesions in the posterior pole and midzone. *(Courtesy of H. Nida Sen, MD/National Eye Institute.)*

PIC	SFU	MEWDS	AZOOR	AIM
Similar to MFCPU; inactive lesions may have posteriorly bowed RPE and outer retinal structures	Variable retinal edema; subretinal fluid and subretinal fibrosis	Abnormal hyperreflectivity and/or disruption of the inner/outer segment line	Loss of the inner/outer segment line (ellipsoid zone)	Subretinal fluid with hyperreflective debris in the subretinal space
ERG: normal	ERG and EOG: markedly attenuated	ERG: diminished a-wave, early receptor potentials (reversible)	ERG, mfERG: abnormal	ERG: normal mfERG: abnormal
VF: enlargement of blind spot (41%)		VF: enlarged blind spot, paracentral scotomas	VF: temporal, superior defects (corresponding to affected retina); enlarged blind spot	VF: central scotoma
Variable	Guarded	Good	Guarded	Variable
Observation; intravitreal anti-VEGF therapy for CNV; local or systemic corticosteroids; IMT	Systemic or local corticosteroids; IMT	Observation	Systemic or local corticosteroids; IMT	Observation; systemic corticosteroids if slow resolution

(continued) angiography; IMT = immunomodulatory therapy; M = male; MD = mean deviation; ME = macular edema; MEWDS = multiple evanescent white dot syndrome; MFCPU = multifocal choroiditis with panuveitis; mfERG = multifocal electroretinogram; OCT = optical coherence tomography; PIC = punctate inner choroiditis; RPE = retinal pigment epithelium; SFU = subretinal fibrosis and uveitis syndrome; SITA = Swedish Interactive Thresholding Algorithm; TB = tuberculosis; VEGF = vascular endothelial growth factor; VA = visual acuity; VF = visual field.

(see Fig 9-3A, C). Enhanced depth imaging OCT may be useful for evaluating choroidal thickening in early disease, and results correlate with hypocyanescent lesions observed on ICGA (see Fig 9-3B, D). In later stages of undertreated BCR, OCT may show macular thinning associated with patchy or diffuse loss of photoreceptors (ie, inner/outer segment line or ellipsoid zone) and chronic diffuse intraretinal cysts (Fig 9-5).

Böni C, Thorne JE, Spaide RF, et al. Choroidal findings in eyes with birdshot chorioretinitis using enhanced-depth optical coherence tomography. *Invest Ophthalmol Vis Sci.* 2016;57(9):591–599.

Le Piffer AL, Boissonnot M, Gobert F, et al. Relevance of wide-field autofluorescence imaging in birdshot retinochoroidopathy: descriptive analysis of 76 eyes. *Acta Ophthalmol.* 2014;92(6):e463–e469.

Differential diagnosis

The differential diagnosis of BCR includes TB, syphilis, multifocal choroiditis with panuveitis (MFCPU), acute posterior multifocal placoid pigment epitheliopathy (APMPPE), multiple

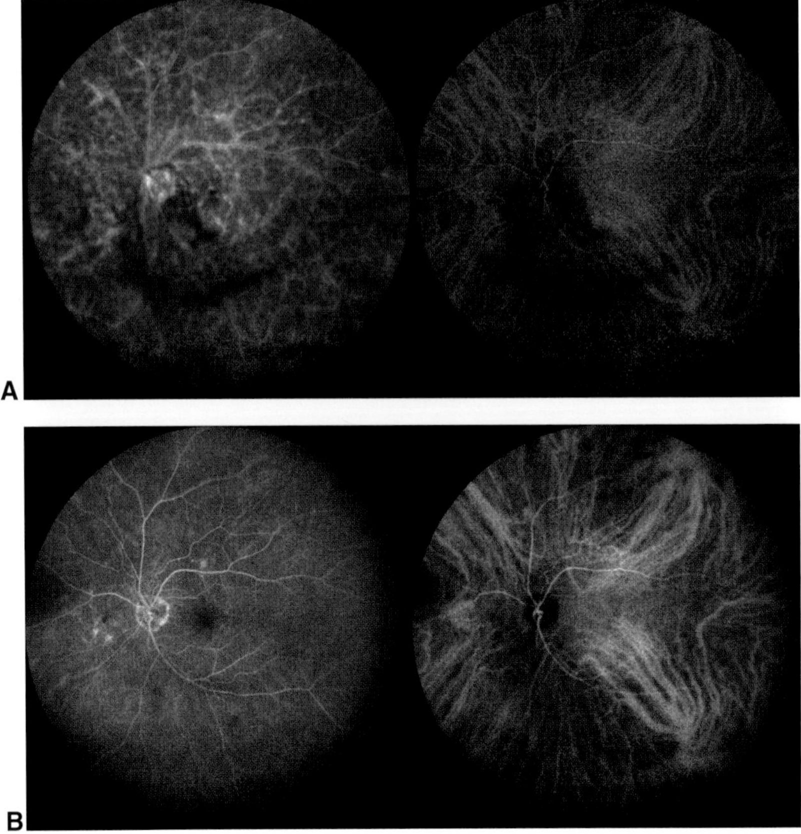

Figure 9-2 Birdshot chorioretinopathy. **A,** Fluorescein angiography (FA) *(left)* shows diffuse retinal vasculitis and shadowing from vitreous debris. Indocyanine green angiography (ICGA) *(right)* shows hypocyanescent lesions. **B,** After systemic immunomodulatory therapy, FA *(left)* shows resolution of the retinal vasculitis and vitreous debris with a few residual hyperfluorescent window defects. A few hypocyanescent lesions remain on ICGA *(right)*. (Courtesy of Wendy M. Smith, MD.)

evanescent white dot syndrome (MEWDS), OHS, autoimmune retinopathy, intraocular lymphoma, and especially sarcoidosis, which may present with chorioretinal lesions of similar morphology and distribution.

Disease course

Although a small subset of patients may have self-limited disease, the clinical course of BCR is characteristically chronic and progressive. Despite good visual acuity and minimal vitreous cells, patients with BCR may still experience progressive, diffuse, inflammatory retinal degeneration that manifests as visual field loss and dysfunction on full-field electroretinogram (ERG). If the clinician simply monitors visual acuity, disease progression will be missed. However, early and aggressive efforts to control inflammation may improve clinical outcomes.

Knickelbein JE, Jeffrey BG, Wei MM, et al. Reproducibility of full-field electroretinogram measurements in birdshot chorioretinopathy patients: an intra- and inter-visit analysis. *Ocul Immunol Inflamm.* 2021;29(5):848–853.

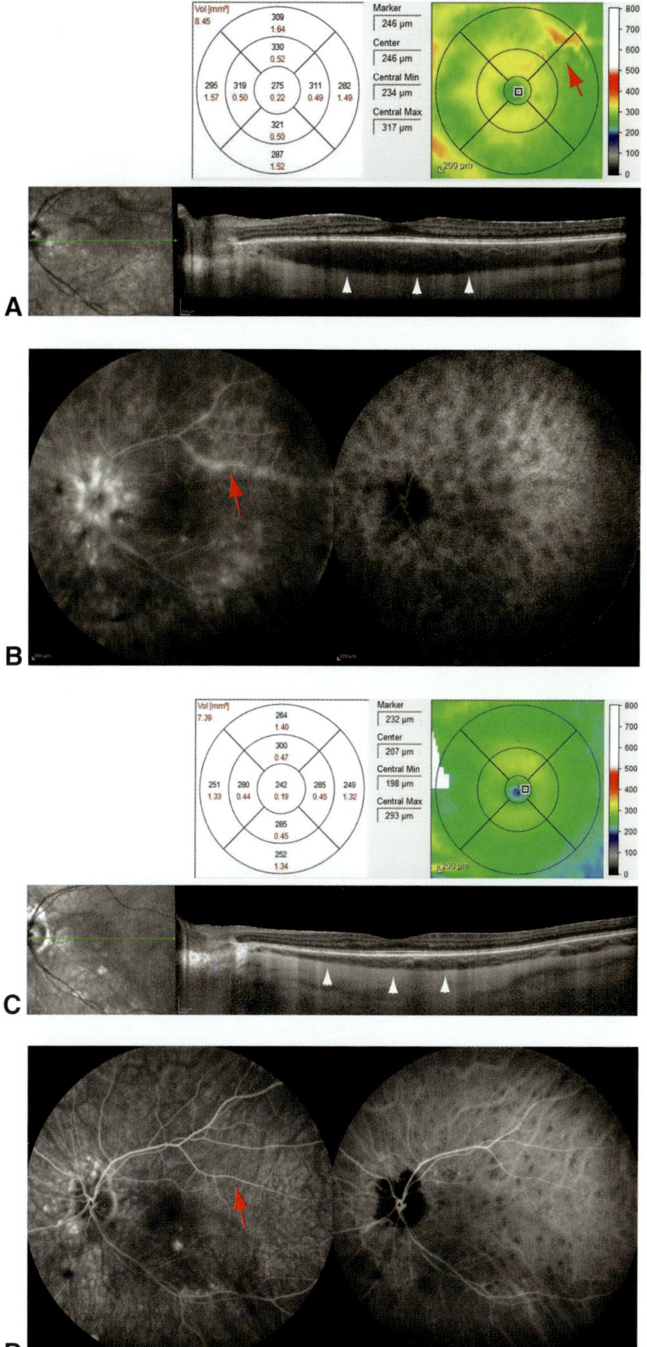

Figure 9-3 Birdshot chorioretinopathy. Multimodal imaging at presentation and after 5 years of systemic immunomodulatory therapy (IMT). **A,** Optical coherence tomography (OCT) heat map shows thickening along a vessel in the superior arcade *(arrow)*. Enhanced depth imaging (EDI) OCT scan shows diffuse choroidal thickening but no intraretinal fluid *(arrowheads)*. **B,** FA *(left)* shows venular arcade leakage *(arrow corresponds to thickening on OCT heat map)* and disc/peripapillary leakage. ICGA *(right)* shows confluent hypocyanescent spots emanating from the optic nerve, most with no correlate on FA. **C,** Five years later, OCT heat map shows mild thinning. EDI-OCT shows significant decrease in choroidal thickness *(arrowheads)*. **D,** FA *(left)* shows resolution of venular and disc leakage *(arrow)* with residual window defects. ICGA *(right)* shows near resolution of the hypocyanescent spots. *(Courtesy of Wendy M. Smith, MD.)*

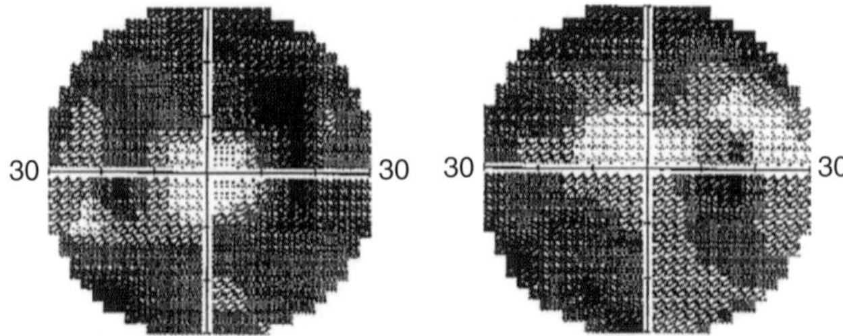

Figure 9-4 Birdshot chorioretinopathy. Visual fields from a 61-year-old woman with extensive visual field loss in both eyes despite 20/20 vision and absence of macular edema. *(Courtesy of Sam S. Dahr, MD, MS.)*

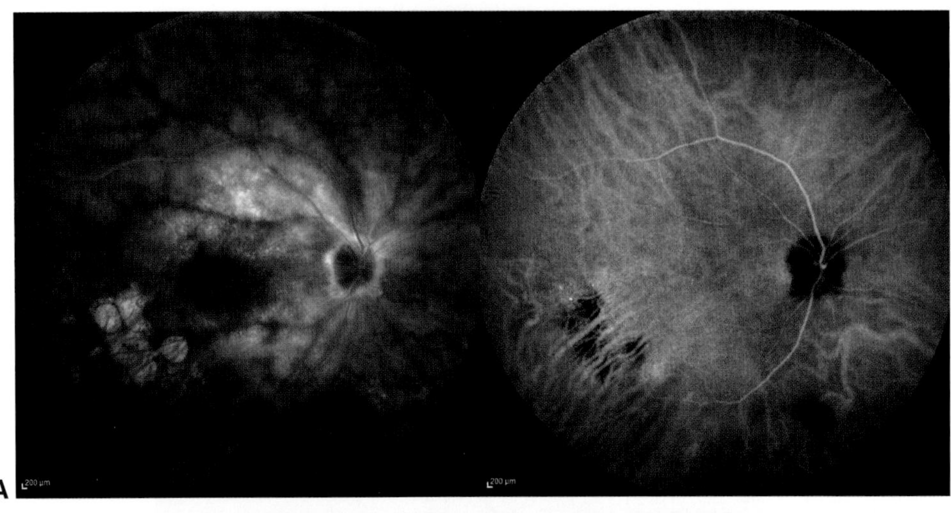

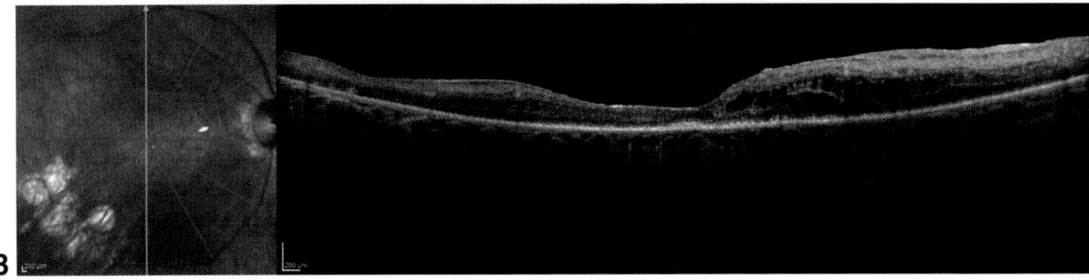

Figure 9-5 Birdshot chorioretinopathy in a patient whose diagnosis and treatment were considerably delayed. **A,** FA *(left)* shows vascular attenuation, diffuse posterior pole small-vessel leakage, and window defects in the inferotemporal macula from chorioretinal scars. The hypocyanescent lesions on ICGA *(right)* correspond to the chorioretinal scars. **B,** OCT shows chronic-appearing intraretinal fluid with loss of outer retinal structures and retinal pigment epithelium (RPE) damage. The choroid (partially visualized) appears thin. *(Courtesy of Wendy M. Smith, MD.)*

Minos E, Barry RJ, Southworth S, et al. Birdshot chorioretinopathy: current knowledge and new concepts in pathophysiology, diagnosis, monitoring and treatment. *Orphanet J Rare Dis.* 2016;11(1):61. doi.org/10.1186/s13023-016-0429-8

Papadia M, Pavésio C, Fardeau C, et al. HLA-A29 birdshot retinochoroiditis in its 5th decade: selected glimpses into the intellectual meanderings and progresses in the knowledge of a long-time misunderstood disease. *Diagnostics (Basel).* 2021;11(7):1291. doi:10.3390/diagnostics11071291

Treatment

Given the chronic nature of BCR, extended immunomodulatory therapy (IMT) is anticipated in most patients and may include methotrexate, mycophenolate mofetil, azathioprine, cyclosporine, tacrolimus, and/or tumor necrosis factor α (TNF-α) inhibitors. Systemic and/or local corticosteroid injections can be used as a bridge until IMT takes effect, typically 2–4 months for some therapeutic improvement and up to 6–12 months for full effect. Depending on individual response, refinement of the IMT regimen may take even longer, and some patients may need combination therapy, typically an antimetabolite and an anti-TNF agent. The long-acting intravitreal fluocinolone acetonide insert (0.18 mg) or implant (0.59 mg) may be used in patients who cannot tolerate systemic therapy (although they may be insufficient as monotherapy) or combined with systemic therapy for breakthrough inflammation. Patients with asymptomatic or minimally symptomatic BCR who lack objective findings such as macular edema, angiographic edema or vasculitis, or visual field/ERG dysfunction may be monitored closely, but the majority of patients with BCR will require corticosteroids and corticosteroid-sparing IMT.

Crowell EL, France R, Majmudar P, Jabs DA, Thorne JE. Treatment outcomes in birdshot chorioretinitis: corticosteroid sparing, corticosteroid discontinuation, remission, and relapse. *Ophthalmol Retina.* 2022;6(7):620–627.

Menezo V, Taylor SR. Birdshot uveitis: current and emerging treatment options. *Clin Ophthalmol.* 2014;8:73–81.

Tomkins-Netzer O, Taylor SRJ, Lightman S. Long-term clinical and anatomic outcome of birdshot chorioretinopathy. *JAMA Ophthalmol.* 2014;132(1):57–62.

Acute Posterior Multifocal Placoid Pigment Epitheliopathy

Acute posterior multifocal placoid pigment epitheliopathy (APMPPE) is an inflammatory disease that manifests as choriocapillaritis with secondary RPE involvement. The disorder presents equally in otherwise healthy men and women, typically before age 50 years.

The etiology of APMPPE is poorly understood, although patients may report a viral prodrome. Infectious associations include group A streptococcus, adenovirus type 5, TB, Lyme disease, and mumps virus. APMPPE has also been reported after vaccination for varicella, hepatitis B, swine flu, and meningococcus. Noninfectious disease associations include erythema nodosum, granulomatosis with polyangiitis, polyarteritis nodosa, scleritis and episcleritis, sarcoidosis, and ulcerative colitis. A rare but potentially life-threatening association also exists between APMPPE and cerebral vasculitis. Therefore, patients with APMPPE and central nervous system (CNS) symptoms such as headache should undergo urgent neurologic evaluation including neuro-imaging and cerebrospinal fluid studies. Although most patients with APMPPE do not experience major extraocular manifestations, the disease associations mentioned here highlight the need for a careful review of patient symptoms, with referral to an appropriate nonophthalmic specialist as required for further assessment.

Manifestations

Patients with APMPPE typically present with sudden-onset unilateral photopsias and vision loss. Involvement of the fellow eye may occur within days to weeks. Anterior segment inflammation is absent or minimal, and vitritis is typically mild. Fundus examination demonstrates large, flat, yellow-white, RPE-involving placoid lesions throughout the posterior pole

(Fig 9-6), with lesion size varying from 1 to 2 disc areas. New peripheral lesions may develop in a linear or radial array. Rapid lesion evolution is a disease hallmark. Papillitis may also occur, but macular edema is uncommon. Other atypical findings include retinal vasculitis, retinal vascular occlusive disease, retinal neovascularization, and exudative retinal detachment. The RPE lesions usually resolve over a period of 2–6 weeks, leaving variable areas of depigmentation and pigment clumping.

In the acute disease phase, FA shows early hypofluorescent lesions (see Fig 9-6C) and late hyperfluorescent staining (see Fig 9-6D). As lesions evolve toward RPE depigmentation and loss, early blockage transitions to transmission hyperfluorescence with late staining. With ICGA, choroidal hypocyanescence with hypervisualization of the underlying choroidal vessels is seen in both the acute and inactive disease stages, with the lesions shrinking in the inactive stages (see Fig 9-6B). On both FA and ICGA, perfusion abnormalities are more numerous than the overlying placoid lesions.

FAF findings lag behind the appearance of clinically evident lesions, and FAF lesions are fewer than the clinical lesions. They are initially hyperautofluorescent and may evolve into areas of hypoautofluorescence over time (Fig 9-7A). OCT of acute lesions shows hyperreflectivity of the outer retinal layers as well as subretinal or intraretinal fluid (Fig 9-7B). As the lesions resolve, outer retinal and photoreceptor loss may be observed.

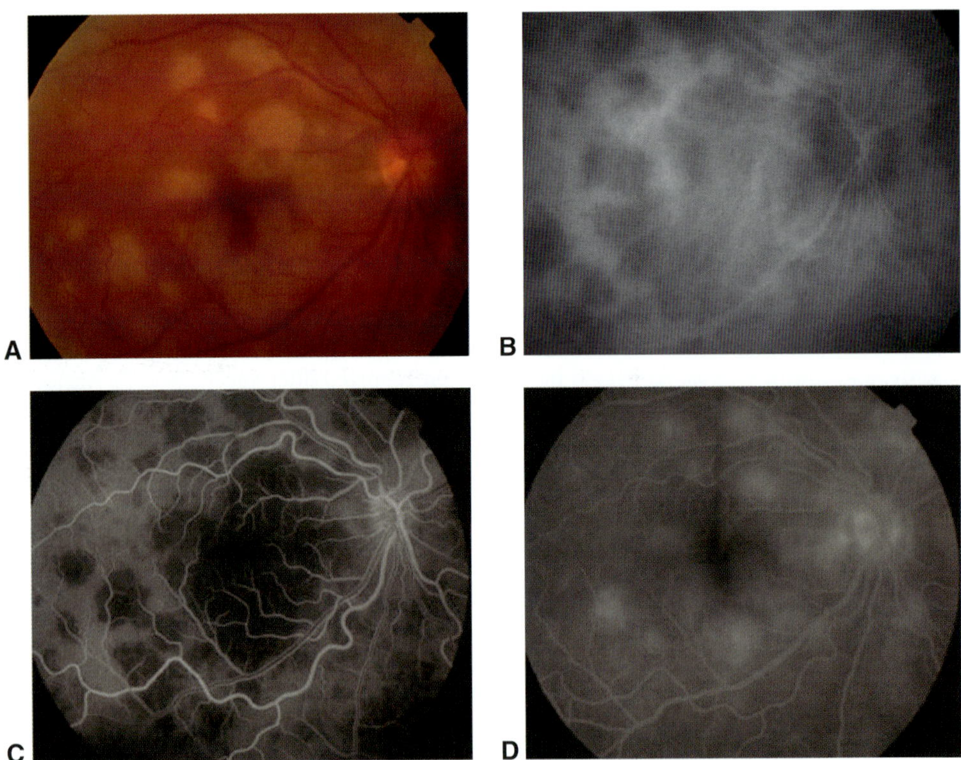

Figure 9-6 Acute posterior multifocal placoid pigment epitheliopathy. **A,** Fundus photograph shows multifocal placoid lesions in the macula. **B,** ICGA shows multiple mid-phase hypocyanescent lesions. **C,** FA shows early hypofluorescent lesions. **D,** FA shows late-phase staining. *(Courtesy of Albert T. Vitale, MD.)*

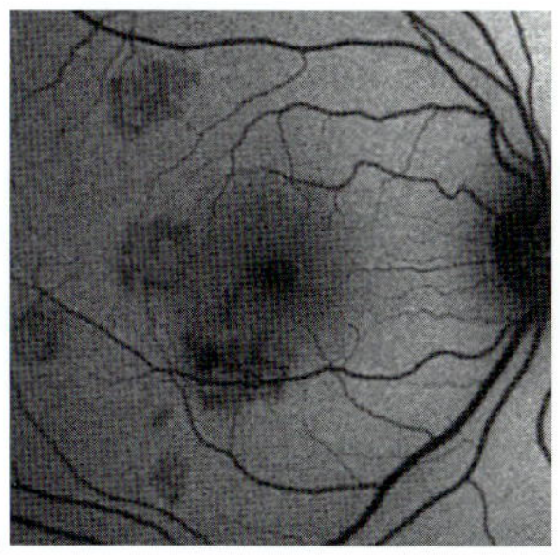

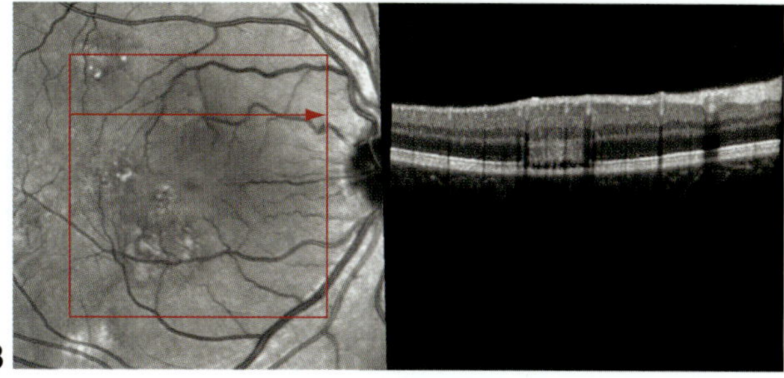

Figure 9-7 Acute posterior multifocal placoid pigment epitheliopathy. **A,** Fundus autofluorescence (FAF) image showing scattered, inactive, hypoautofluorescent lesions. **B,** OCT through an active lesion *(red horizontal arrow),* demonstrating hyperreflectivity of the outer retina and RPE, a sliver of subretinal fluid, and focal disruption of the photoreceptor layer. *(Courtesy of Bryn M. Burkholder, MD.)*

Differential diagnosis

APMPPE is a clinical diagnosis based on examination findings and ancillary studies such as FA, ICGA, FAF, and OCT. The differential diagnosis of active APMPPE includes syphilis, TB, pneumocystis choroiditis, endogenous fungal endophthalmitis, sarcoidosis, and choroidal metastasis or lymphoma. Although active lesions in APMPPE, ampiginous choroiditis, and serpiginous choroiditis may have similar appearances, APMPPE is usually an acute, nonrecurring disease, unlike ampiginous and serpiginous choroiditis, which are insidious and progressive. The OCT findings in active APMPPE can resemble the serous retinal detachments in Vogt-Koyanagi-Harada syndrome, but other clinical features should differentiate the two entities. (See Chapter 10 for further discussion of Vogt-Koyanagi-Harada syndrome.) While inactive APMPPE scars can look similar to the lesions in MFCPU and punctate inner choroiditis, these entities are usually not included in the differential diagnosis of active APMPPE.

Prognosis

Most patients with APMPPE have a good prognosis, with visual acuity returning to 20/40 or better within 6 months. However, 20% are left with residual visual dysfunction. Risk factors for vision loss include foveal involvement at presentation, older age at presentation, unilateral disease, a longer interval between initial and fellow eye involvement, and recurrence. Although patients with APMPPE are often simply observed, corticosteroid therapy may be considered to hasten lesion resolution, especially in those with extensive macular involvement. In patients with APMPPE and concurrent CNS vasculitis, prompt systemic corticosteroid treatment is indicated to reduce CNS morbidity and mortality.

Li AL, Palejwala NV, Shantha JG, et al. Long-term multimodal imaging in acute posterior multifocal placoid pigment epitheliopathy and association with coxsackievirus exposure. *PLoS One.* 2020;15(8):e0238080. doi:10.1371/journal.pone.0238080

Papasavvas I, Mantovani A, Herbort CP Jr. Acute posterior multifocal placoid pigment epitheliopathy (APMPPE): a comprehensive approach and case series: systemic corticosteroid therapy is necessary in a large proportion of cases. *Medicina (Kaunas).* 2022;58(8):1070. doi:10.3390/medicina58081070

Testi I, Vermeirsch S, Pavesio C. Acute posterior multifocal placoid pigment epitheliopathy (APMPPE). *J Ophthalmic Inflamm Infect.* 2021;11(1):31. doi:10.1186/s12348-021-00263-1

Serpiginous Choroiditis

Serpiginous choroiditis, also known as *geographic* or *helicoid choroidopathy,* is a rare, chronic, relentlessly progressive posterior uveitis that affects adult men and women equally. It is hypothesized to be an immune-mediated occlusive vasculitis. Although associations between serpiginous choroiditis and systemic diseases have been inconsistent, the disorder has been reported in patients with Crohn disease, sarcoidosis, and polyarteritis nodosa. TB can cause a serpiginous-like choroiditis; thus, all patients with suspected serpiginous choroiditis should be tested for TB exposure.

Manifestations

Patients with serpiginous choroiditis present with decreased vision, painless paracentral scotomas, a quiet anterior chamber, and minimal to no vitreous cells. The disease is usually bilateral but may be asymmetric. Active gray-white or creamy yellow RPE-level lesions originate in the peripapillary region and progress in a serpentine or pseudopodial manner (Fig 9-8A). However, one-third of patients may have macular serpiginous choroiditis, in which the serpentine lesions arise principally within the macula rather than the peripapillary region. Without treatment, serpiginous lesions evolve slowly into areas of atrophic retina, RPE, and choriocapillaris, often with fibrosis and/or hyperpigmentation. New activity usually occurs at the edge of a scarred lesion and may have associated shallow subretinal fluid. In up to 25% of patients, CNV develops at the border of an old serpiginous scar.

On FA, active serpiginous choroiditis lesions or lesion edges show early hypofluorescence of the entire active area, followed by late hyperfluorescent staining (Fig 9-8B, C). In contrast, scarred lesions show sharp margins and areas of hypofluorescence (secondary to loss of choriocapillaris and blocking by RPE hyperplasia) and transmission hyperfluorescence (due to atrophic RPE) on early FA. Later FA images of scarred lesions show staining of atrophic and hyperplastic RPE and fibrosis that has well-defined borders (versus the fuzzier borders of active staining/leaking lesions). ICGA of both acute and old lesions reveals hypocyanescence throughout all phases and may reveal more extensive involvement than seen on FA. In patients with active CNV, early hyperfluorescence with late leakage is seen on FA, whereas hypercyanescence is seen on ICGA. FAF is also very useful for monitoring serpiginous choroiditis, with inactive scarred lesions appearing hypoautofluorescent and newly active lesions appearing hyperautofluorescent (Fig 9-9A).

Findings on OCT also vary depending on disease stage. OCT of active lesions shows normal or slightly increased retinal thickness due to hyperreflective, blurred, and thickened outer retinal structures (Fig 9-9B). The underlying choroid is usually thickened, and there may be associated shallow subretinal fluid. In contrast, scarred lesions are characterized by retinal thinning with loss of outer retinal structures and a deeper, patchy hyperreflectivity of the choroid from enhanced light transmission through atrophic RPE.

Bansal R, Gupta A, Gupta V. Imaging in the diagnosis and management of serpiginous choroiditis. *Int Ophthalmol Clin.* 2012;52(4):229–236.

Treatment

The course of serpiginous choroiditis involves centrifugal extension, progressive chorioretinal scarring, and often a poor visual outcome. Initial treatment of serpiginous choroiditis usually requires systemic and/or local corticosteroids to quiet active lesions, particularly those

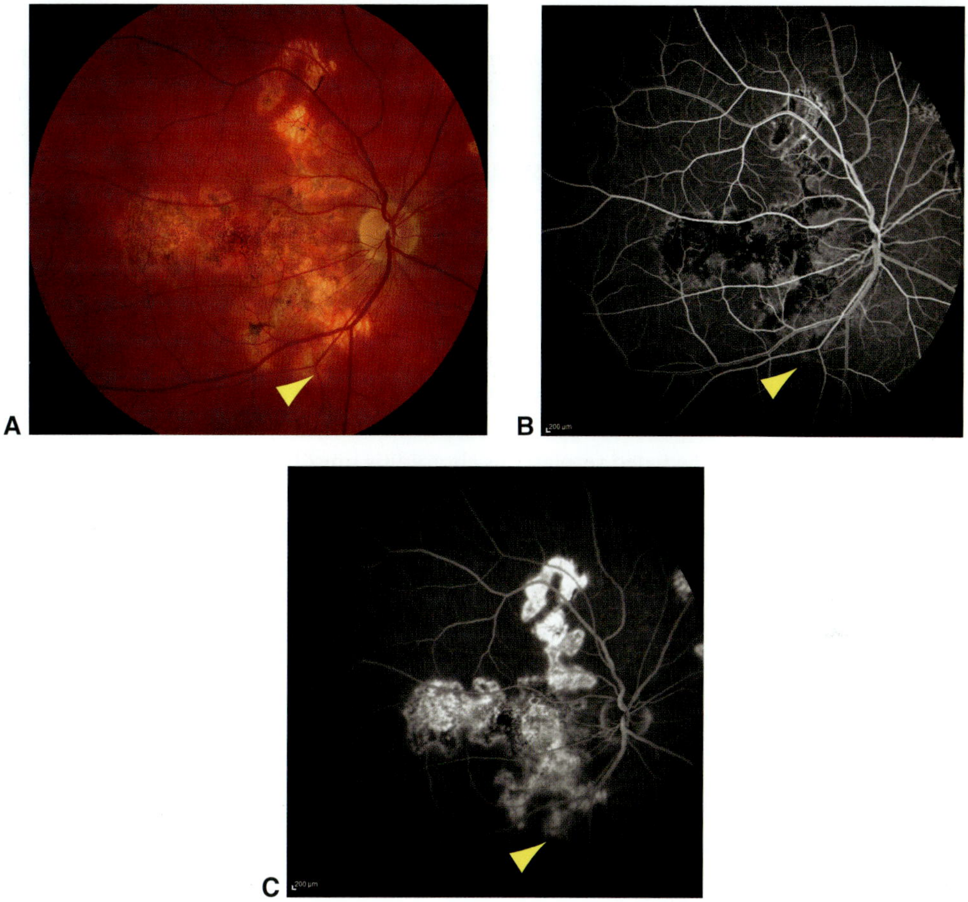

Figure 9-8 Serpiginous choroiditis. **A,** Color fundus photograph shows areas of active choroiditis at the inferior border of the macular lesion *(arrowhead)*. **B,** Early FA shows blocked fluorescence *(arrowhead)*. **C,** Late FA shows late staining and leakage at the active border of the lesion *(arrowhead)*. *(Courtesy of Wendy M. Smith, MD.)*

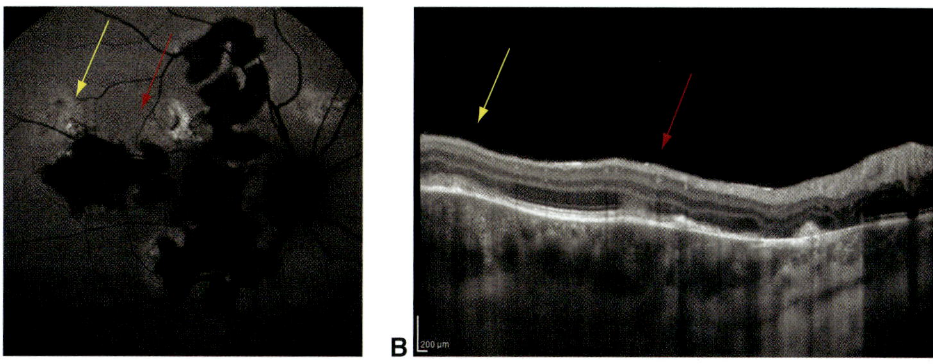

Figure 9-9 Serpiginous choroiditis. **A,** FAF shows areas of hyperautofluorescence *(yellow and red arrows)* signifying new or recent activity. **B,** OCT scan through active lesions demonstrates outer retinal blurring and hyperreflectivity *(yellow and red arrows)* and thickening of the underlying choroid. *(Courtesy of Wendy M. Smith, MD.)*

threatening the fovea. Early addition of systemic IMT improves the long-term prognosis of patients with serpiginous choroiditis by reducing progression and recurrence. Options for systemic IMT include the following medications:

- combination therapy with an antimetabolite and a T-cell inhibitor
- cytotoxic therapy with cyclophosphamide or chlorambucil. Although the associated adverse effects are more severe than those associated with other systemic IMT, this class of agents has been shown to induce long, drug-free remissions in serpiginous choroiditis.
- TNF inhibitors (may be considered as long as TB test results are negative and/or TB has been treated)

Adjunctive treatment for inflammatory CNV can involve anti-vascular endothelial growth factor (anti-VEGF) agents and/or intravitreal corticosteroids.

Presumed immune-mediated serpiginous choroiditis must be distinguished from infectious diseases that can simulate it. Rare mimics of serpiginous choroiditis include herpetic or syphilitic choroiditis as well as TB. As noted previously, tuberculous uveitis may also present as a *multifocal serpiginoid choroiditis* or *serpiginous-like choroiditis;* therefore, all patients with features of serpiginous uveitis should have TB screening tests (see Chapter 11). TB-associated serpiginous-like choroiditis requires treatment with quadruple drug therapy and may also require corticosteroids and IMT for post-infection inflammation.

Dutta Majumder P, Biswas J, Gupta A. Enigma of serpiginous choroiditis. *Indian J Ophthalmol.* 2019;67(3):325–333.

Ebrahimiadib N, Modjtahedi BS, Davoudi S, Foster CS. Treatment of serpiginous choroiditis with chlorambucil: a report of 17 patients. *Ocul Immunol Inflamm.* 2018;26(2):228–238.

Papasavvas I, Jeannin B, Herbort CP Jr. Tuberculosis-related serpiginous choroiditis: aggressive therapy with dual concomitant combination of multiple anti-tubercular and multiple immunosuppressive agents is needed to halt the progression of the disease. *J Ophthalmic Inflamm Infect.* 2022;12(1):7.

Ampiginous Choroiditis, or Relentless Placoid Chorioretinitis

Ampiginous choroiditis, also called *relentless placoid chorioretinitis,* is an uncommon entity that has features of both serpiginous choroiditis and APMPPE. Affected men and women, typically between 10 and 50 years of age, present with floaters, photopsias, paracentral scotomas, and decreased vision, as well as variable degrees of anterior segment inflammation and vitritis.

The creamy-white placoid lesions of acute ampiginous choroiditis are clinically and angiographically similar to the active lesions of serpiginous choroiditis and APMPPE. Similar to serpiginous choroiditis lesions, ampiginous choroiditis abnormalities may develop at the border of a scarred lesion as well as de novo. In addition, untreated lesions evolve into chorioretinal atrophy, and advanced disease may be clinically indistinguishable from that of serpiginous choroiditis, including the development of CNV. Moreover, active and scarred lesions in ampiginous choroiditis are essentially identical to those of serpiginous choroiditis on FA (Fig 9-10). However, the clinical courses of the two diseases differ. For example, the active

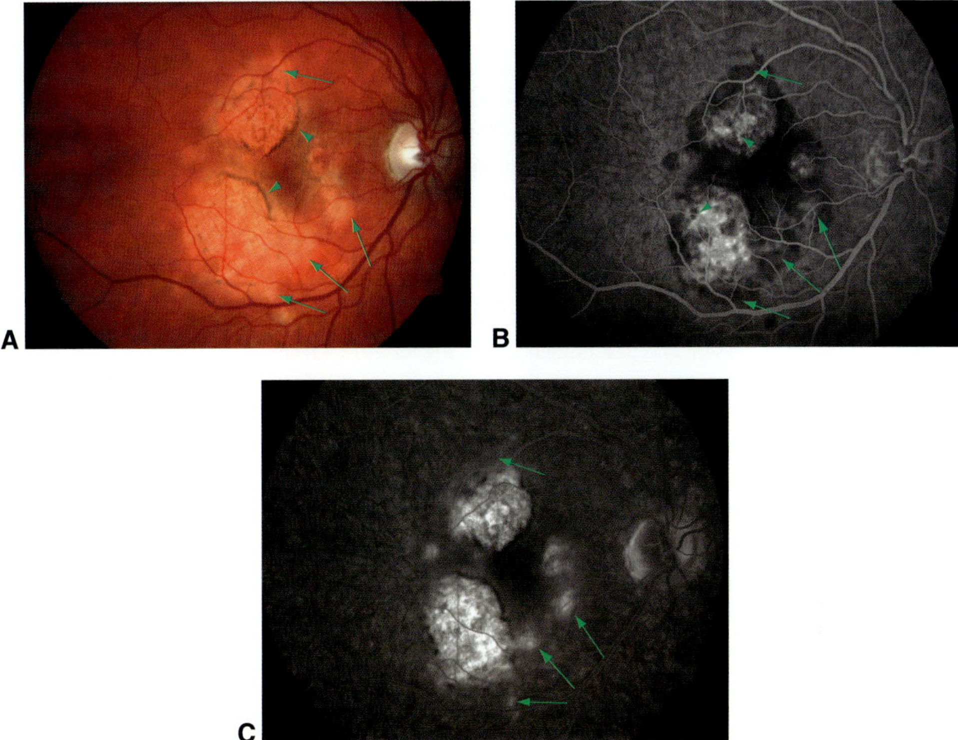

Figure 9-10 Ampiginous choroiditis, subacute lesion. **A,** Fundus photograph shows a white placoid lesion with active edges *(arrows)* and older pigmented edges *(arrowheads)*. **B,** Early-phase FA shows mixture of early blockage within newer parts of the lesion *(arrows)* and transmission within older parts of the lesion *(arrowheads)*. **C,** Late-phase FA shows staining throughout the lesion, although staining of the active edges is more subtle *(arrows)* than staining of the older central portion of the lesion. *(Courtesy of Sam S. Dahr, MD, MS.)*

lesions of ampiginous choroiditis are often multifocal and distinctly separate, unlike those of serpiginous choroiditis, which arise from a single location and are clustered. In addition, lesions of ampiginous choroiditis occur in the periphery and may predate those in the posterior pole, and macular lesions do not radiate from the peripapillary area as they do in serpiginous choroiditis.

In patients with ampiginous choroiditis, prolonged periods of chronic disease activity may be characterized by the appearance of more than 50 multifocal lesions, which appear throughout the fundus and progress over a 2-year period. Depending on disease severity and clinical course, treatment may include systemic and/or local corticosteroids, systemic IMT, and/or anti-VEGF therapy. As with all diseases characterized by chorioretinal lesions, TB-associated serpiginous-like choroiditis should be ruled out in patients with suspected ampiginous choroiditis.

Jones BE, Jampol LM, Yannuzzi LA, et al. Relentless placoid chorioretinitis: a new entity or an unusual variant of serpiginous chorioretinitis? *Arch Ophthalmol.* 2000;118(7):931–938.

Jyotirmay B, Jafferji SS, Sudharshan S, Kalpana B. Clinical profile, treatment, and visual outcome of ampiginous choroiditis. *Ocul Immunol Inflamm.* 2010;18(1):46–51.

Multifocal Choroiditis With Panuveitis, Punctate Inner Choroiditis, and Subretinal Fibrosis and Uveitis Syndrome

Multifocal choroiditis with panuveitis (MFCPU), punctate inner choroiditis (PIC), and subretinal fibrosis and uveitis syndrome (SFU) are a subset of white dot syndromes with similar features. Some authorities have traditionally defined them as discrete disorders; however, others consider them to be a single disease (often called *multifocal choroiditis*) that falls along a continuum, with the presence of fibrosis or panuveitis described separately. For this discussion, MFCPU, PIC, and SFU are considered discrete disorders.

Essex RW, Wong J, Jampol LM, Dowler J, Bird AC. Idiopathic multifocal choroiditis: a comment on present and past nomenclature. *Retina.* 2013;33(1):1–4.

Multifocal choroiditis with panuveitis

MFCPU is an idiopathic inflammatory disorder that affects the choroid, retina, and vitreous, most often in young (average age is approximately 30 years but ranges from 10 to 70 years) women with myopia. MFCPU is considered a posterior uveitis because the primary inflammation is in the choroid, and any associated anterior chamber or vitreous inflammation is usually mild. The disease is typically bilateral but may be asymmetric. Although a viral etiology has not been proven for MFCPU, herpes simplex and Epstein-Barr viruses have been implicated in some cases, possibly as triggers of an autoimmune process. Variable findings on histologic examination of affected eyes, such as increased choroidal B and/or T lymphocytes, suggest that different immune pathways may produce similar disease phenotypes.

Manifestations Symptoms of MFCPU include floaters, photopsias, blind-spot enlargement, and decreased vision. Clinical examination shows multiple oval or round lesions typically >125 μm at the level of the RPE or inner choroid in any zone of the fundus, although most are peripapillary. Acute lesions have a white-yellow, opaque appearance. As the lesions transition to atrophic scars, they develop a "punched-out appearance" with a white center and a discrete border that may become pigmented (Fig 9-11). Peripheral streaks or linear arrays of lesions and peripapillary pigmentary atrophy may also occur. In some patients, the disease resembles PIC in one eye and MFCPU in the other. Complications include macular edema, CNV, epiretinal membrane, and macular subretinal fibrosis.

Multimodal imaging is used to assess MFCPU. FA of acute active lesions shows early hypofluorescence with late staining (Fig 9-12). Atrophic scars produce transmission defects (early hyperfluorescence that fades in the late phases of the angiogram). Early hyperfluorescence and late leakage may represent macular edema or CNV.

As with BCR, ICGA of active MFCPU reveals more mid-phase hypocyanescent lesions than are seen on clinical examination or FA (see Fig 9-12). The lesions frequently cluster around the optic nerve and correlate with an enlarged blind spot on visual fields. Most of these hypofluorescent spots fade with resolution of inflammation.

FAF findings in MFCPU vary and are often most useful when correlated with other imaging modalities and followed longitudinally. In active disease, FAF may show fully *hyper*autofluorescent lesions, *hyper*autofluorescent edges associated with *hypo*autofluorescent central lesions, or increase in size of *hypo*autofluorescent lesions compared with their size in the inactive phase. In general, FAF lesions are often smaller and more numerous than those

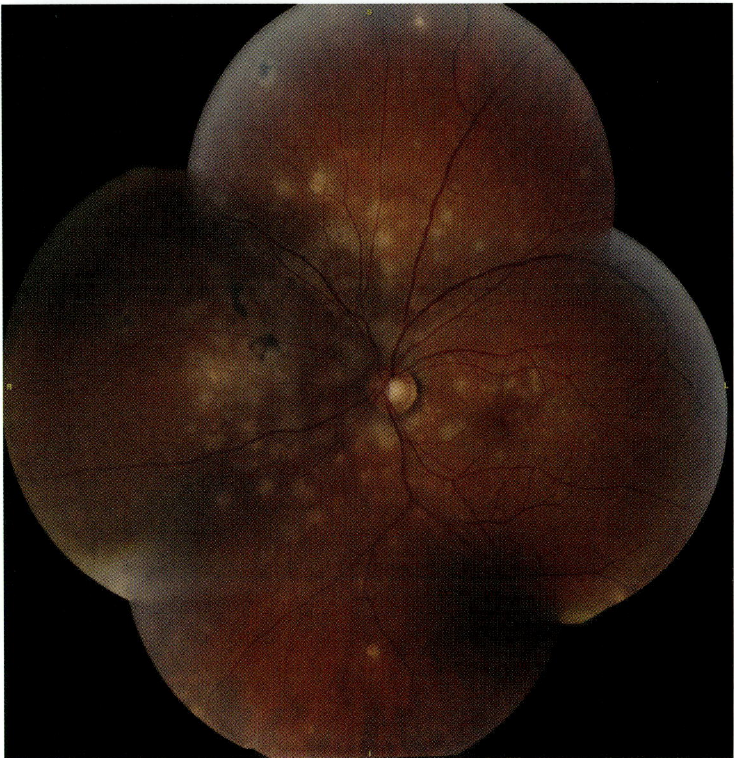

Figure 9-11 Multifocal choroiditis with panuveitis. Montage of color fundus photographs shows multiple active creamy lesions emanating from the optic nerve. *(Courtesy of Wendy M. Smith, MD.)*

noted on clinical examination (Fig 9-13A, C). OCT of active lesions may show RPE elevation, disruption of the overlying outer retina, subretinal hyperreflective material, and hyperreflectivity of the underlying choroid (Fig 9-13B, D).

Spaide RF, Goldberg N, Freund KB. Redefining multifocal choroiditis and panuveitis and punctate inner choroidopathy through multimodal imaging. *Retina.* 2013;33(7): 1315–1324.

Diagnosis The differential diagnosis of MFCPU includes sarcoidosis, syphilis, OHS, TB, PIC, and BCR. MFCPU lesions are larger than PIC lesions, and PIC usually lacks anterior chamber and vitreous inflammation. Compared with birdshot lesions, those of MFCPU are smaller and more discrete or "punched out"; in addition, patients with MFCPU are typically younger than those with BCR and do not have HLA-A29–positive test results. Similar to OHS, MFCPU may produce peripheral chorioretinal streaks and peripapillary pigment atrophy and hyperplasia; however, OHS typically does not cause anterior segment or vitreous inflammation or substantial subretinal fibrosis unless it is associated with CNV.

Treatment In the typically young patient with MFCPU, the goal of treatment is to minimize the progressive RPE atrophy and macular subretinal fibrosis that leads to vision loss. Because the natural history of untreated disease is poor, an aggressive approach is warranted,

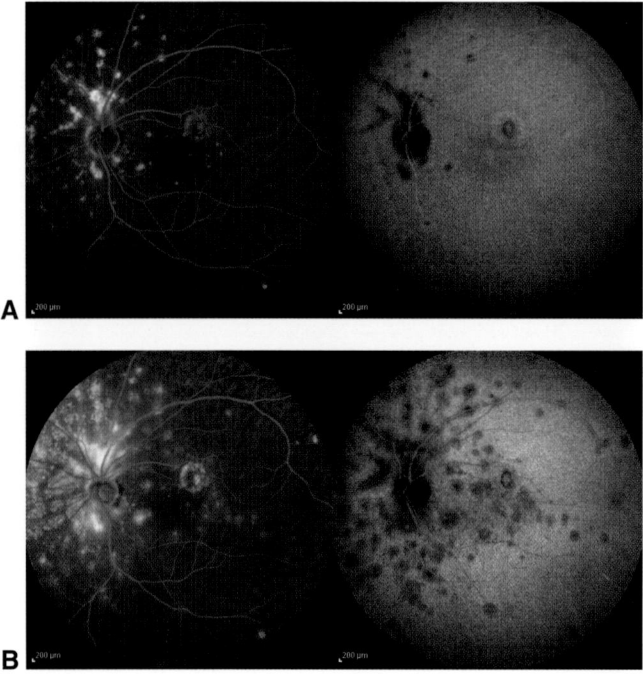

Figure 9-12 Multifocal choroiditis with panuveitis. **A,** Inactive lesions after initiation of systemic IMT. FA *(left)* shows hyperfluorescent window defects. The lesions are hypocyanescent on ICGA *(right)*. Central macular choroidal neovascularization has a hypercyanescent center surrounded by hypocyanescence. **B,** Breakthrough inflammation. FA *(left)* shows increased hyperfluorescent lesions, some leaking on late images. On ICGA *(right)*, the preexisting hypocyanescent lesions are larger, and numerous new hypocyanescent lesions are visible. *(Courtesy of Wendy M. Smith, MD.)*

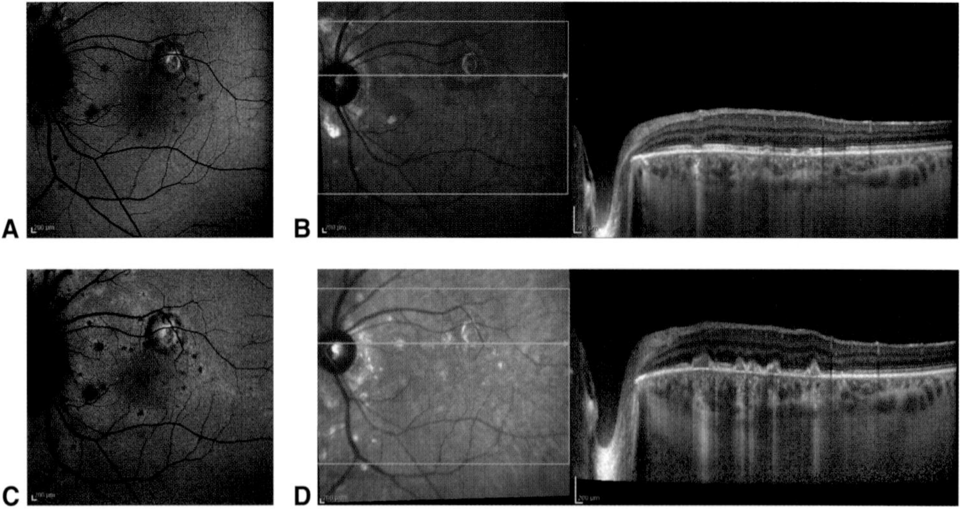

Figure 9-13 Multifocal choroiditis with panuveitis. **A,** Inactive lesions during systemic IMT. FAF shows hypoautofluorescent lesions. Choroidal neovascularization in superior macula has central hyperautofluorescence. **B,** OCT shows irregular patchy outer retinal structures of inactive lesions. **C,** Breakthrough inflammation. FAF shows increased size of hypoautofluorescent lesions compared with that of lesions shown in part A and intervening hyperautofluorescence. **D,** OCT through active lesions shows elevations of the outer retina and thickening of the underlying choroid. *(Courtesy of Wendy M. Smith, MD.)*

including use of systemic IMT. In a large retrospective cohort study of patients with MFCPU, IMT was associated with an 83% reduction in the risk of posterior pole complications and a 92% reduction in the risk of 20/200 vision or worse. Systemic, periocular, and intravitreal corticosteroids often quiet active lesions in the short term; however, antimetabolites, T-cell inhibitors, and/or TNF inhibitors are commonly required for long-term disease control. In some cases, an intravitreal fluocinolone implant may be effective for long-term control of inflammation. Intravitreal anti-VEGF therapy may be used as adjunctive treatment for inflammatory CNV, although use of corticosteroids and/or systemic IMT to control uveitis activity may eliminate the need for ongoing anti-VEGF injections.

de Groot EL, Ten Dam-van Loon NH, de Boer JH, Ossewaarde-van Norel J. The efficacy of corticosteroid-sparing immunomodulatory therapy in treating patients with central multifocal choroiditis. *Acta Ophthalmol.* 2020;98(8):816–821.

Erba S, Cozzi M, Xhepa A, Cereda M, Staurenghi G, Invernizzi A. Distribution and progression of inflammatory chorioretinal lesions related to multifocal choroiditis and their correlations with clinical outcomes at 24 months. *Ocul Immunol Inflamm.* 2022;30(2):409–416.

Papasavvas I, Neri P, Mantovani A, Herbort CP Jr. Idiopathic multifocal choroiditis (MFC): aggressive and prolonged therapy with multiple immunosuppressive agents is needed to halt the progression of active disease. An offbeat review and a case series. *J Ophthalmic Inflamm Infect.* 2022;12(1):2.

Standardization of Uveitis Nomenclature (SUN) Working Group. Classification Criteria for Multifocal Choroiditis With Panuveitis. *Am J Ophthalmol.* 2021;228:152–158.

Thorne JE, Wittenberg S, Jabs DA, et al. Multifocal choroiditis with panuveitis: incidence of ocular complications and loss of visual acuity. *Ophthalmology.* 2006;113(12): 2310–2316.

Punctate inner choroiditis

Punctate inner choroiditis (PIC) is an idiopathic multifocal chorioretinopathy of the outer retina, RPE, and inner choroid that predominantly affects women with myopia. The median age at disease onset is approximately 30 years.

Manifestations Patients with PIC present with metamorphopsia, paracentral scotomas, photopsias, and vision loss. The disease is usually bilateral but often asymmetric. The yellow-white spots of PIC are typically smaller (100–300 μm) than those of MFCPU and are mostly confined to the posterior pole (Fig 9-14). Although inactive lesions may be very subtle on clinical examination, some transition to well-defined, atrophic, variably hyperpigmented chorioretinal scars. In addition, patients with PIC are more likely than those with MFCPU to present with CNV, although they are less likely to have bilateral vision loss.

In patients with active inflammatory lesions of PIC, FA shows hypofluorescence or hyperfluorescence in the early phase and subsequently displays late staining (Fig 9-15). Inactive lesions show transmission hyperfluorescence. CNV produces a zone of early hyperfluorescence, often with a surrounding zone of hypofluorescence. On ICGA, active and inactive lesions are hypocyanescent; during active inflammation, hypocyanescent lesions increase in size, and hypocyanescent mottling may be observed between lesions (see Fig 9-15). On FAF, PIC lesions are *hypo*autofluorescent; when active, they may show a subtle increase in size and/or develop a *hyper*autofluorescent border or halo that recedes as activity resolves.

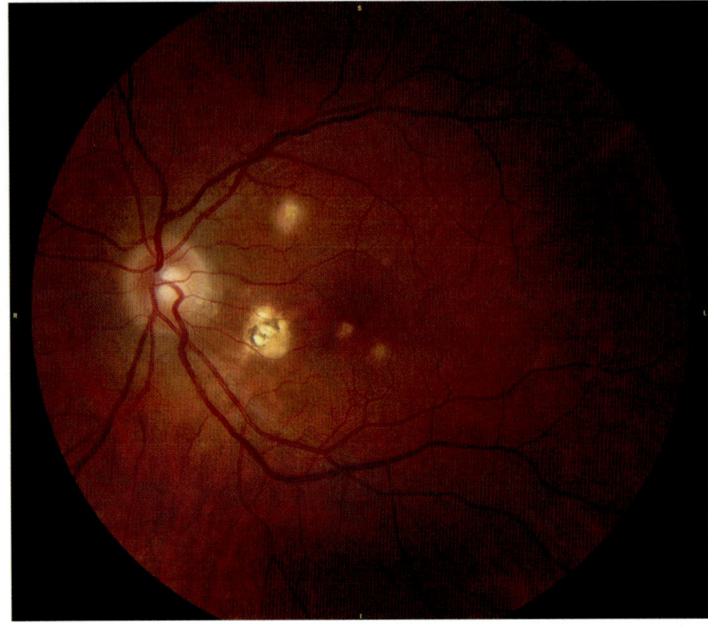

Figure 9-14 Fundus photograph showing punctate inner choroiditis. *(Courtesy of Wendy M. Smith, MD.)*

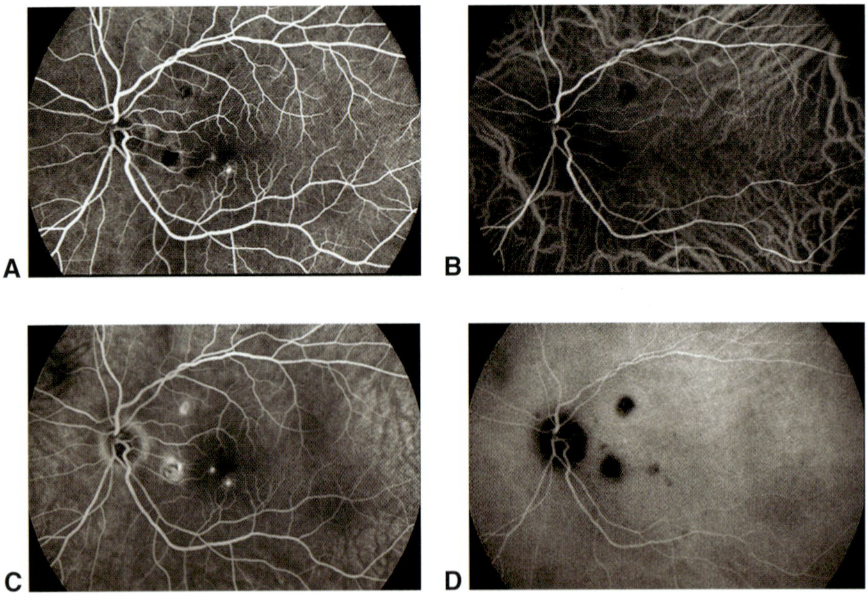

Figure 9-15 Punctate inner choroiditis (PIC). Fluorescein angiograms demonstrating early hyperfluoresence **(A)** and late staining **(C)** of PIC lesions. Corresponding early **(B)** and late **(D)** ICG angiograms demonstrating multiple hypocyanescent spots. *(Courtesy of Wendy M. Smith, MD.)*

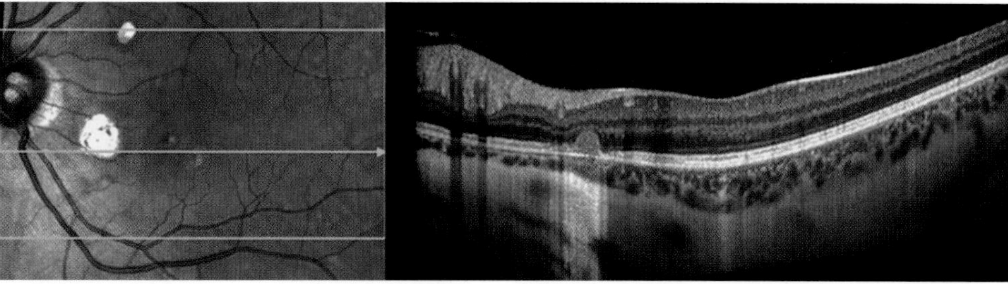

Figure 9-16 Punctate inner choroiditis. OCT scan through an active lesion. *(Courtesy of Wendy M. Smith, MD.)*

OCT of an early, active PIC lesion shows focal hyperreflective elevation of the RPE, often with disruption of the overlying outer retina. The lesion may break through the RPE and form a hump-shaped nodule beneath the outer plexiform layer (Fig 9-16). As the acute lesion regresses, OCT shows tissue loss within the outer retina and inner choroid. A focal choroidal excavation may develop, with V-shaped herniation of the outer plexiform layer and inner retina into the choroid. Active CNV lesions have associated subretinal and intraretinal fluid on OCT. OCT angiography may also help identify CNV lesions.

Ahnood D, Madhusudhan S, Tsaloumas MD, Waheed NK, Keane PA, Denniston AK. Punctate inner choroidopathy: a review. *Surv Ophthalmol.* 2017;62(2):113–126.

Kim H, Woo SJ, Kim Y-K, Lee SC, Lee CS. Focal choroidal excavation in multifocal choroiditis and punctate inner choroidopathy. *Ophthalmology.* 2015;122(7):1534–1535.

Levison AL, Baynes KM, Lowder CY, Kaiser PK, Srivastava SK. Choroidal neovascularisation on optical coherence tomography angiography in punctate inner choroidopathy and multifocal choroiditis. *Br J Ophthalmol.* 2017;101(5):616–622.

Spaide RF, Goldberg N, Freund KB. Redefining multifocal choroiditis and panuveitis and punctate inner choroidopathy through multimodal imaging. *Retina.* 2013;33(7): 1315–1324.

Treatment In some cases, active PIC lesions may regress without anti-inflammatory therapy, and treatment may be limited to intermittent intravitreal anti-VEGF. Indications for corticosteroids and/or systemic IMT include new or persistently active inflammatory lesions in vision-threatening locations or incomplete response to intravitreal anti-VEGF therapy. When inflammatory activity in PIC is controlled with systemic IMT, retinal function and visual acuity may improve even in the presence of perifoveal CNV.

Subretinal fibrosis and uveitis syndrome

Subretinal fibrosis and uveitis (SFU) syndrome is an extremely rare idiopathic panuveitis that has been described in otherwise healthy 20- to 40-year-old women with myopia.

Manifestations and differential diagnosis SFU syndrome is typically bilateral with high-grade anterior chamber inflammation and mild to moderate vitritis. Acute lesions resemble those of early MFCPU: white-yellow lesions (50–500 μm) at the level of the RPE, located from the posterior pole to the midperiphery. Acute lesions may fade with minimal RPE disruption, become atrophic, or coalesce to form multiple large areas of subretinal fibrosis

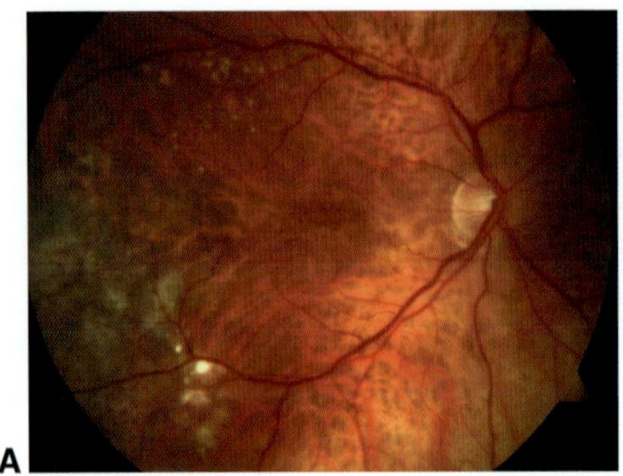

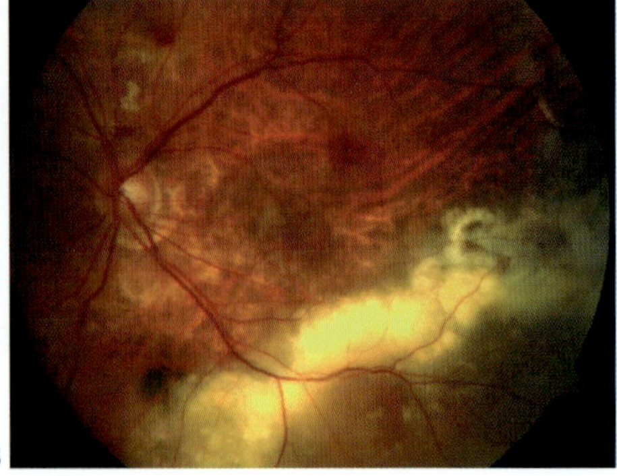

Figure 9-17 Subretinal fibrosis and uveitis syndrome. **A,** Right eye, with white-yellow lesions at the level of the RPE. **B,** Left eye, with confluent lesions signifying more advanced disease. *(Courtesy of Sam S. Dahr, MD, MS.)*

(Fig 9-17). Serous and hemorrhagic retinal detachment, macular edema, and CNV may also occur. Histologic studies reveal a lymphocytic granulomatous infiltration of the choroid with marked gliosis of the retina and subretinal fibrosis, suggesting immune-mediated destruction of the RPE and subsequent fibrosis.

Both FA and OCT are useful for diagnosing SFU. FA may show early alternating areas of blocked choroidal fluorescence and hyperfluorescence, with subsequent late staining, and OCT may show retinal edema, subretinal fluid, and subretinal fibrosis. The differential diagnosis of SFU includes syphilis, TB, sarcoidosis, APMPPE, ampiginous choroiditis, serpiginous choroiditis, sympathetic ophthalmia, toxoplasmosis, OHS, and pathologic myopia.

Treatment SFU may progress over months to years. The prognosis is guarded, but early and aggressive intervention with IMT may slow or stop progression. In recent reports, biologic agents such as rituximab have shown some efficacy in treating SFU.

Adán A, Sanmarti R, Burés A, Casaroli-Marano RP. Successful treatment with infliximab in a patient with diffuse subretinal fibrosis syndrome. *Am J Ophthalmol.* 2007;143(3):533–534.

Cornish KS, Kuffova L, Forrester JV. Treatment of diffuse subretinal fibrosis uveitis with rituximab. *Br J Ophthalmol.* 2015;99(2):153–154.

Kim MK, Chan CC, Belfort R Jr, et al. Histopathologic and immunohistopathologic features of subretinal fibrosis and uveitis syndrome. *Am J Ophthalmol.* 1987;104(1):15–23.

Multiple Evanescent White Dot Syndrome

Multiple evanescent white dot syndrome (MEWDS) is a rare idiopathic posterior uveitis that affects the outer retina and RPE. The typical patient is a young female (mean age at onset, 28 years) with moderate myopia. Patients may report a preceding viral illness.

Manifestations

Presenting symptoms include photopsias, paracentral scotoma, and decreased vision that may be as poor as 20/200. A relative pupillary afferent defect may also be observed.

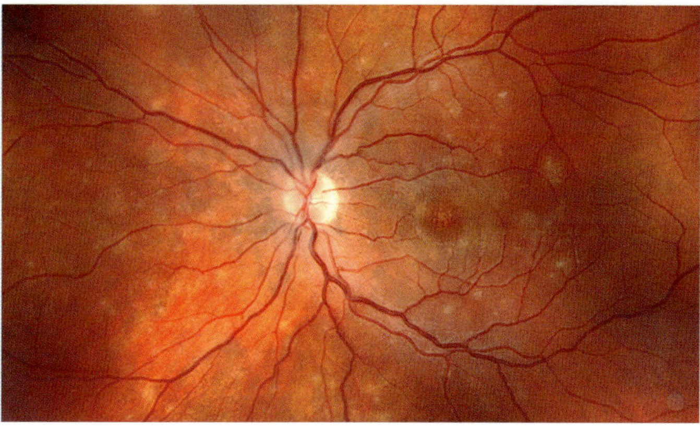

Figure 9-18 Multiple evanescent white dot syndrome. Fundus photograph shows multiple discrete, punctate, yellowish perifoveal dots. *(Courtesy of Wendy M. Smith, MD.)*

Examination may show discrete, white-to-orange spots (100–200 μm) at the deep retina or RPE (Fig 9-18). These lesions, which are transitory and may be subtle, are typically perifoveal and peripapillary, but they may also extend to the periphery. The fovea often has a granular, stippled appearance, termed *peau d'orange.* This appearance may persist even after the retinal lesions have faded. Anterior segment inflammation is minimal or absent, and mild degrees of vitreous cell, optic nerve edema, and vascular sheathing may be present. The lesions and foveal granularity usually resolve over several weeks as vision recovers.

MEWDS lesions are often described as *wreathlike.* For example, when the late-staining punctate hyperfluorescent lesions (Fig 9-19) are viewed under high magnification on FA, the individual lesions look like tiny "wreaths," consistent with the original description of this entity in the literature. In addition, the lesions are often arranged in a wreathlike configuration within the posterior pole. Even when the lesions are very subtle or have resolved on clinical examination, they may still be visualized on FAF (hyperautofluorescence; Fig 9-20) and ICGA (hypocyanescent; see Fig 9-19). ICGA also shows areas of hypocyanescence that are larger and more numerous than the hyperfluorescent lesions seen on FA.

Visual field abnormalities include generalized depression, paracentral or peripheral scotomas, and/or an enlarged blind spot. ERG reveals diminished a-wave and early receptor potential amplitudes, both of which are reversible. Multifocal ERG and electro-oculogram (EOG) localize the disease to the RPE–photoreceptor complex, not the choroid. OCT through the lesions shows photoreceptor inner/outer segment line hyperreflectivity and/or disruption, which also resolves over time (Fig 9-21). In addition, the foveal granularity corresponds to outer retinal structure disruption, and reconstitution of the retinal structures correlates with improvement in vision.

Papasavvas I, Mantovani A, Tugal-Tutkun I, Herbort CP Jr. Multiple evanescent white dot syndrome (MEWDS): update on practical appraisal, diagnosis and clinicopathology; a review and an alternative comprehensive perspective. *J Ophthalmic Inflamm Infect.* 2021; 11(1):45.

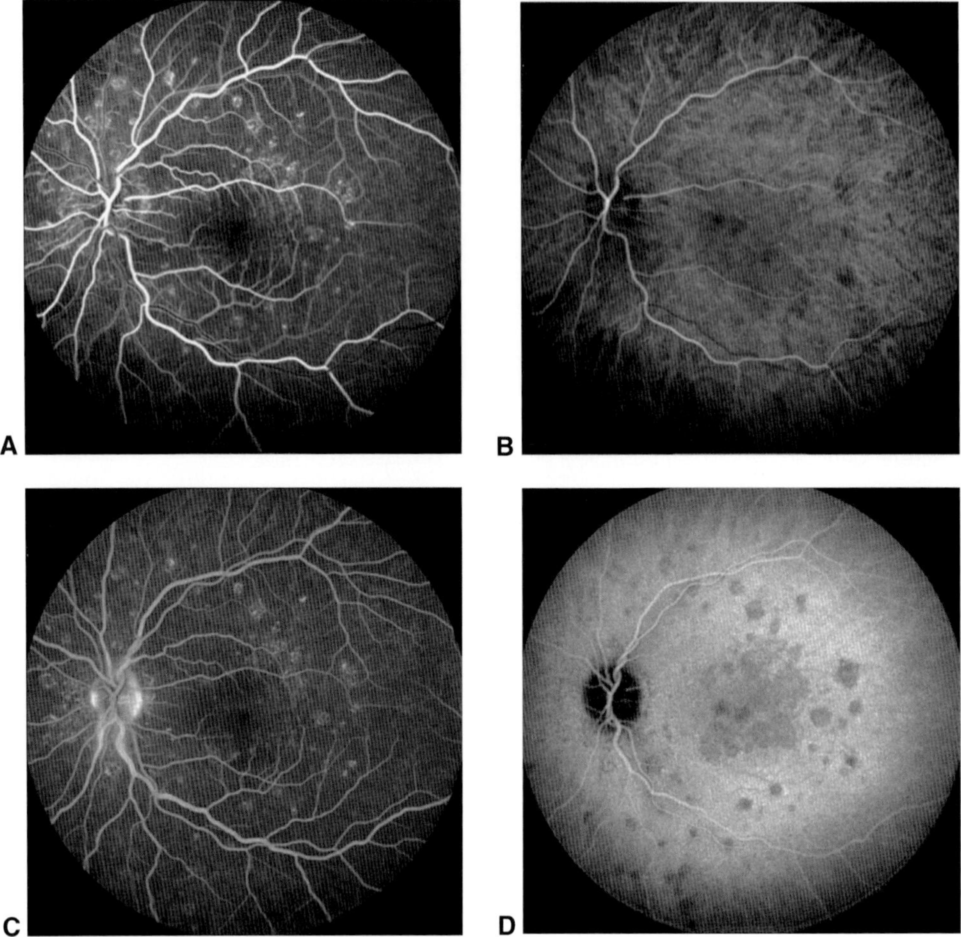

Figure 9-19 Multiple evanescent white dot syndrome (MEWDS). Fluorescein angiograms demonstrating early hyperfluoresence **(A)** and late staining **(C)** of MEWDS lesions. Corresponding early **(B)** and late **(D)** ICG angiograms demonstrating multiple hypocyanescent lesions. *(Courtesy of Wendy M. Smith, MD.)*

Prognosis

No treatment is usually required for MEWDS. After 1 to 2 months, vision typically returns to baseline, and imaging abnormalities mostly resolve, although residual photopsias and blind-spot enlargement may persist for months. Recurrences are rare. When central macular involvement is substantial or multiple recurrences occur, local or systemic treatment or an alternative diagnosis may be considered.

Disease associations

MEWDS has been associated with MFCPU, acute zonal occult outer retinopathy, and acute macular neuroretinopathy (AMN). AMN was previously considered a white dot syndrome because the demographics and symptoms of affected patients matched those of the syndrome. However, multimodal imaging techniques suggest that AMN is a microvascular event in the

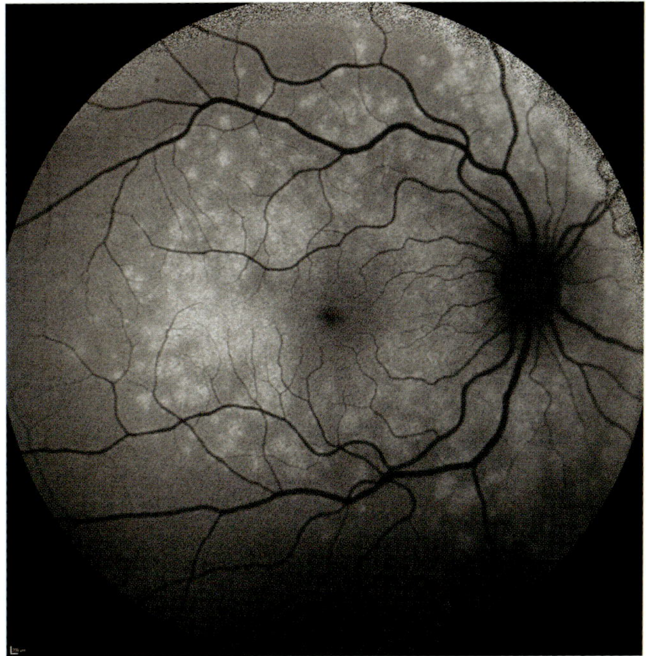

Figure 9-20 Multiple evanescent white dot syndrome. FAF image shows multiple hyperautofluorescent spots. *(Courtesy of Bryn M. Burkholder, MD.)*

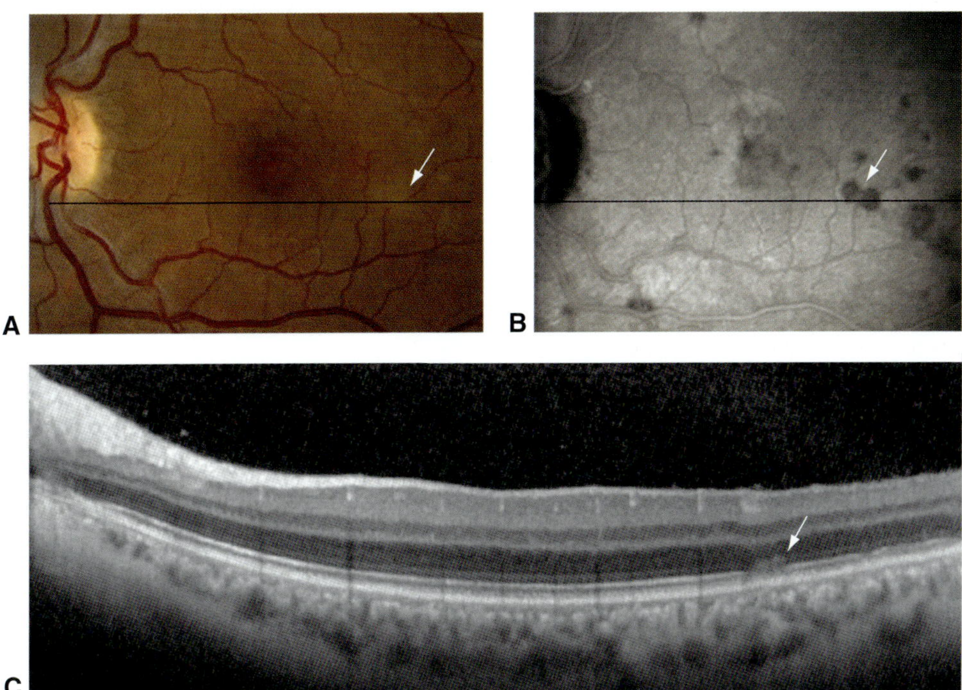

Figure 9-21 Multiple evanescent white dot syndrome. **A,** Color fundus photograph shows subtle spots *(arrow)* and foveal granularity. **B,** ICG angiogram shows more spots *(arrow)* than are apparent on the color photograph. **C,** OCT of the spots (positioned at horizontal lines in **A** and **B**) shows disruption of the inner/outer segment line (ellipsoid zone) *(arrow)*. *(Courtesy of Janet L. Davis, MD, and Charles Wycoff, MD.)*

deep capillary plexus of the macula, not a primary inflammatory process. See BCSC Section 12, *Retina and Vitreous*, for further discussion about AMN.

Acute Retinal Pigment Epitheliitis

Acute retinal pigment epitheliitis (ARPE), or Krill disease, is a benign, self-limited inflammation of the RPE with acute onset. ARPE is one of the rarest white dot syndromes. Males and females are affected equally. Affected individuals aged 15–40 years present with vision loss, central metamorphopsia, and scotomas, usually unilaterally (75%). The lesions resolve spontaneously over 6–12 weeks, so patients are usually observed without treatment. The visual prognosis is good.

Manifestations

In patients with ARPE, clusters of small dark-gray or black spots (100–200 μm) with a yellow halo or rim appear in the deep retina, within the posterior pole. Over time, the halo disappears, and pigment clumping may develop. There is mild or no vitritis. FA performed soon after initial onset shows central hypofluorescence of the lesions with a lacy hyperfluorescent rim that creates a honeycomb effect (Fig 9-22). Older lesions may show early and late fluorescein hyperfluorescence without leakage. FAF findings are variable, but hyperautofluorescent lesions are often depicted. ICGA shows early- and mid-phase patchy macular hypercyanescence and a late hypercyanescent halo in the macula. OCT shows transient disruption of the ellipsoid zone and the inner layer of the RPE. Visual field testing reveals a central scotoma. An abnormal EOG after a normal ERG suggests that the disease originated within the RPE.

Baillif S, Wolff B, Paoli V, Gastaud P, Mauget-Faÿsse M. Retinal fluorescein and indocyanine green angiography and spectral-domain optical coherence tomography findings in acute retinal pigment epitheliitis. *Retina.* 2011;31(6):1156–1163.

Cho HJ, Han SY, Cho SW, et al. Acute retinal pigment epitheliitis: spectral-domain optical coherence tomography findings in 18 cases. *Invest Ophthalmol Vis Sci.* 2014;55(5): 3314–3319.

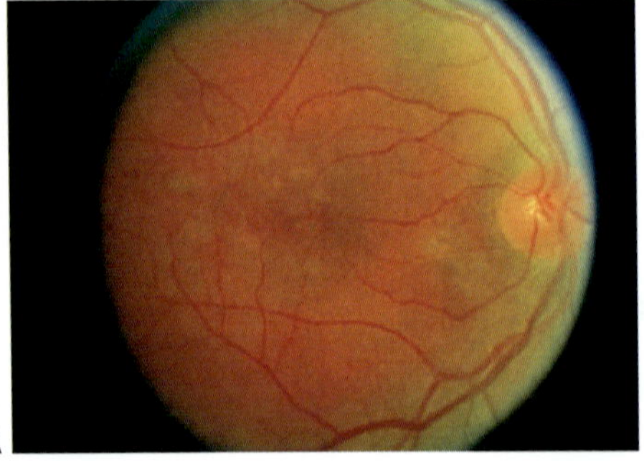

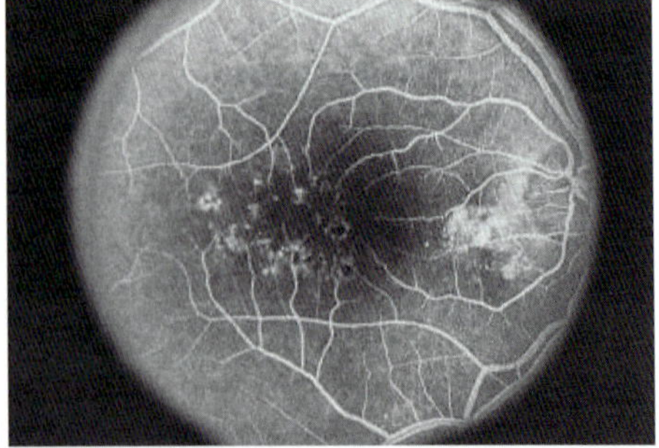

Figure 9-22 Acute retinal pigment epitheliitis. **A,** Fundus photograph shows small yellow-gray lesions in the deep retina. **B,** FA demonstrates honeycomb lesions at the level of the RPE. *(Courtesy of E. Mitchel Opremcak, MD.)*

Acute Zonal Occult Outer Retinopathy

Acute zonal occult outer retinopathy (AZOOR) is an inflammatory outer retinal degeneration that often presents with a clinically normal-appearing fundus. Photopsias are usually prominent and are described as pulsations, windmills, bubbles, sprays, or sparkles. The mean age at disease onset is 37 years, and 76% of patients are female. Diagnosis is often delayed, however, because findings on clinical examination are limited in early disease. At presentation, the disease is commonly unilateral, but fellow eye involvement eventually develops in most cases. Early in the disease, the differential diagnosis of AZOOR includes optic neuritis, optic nerve compressive lesion, a pituitary or intracranial tumor, and paraneoplastic and nonparaneoplastic autoimmune retinopathy. The differential diagnosis also includes MEWDS, DUSN, and inherited retinal degenerations.

Manifestations

In the initial stage of AZOOR, visual acuity is good. Anterior segment inflammation is absent, and mild vitreous cells may occur. The fundus examination is grossly unremarkable at presentation, but eventually a white annular ring (diameter, 3–5 mm) involving the outer retina and centered on the optic disc may be visualized. Later, islands of subtle RPE granularity and/or depigmentation develop in the posterior and midzones of the fundus, sometimes with vessel attenuation or sheathing (Fig 9-23A). FAF shows hypoautofluorescence in zones of RPE and choriocapillary atrophy. Persistent or progressive activity at the lesion border may be hyperautofluorescent secondary to lipofuscin-laden cells that precede RPE cell death (Fig 9-23B). In addition, areas of subacute disease activity may show speckled hyperautofluorescence that evolves into hypoautofluorescence as atrophic changes develop.

Early in the disease, findings on FA are usually normal, but eventually the affected RPE is highlighted as hyperfluorescent window defects. OCT of the involved zones demonstrates

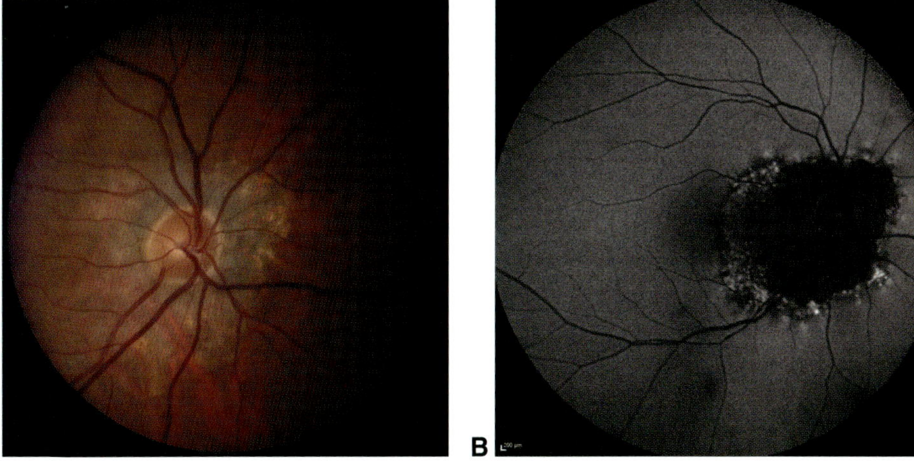

Figure 9-23 Acute zonal occult outer retinopathy. **A,** Fundus photograph demonstrates peripapillary atrophy of the RPE and choriocapillaris. **B,** FAF shows a broad area of peripapillary hypoautofluorescence with a stippled hyperautofluorescent border. *(Courtesy of Bryn M. Burkholder, MD.)*

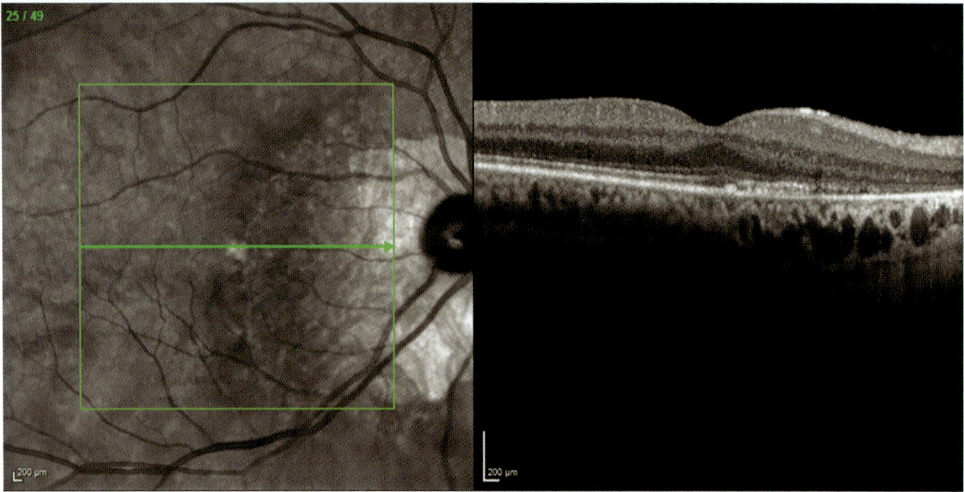

Figure 9-24 Acute zonal occult outer retinopathy. OCT image from the patient in Figure 9-23 demonstrates loss of the peripapillary ellipsoid zone. *(Courtesy of Bryn M. Burkholder, MD.)*

areas of ellipsoid zone loss or irregularity (Fig 9-24). ERG shows dysfunction at both the photoreceptor–RPE complex and the inner retina, including a delayed 30-Hz flicker ERG and a reduction in the EOG light rise. Visual field deficits correspond to the zone of affected retina and may manifest as central, arcuate, or ring scotoma; horizontal or vertical hemianopias; or any combination of these.

Prognosis and treatment

AZOOR evolves over months to years, but visual field loss often stabilizes in approximately 75% of patients. A large case review of long-term outcomes suggests that 68% of eyes retained 20/40 or better vision, but 27% developed 20/200 vision or worse. It is unclear whether treatment with systemic corticosteroids or IMT alters the disease course or visual outcome. However, for a patient with progressive RPE or visual field loss, long-term IMT and/or extended-duration steroid implants may be considered.

Francis PJ, Marinescu A, Fitzke FW, Bird AC, Holder GE. Acute zonal occult outer retinopathy: towards a set of diagnostic criteria. *Br J Ophthalmol.* 2005;89(1):70–73.

Gass JD, Agarwal A, Scott IU. Acute zonal occult outer retinopathy: a long-term follow-up study. *Am J Ophthalmol.* 2002;134(3):329–339.

Monson DM, Smith JR. Acute zonal occult outer retinopathy. *Surv Ophthalmol.* 2011; 56(1):23–35.

Mrejen S, Khan S, Gallego-Pinazo R, Jampol LM, Yannuzzi LA. Acute zonal occult outer retinopathy: a classification based on multimodal imaging. *JAMA Ophthalmol.* 2014;132(9):1089–1098.

Acute Idiopathic Maculopathy

Acute idiopathic maculopathy (AIM) is typically a unilateral disease (unilateral AIM) that presents with acute central vision loss (ie, 20/200) associated with macular subretinal fluid. Patients are typically aged 20–40 years and may have a viral prodrome. Some patients concurrently experience hand-foot-and-mouth disease, which is linked to coxsackievirus. Adult patients with AIM may also have a history of exposure to a child with hand-foot-and-mouth disease.

Manifestations and differential diagnosis

Clinical examination of a patient with suspected AIM is notable for turbid yellow subretinal fluid in the macula (Fig 9-25A). The underlying RPE may appear yellow-white-gray and thickened. Minimal intraretinal hemorrhages may also be present, and anterior chamber and vitreous cells are minimal or absent. OCT shows subretinal fluid with hyperreflective debris in the subretinal space (Fig 9-25B). FA of the central lesion shows early hypofluorescence or hyperfluorescence followed by late stippled hyperfluorescent staining of the RPE and pooling of dye in the subretinal space (Fig 9-25C, D). ICGA of the lesion is hypocyanescent.

The differential diagnosis of AIM includes central serous chorioretinopathy, choroidal infarction, CNV, Vogt-Koyanagi-Harada syndrome, sympathetic ophthalmia, serpiginous choroiditis, APMPPE, posterior scleritis, and syphilis.

Prognosis and treatment

The prognosis is variable based on the degree of RPE damage. Macular subretinal fluid typically resolves spontaneously and fairly rapidly. After lesion resolution, residual RPE hypopigmentation and granularity within the macula or a bull's-eye RPE pattern of central

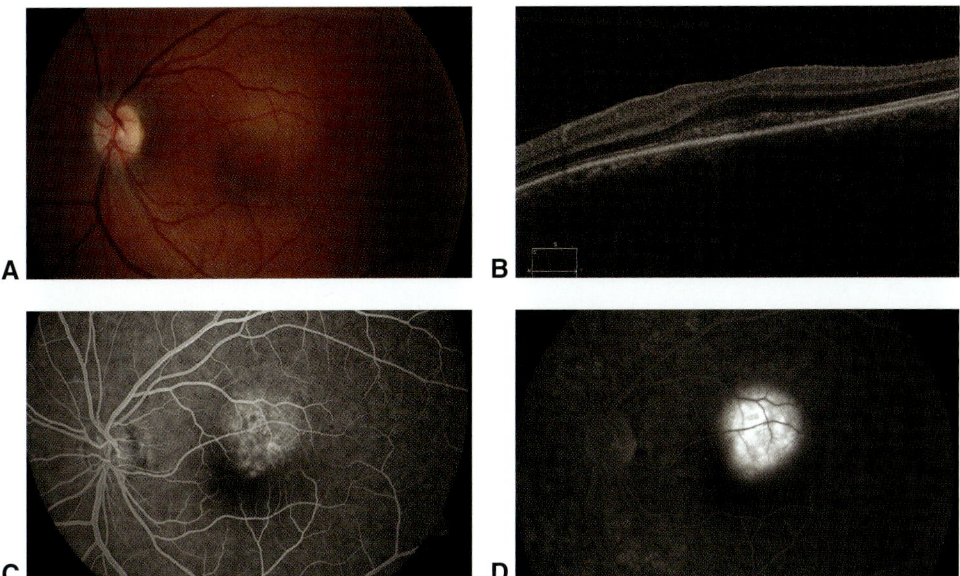

Figure 9-25 Images from a 27-year-old woman with unilateral acute idiopathic maculopathy. **A,** Color fundus photograph shows grayish-yellow discoloration of the RPE. **B,** OCT shows shallow subretinal fluid with hyperreflective material. **C,** FA shows a mixed pattern of early hypofluorescence and hyperfluorescence. **D,** Late FA shows RPE staining and pooling within the neurosensory detachment. *(Courtesy of Sam S. Dahr, MD, MS.)*

hyperpigmentation surrounded by hypopigmentation is typically seen. If subfoveal RPE degeneration or CNV develops, the visual outcome may be poor. Patients are usually monitored without therapy, although oral corticosteroids may be considered in patients with significant vision loss or slow lesion resolution.

Pajtler Rosar A, Casalino G, Cozzi M, et al. Acute idiopathic maculopathy: a proposed disease staging based on multimodal imaging. *Retina*. 2021;41(12):2446–2455.

Autoimmune Retinopathy

Autoimmune retinopathy (AIR) is a rare, presumably immune-mediated retinal degeneration characterized by visual field deficits and photoreceptor dysfunction on ERG. Paraneoplastic AIR (pAIR) encompasses cancer-associated retinopathy (CAR) and melanoma-associated retinopathy (MAR). In contrast, nonparaneoplastic AIR (npAIR) occurs in the absence of any malignancy and is more common in females than in males (ratio 2:3), typically aged 40–60 years. Approximately 50% of patients with npAIR have a systemic autoimmune disease.

Manifestations

Autoimmune retinopathy presents with progressive, bilateral vision loss; photopsias; scotomas; dyschromatopsia; photoaversion; and nyctalopia. Ophthalmic examination may demonstrate normal findings initially, but vessel attenuation, RPE disruption, optic nerve pallor, and/or diffuse retinal atrophy may develop over time (Fig 9-26). Anterior chamber and vitreous inflammation is absent or very minimal. FA may show macular leakage, whereas OCT reveals macular thinning with ellipsoid zone disruption and thinned outer nuclear and photoreceptor layers (Fig 9-27). FAF may show a parafoveal ring of hyperautofluorescence.

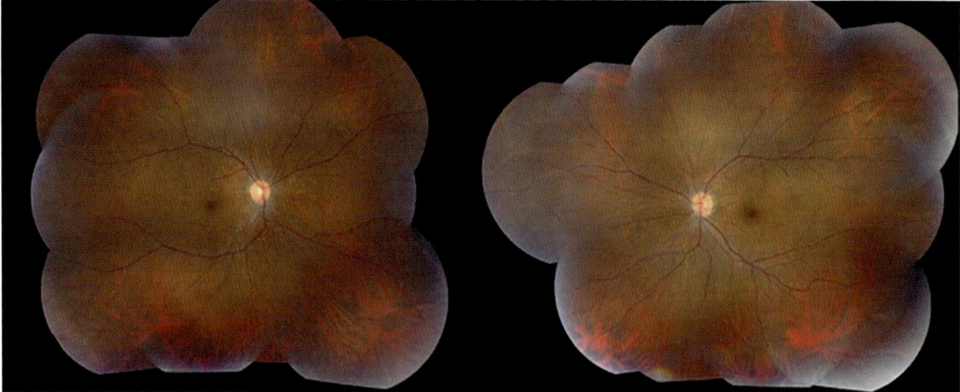

Figure 9-26 Nonparaneoplastic autoimmune retinopathy in a 39-year-old patient. The photographs show mild vascular attenuation, diminished foveal reflex, and mild optic nerve pallor. The electroretinogram (not shown) showed diminished cone and rod responses. *(Courtesy of H. Nida Sen, MD. Autoimmune retinopathy: current concepts and practices (an American Ophthalmological Society thesis).* Trans Am Ophthalmol Soc. *2017;115:T8(1–13). Published with permission of the American Ophthalmological Society.)*

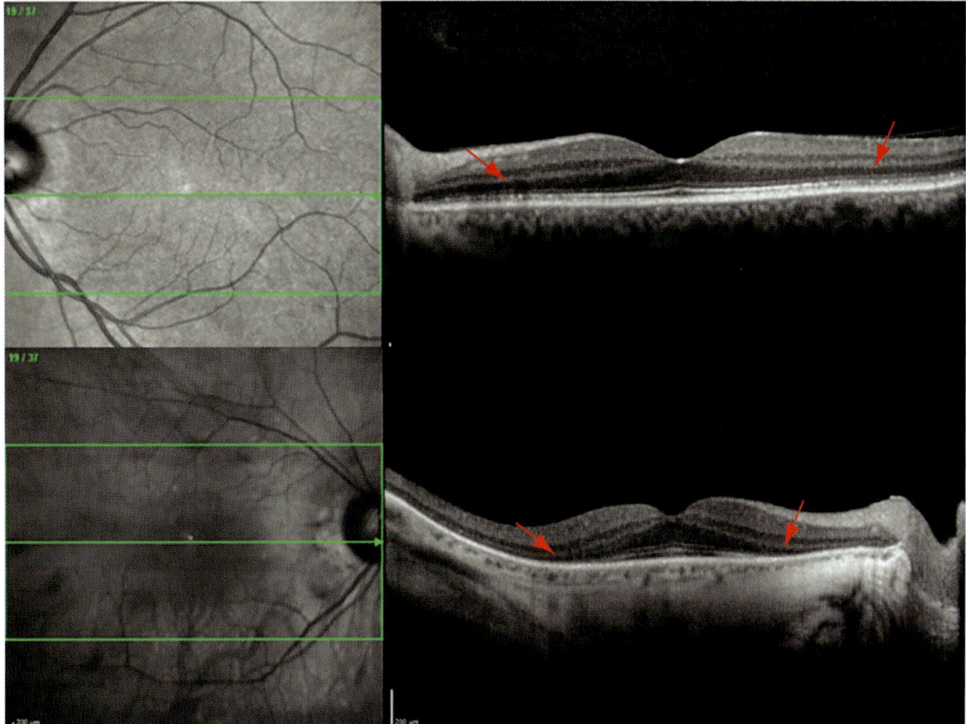

Figure 9-27 Optical coherence tomography images from 2 patients with nonparaneoplastic autoimmune retinopathy. *Top,* Patient with mild disruption of the photoreceptors *(red arrows). Bottom,* Patient with more severe photoreceptor loss *(red arrows). (Courtesy of H. Nida Sen, MD. Autoimmune retinopathy: current concepts and practices (an American Ophthalmological Society thesis).* Trans Am Ophthalmol Soc. *2017;115:T8(1–13). Published with permission of the American Ophthalmological Society.)*

Visual field changes include central scotoma, paracentral scotoma, or constricted fields. ERG findings may be markedly abnormal: In patients with CAR, cone responses are typically depressed, whereas in those with MAR, the photoreceptor response is normal followed by an attenuated b-wave, representing on-bipolar cell dysfunction.

Diagnosis

Diagnosis of AIR is challenging. Traditionally, the major biomarker in diagnosing and managing this disease has been the presence of serum anti-retinal antibodies (ARAs). However, recent research indicating a poor correlation between most serum ARAs and disease phenotype has raised questions about whether the antibodies are a cause or a consequence of retinal degeneration in AIR. Concerns have also arisen with detection of ARAs in healthy controls as well as in patients with systemic autoimmune disease, other uveitic entities such as BCR and AZOOR, age-related macular degeneration, and diabetic retinopathy. Conversely, there are reports of negative serum ARA test results in patients with clinical and ERG findings consistent with AIR. Further complicating diagnosis, techniques for detecting ARAs have not been standardized, leading to widely variable results between laboratories. Taken together, these findings have led many to conclude that the presence of serum ARAs cannot be automatically equated with the diagnosis of AIR.

Ultimately, the diagnosis of AIR is one of exclusion, with the following criteria warranting consideration:

- compatible symptoms
- positive serum ARA test results
- abnormal ERG results with or without visual field loss
- absence of overt (>1+ grade) intraocular inflammation
- absence of fundus findings or an alternative uveitic diagnosis that explains visual field or ERG loss
- absence of inherited retinal degeneration such as retinitis pigmentosa or cone dystrophy
- absence of malignancy (ie, to diagnose npAIR)

When pAIR is suspected, testing for the presence of anti-recoverin antibodies, which are strongly associated with CAR, can be considered. The most common CAR-associated malignancy is small cell lung cancer. Autoantibodies to transient receptor potential cation channel (TRMP1; expressed in both melanocytes and retinal on-bipolar cells) strongly support a diagnosis of MAR in a compatible clinical context. Nevertheless, the absence of these autoantibodies does not rule out pAIR. When there is strong clinical suspicion for pAIR, obtaining age-, sex-, and risk factor–appropriate cancer screenings may be most expeditious.

Treatment

In addition to uncertainty surrounding the diagnosis of AIR, treatment may also be challenging because the systemic and local strategies used for other types of ocular inflammation may not be as effective for AIR. For patients with npAIR, corticosteroids (local or systemic), conventional IMT, or biologic agents (ie, rituximab) may be considered. In patients with pAIR, therapy for the underlying malignancy is the first step in treatment; additional measures may include systemic or local corticosteroids, intravenous immunoglobulin, and/or plasmapheresis. Treatment response may be assessed with OCT, FAF, visual field evaluations, and ERG. Unfortunately, reversal of retinal damage is unlikely, although stabilization may be possible. See BCSC Section 5, *Neuro-Ophthalmology*, for additional discussion on AIR.

Adamus G. Are anti-retinal autoantibodies a cause or a consequence of retinal degeneration in autoimmune retinopathies? *Front Immunol.* 2018;9:765.

Chen JJ, McKeon A, Greenwood TM, et al. Clinical utility of antiretinal antibody testing. *JAMA Ophthalmol.* 2021;139(6):658–662.

Faez S, Loewenstein J, Sobrin L. Concordance of antiretinal antibody testing results between laboratories in autoimmune retinopathy. *JAMA Ophthalmol.* 2013;131(1):113–115.

Fox AR, Gordon LK, Heckenlively JR, et al. Consensus on the diagnosis and management of nonparaneoplastic autoimmune retinopathy using a modified Delphi approach. *Am J Ophthalmol.* 2016;168:183–190.

Sen HN, Grange L, Akanda M, Fox A. Autoimmune retinopathy: current concepts and practices (an American Ophthalmological Society thesis). *Trans Am Ophthalmol Soc.* 2018;115:T8(1–13).

CHAPTER 10

Posterior Uveitis and Panuveitis With Possible Systemic Manifestations

Highlights

- Posterior uveitis and panuveitis can be isolated to the eye(s), or they may be associated with systemic infectious or inflammatory disease.
- The diagnosis of many systemic inflammatory diseases (ie, systemic lupus erythematosus, Behçet disease, and Vogt-Koyanagi-Harada syndrome) is based on a combination of clinical findings, not a single diagnostic test.
- Diagnostic ambiguity within the noninfectious uveitic entities should not preclude or delay appropriate therapy once infectious uveitis has been ruled out.
- Many patients with noninfectious posterior uveitis or panuveitis require systemic immunomodulatory therapy (IMT), and systemic and/or local corticosteroids are used as a bridge while IMT takes effect. Further details of the approach to systemic treatment are discussed in Chapter 6.

Introduction

Posterior uveitis is defined as intraocular inflammation that involves primarily the retina and/or choroid. Occlusive retinal vasculitis is also classified as posterior uveitis. In panuveitis, inflammation is present in all anatomical compartments of the eye without a single dominant site. Chapter 9 discusses the white dot syndromes, a group of noninfectious posterior uveitis entities that typically have no associated systemic inflammatory disease. This chapter discusses types of posterior uveitis and panuveitis that can occur as an isolated ophthalmic disorder or may have a systemic disease association. Such diseases include systemic lupus erythematosus, polyarteritis nodosa, granulomatosis with polyangiitis (antineutrophil cytoplasmic antibodies–associated vasculitis), sarcoidosis, Vogt-Koyanagi-Harada (VKH) syndrome, and Behçet disease. Ocular disease may be the first clue to a systemic diagnosis. Because untreated systemic inflammation may result in major morbidity and even mortality, proper ophthalmic evaluation leading to appropriate and early diagnosis can positively affect patient outcomes. In some cases, diagnostic ambiguity may make it challenging to establish a specific uveitis diagnosis. As long as infectious causes have been sufficiently investigated, treatment should not be delayed because of the inability to make an exact diagnosis.

Posterior Uveitis With Possible Systemic Manifestations

Systemic Lupus Erythematosus

Systemic lupus erythematosus (SLE) is a multisystem inflammatory disorder that affects primarily women of childbearing age, with higher incidence among Black and Hispanic women in the United States. Although incompletely understood, SLE is considered an autoimmune disorder that features B-lymphocyte hyperactivity, polyclonal B-lymphocyte activation, hypergammaglobulinemia, autoantibody formation, and T-lymphocyte autoreactivity with immune complex deposition, leading to end-organ damage. Autoantibodies associated with SLE include antinuclear antibodies (ANAs), antibodies to both single- and double-stranded DNA, antibodies to cytoplasmic components (eg, anti-Sm, anti-Ro, and anti-La), and antiphospholipid antibodies.

SLE is a clinical diagnosis based on criteria established by the European League Against Rheumatism/American College of Rheumatology. According to the literature, the association between SLE and uveitis is low. Recent analysis of laboratory tests typically used for uveitis shows a low (4.4%) positive predictive value of ANA testing in the context of intraocular inflammation. Thus, ANA testing should be limited to patients with signs or symptoms suggestive of SLE or to patients with juvenile idiopathic arthritis (JIA), for whom such testing helps determine the risk of uveitis. See BCSC Section 1, *Update on General Medicine,* for diagnostic criteria for SLE and for more information on interpreting diagnostic and screening tests.

Aringer M, Costenbader K, Daikh D, et al. 2019 European League Against Rheumatism/American College of Rheumatology classification criteria for systemic lupus erythematosus. *Arthritis Rheumatol.* 2019;71(9):1400–1412.

McKay KM, Lim LL, Van Gelder RN. Rational laboratory testing in uveitis: a Bayesian analysis. *Surv Ophthalmol.* 2021;66(5):802–825.

Manifestations

Systemic manifestations of SLE include acute cutaneous diseases (eg, malar rash, discoid lupus, photosensitivity, and mucosal lesions) in approximately 70%–80% of patients, arthritis in 80%–85%, renal disease in 50%–75%, Raynaud phenomenon in 30%–50%, and neurologic involvement in 35%. Cardiac, pulmonary, hepatic, and hematologic abnormalities may also develop.

Ocular manifestations occur in 50% of patients with SLE and include cutaneous lesions on the eyelids (discoid lupus erythematosus), secondary Sjögren syndrome, scleritis, cranial nerve palsies, optic neuropathy, and retinal and choroidal vasculopathy. As mentioned previously, uveitis is only rarely associated with SLE.

Lupus retinopathy (a non-uveitic marker for systemic SLE activity) is the most well-known posterior segment manifestation of SLE. Prevalence ranges from 3% among patients with mild systemic SLE to 29% among those with more active systemic disease. Fundamentally a vasculopathy, lupus retinopathy may produce cotton-wool spots and retinal nonperfusion (Fig 10-1) or infarction (Fig 10-2). In patients with lupus retinopathy, a hypercoagulable state caused by autoantibodies (rather than an inflammatory retinal vasculitis) provokes arterial and/or venous thrombosis. Although lupus retinopathy has similarities to hypertensive retinopathy secondary to SLE-induced hypertension and nephritis, the latter conditions may also result in arteriolar narrowing, retinal hemorrhage, and disc edema.

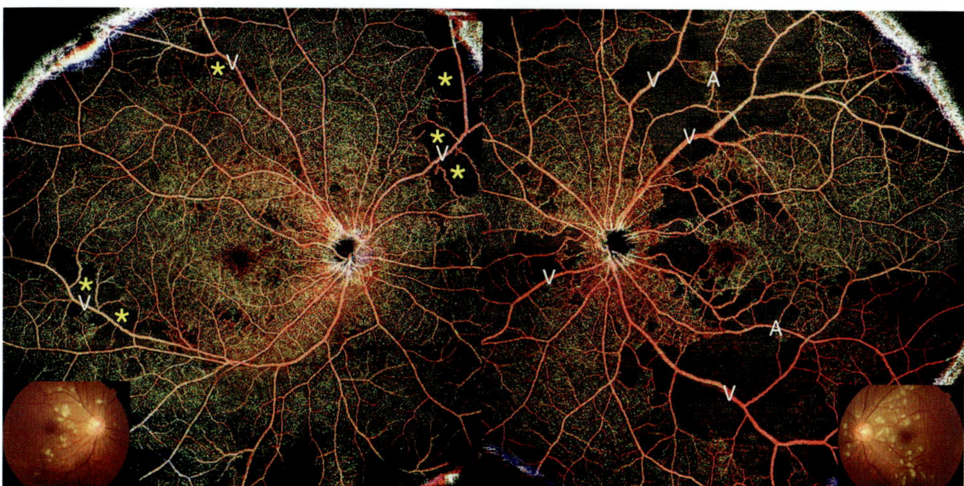

Figure 10-1 Systemic lupus erythematosus. Color fundus photographs *(lower left and right insets)* show multiple cotton-wool spots in both eyes. Optical coherence tomography (OCT) angiography shows multiple areas of capillary nonperfusion *(yellow asterisks)* associated with retinal veins *(V)* and arteries *(A)*. *(From Ishibashi T, Wakabayashi T, Nishida K. Purtscher-like retinopathy associated with systemic lupus erythematosus observed using wide-field OCT angiography.* Ophthalmol Retina. *2019;3(1):76.)*

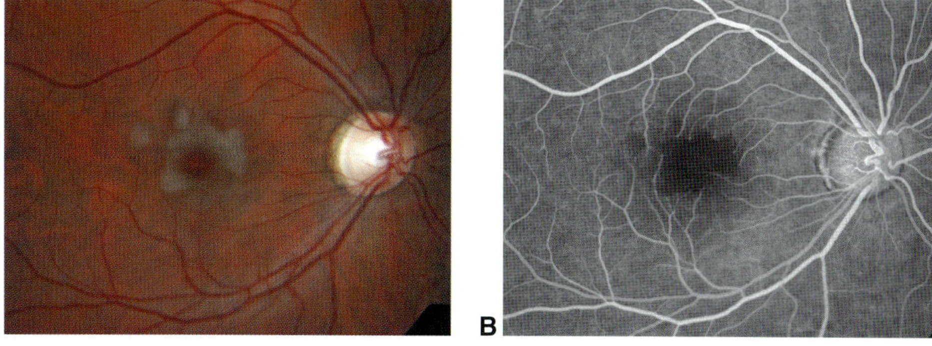

Figure 10-2 Systemic lupus erythematosus, initial presentation. **A,** Fundus photograph shows macular infarction in a 30-year-old woman who presented with diminished vision (counting fingers) and 1 week of myalgias. Laboratory test results were notable for positive antinuclear antibodies and double-stranded DNA. **B,** Early-phase fluorescein angiogram (FA). *(Courtesy of Sam S. Dahr, MD, MS.)*

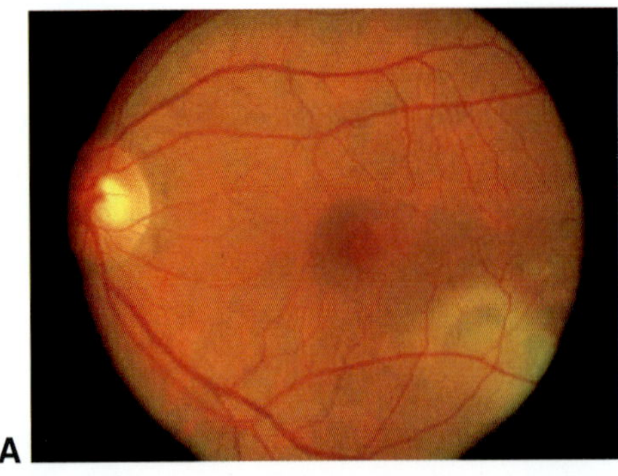

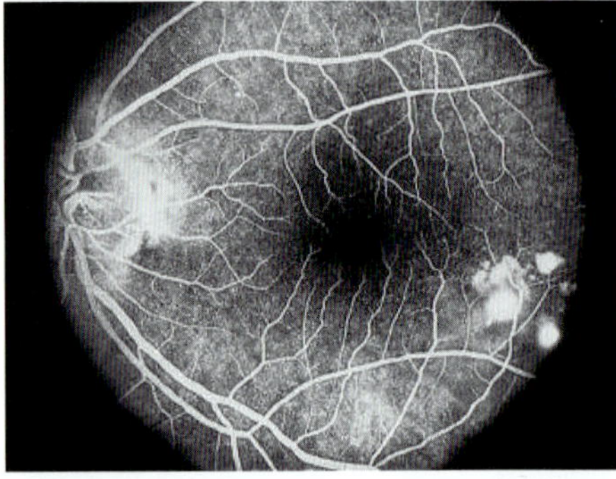

Figure 10-3 Systemic lupus erythematosus (SLE). **A,** Fundus photograph of multifocal choroiditis in a patient with SLE. **B,** FA showing multifocal areas of hyperfluorescence. *(Courtesy of E. Mitchel Opremcak, MD.)*

Retinal ischemia and nonperfusion may be extensive in lupus retinopathy, resulting in retinal neovascularization and vitreous hemorrhage. Severe retinal vascular occlusive disease can be associated with central nervous system (CNS) lupus and the presence of antiphospholipid antibodies (see BCSC Section 1, *Update on General Medicine,* for more information on antiphospholipid antibodies).

Autoantibodies associated with SLE also may trigger a *lupus choroidopathy* (Fig 10-3). Choroidal thrombosis may produce choroidal infarction, multifocal retinal pigment epithelium (RPE) detachments, and subretinal fluid.

Jabs DA, Fine SL, Hochberg MC, Newman SA, Heiner GG, Stevens MB. Severe retinal vaso-occlusive disease in systemic lupus erythematosus. *Arch Ophthalmol.* 1986;104(4):558–563.

Nguyen QD, Uy HS, Akpek EK, Harper SL, Zacks DN, Foster CS. Choroidopathy of systemic lupus erythematosus. *Lupus.* 2000;9(4):288–298.

Papagiannuli E, Rhodes B, Wallace GR, Gordon C, Murray PI, Denniston AK. Systemic lupus erythematosus: an update for ophthalmologists. *Surv Ophthalmol.* 2016;61(1):65–82.

Treatment

Management of ophthalmic SLE focuses on treating the underlying systemic disease, which may involve corticosteroids and immunomodulatory therapy (IMT), including hydroxychloroquine. Patients with severe vaso-occlusive disease or antiphospholipid antibodies may require antiplatelet therapy or systemic anticoagulation, whereas those with severe sight-threatening disease may require aggressive therapy with intravenous immunoglobulin, cyclophosphamide, and/or plasma exchange. Ischemic complications, including proliferative retinopathy and vitreous hemorrhage, can be managed with panretinal photocoagulation, intravitreal anti–vascular endothelial growth factor, and vitrectomy.

Patients taking hydroxychloroquine should be counseled on the need for regular ophthalmic examinations to screen for retinal toxicity. For further information, see BCSC Section 12, *Retina and Vitreous.*

Rosenbaum JT, Costenbader KH, Desmarais J, et al. American College of Rheumatology, American Academy of Dermatology, Rheumatologic Dermatology Society, and American Academy of Ophthalmology 2020 joint statement on hydroxychloroquine use with respect to retinal toxicity. *Arthritis Rheumatol.* 2021;73(6):908–911.

Polyarteritis Nodosa

Polyarteritis nodosa (PAN) is a rare systemic vasculitis (annual incidence, 0.7 per 100,000 individuals) that involves subacute or chronic focal, necrotizing inflammation of medium-sized and small arteries. The disease affects patients aged 40 to 60 years and occurs 1.5 times more frequently in men than in women. Hepatitis B and hepatitis C infection may play a pathogenic role in some cases of PAN, but most cases are idiopathic.

Manifestations and diagnosis

PAN vasculitis may affect multiple organ systems but characteristically spares the lungs. Skin features include subcutaneous nodules, purpura, livedo reticularis, and Raynaud phenomenon. Mononeuropathy multiplex with motor and sensory deficits affects up to 70% of patients. In approximately one-third of patients, kidney disease causes secondary hypertension. Gastrointestinal disease may result in small bowel ischemia and infarction, and cardiac manifestations include coronary arteritis and pericarditis.

Ocular involvement occurs in up to 20% of patients with PAN, with varying posterior segment manifestations. Retinal vasculitis may provoke amaurosis fugax or branch or central retinal artery occlusion (Fig 10-4). Choroidal or posterior ciliary artery vasculitis may cause lobular choroidal ischemia and infarcts, initially presenting as exudative retinal detachments and later resulting in *Elschnig spots* (focal areas of choroidal hyperpigmentation with margins of hypopigmentation; see BCSC Section 12, *Retina and Vitreous*). Systemic hypertension associated with kidney disease may cause hypertensive retinopathy. Neuro-ophthalmic manifestations include cranial nerve palsies, homonymous hemianopia, Horner syndrome, and ischemic optic neuropathy. In addition, scleral inflammatory diseases of all types, including necrotizing and posterior scleritis, have been reported. Peripheral ulcerative keratitis, often accompanied by scleritis, may be an early manifestation of PAN.

There is no definitive laboratory test for PAN, so laboratory evaluation is directed at ruling out other causes of systemic vasculitis. Unlike granulomatosis with polyangiitis (GPA; previously known as *Wegener granulomatosis*), PAN is *not* associated with antineutrophil

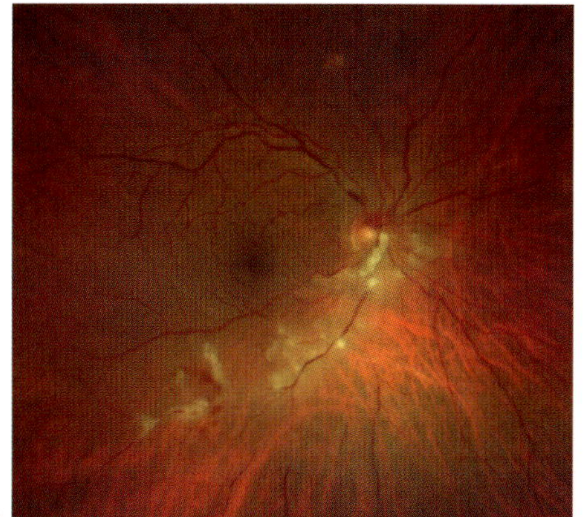

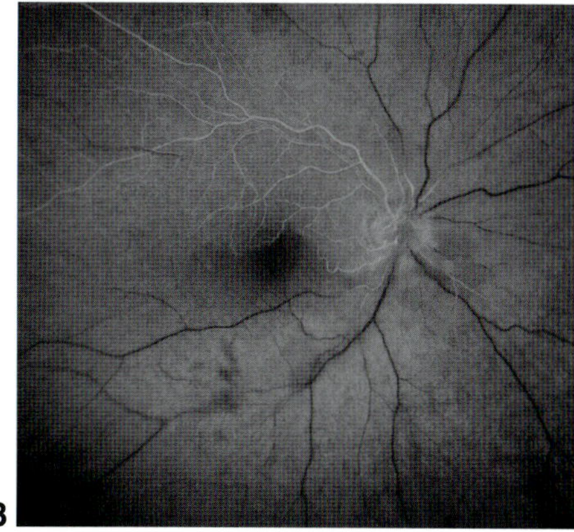

Figure 10-4 Polyarteritis nodosa. **A,** Fundus photograph indicates retinal vasculitis associated with vascular sheathing and intraretinal hemorrhage. **B,** Early-phase FA shows retinal infarction due to a hemiretinal artery occlusion. *(Courtesy of Sam S. Dahr, MD, MS.)*

cytoplasmic antibodies (ANCAs). The tissue biopsy (often skin or kidney) result may be confirmatory, but often the diagnosis is clinical and based on the presence of at least 3 of the following 10 criteria:

- weight loss >4 kg
- livedo reticularis
- testicular pain or tenderness
- diffuse myalgias (excluding shoulder and hip girdle) or weakness of muscles or tenderness of leg muscles
- development of mononeuropathy or multiple mononeuropathies or polyneuropathy
- development of hypertension with diastolic blood pressure >90 mm Hg
- elevation of blood urea nitrogen level >40 mg/dL or creatinine value >1.5 mg/dL, not due to dehydration or obstruction
- presence of hepatitis B surface antigen or antibody in the serum
- arteriogram showing aneurysms or occlusions of the visceral arteries, not due to arteriosclerosis, fibromuscular dysplasia, or other noninflammatory causes
- biopsy of small or medium-sized artery showing the presence of granulocytes or granulocytes and mononuclear leukocytes in the artery wall

Hočevar A, Tomšič M, Perdan Pirkmajer K. Clinical approach to diagnosis and therapy of polyarteritis nodosa. *Curr Rheumatol Rep.* 2021;23(3):14. doi:10.1007/s11926-021-00983-2

Rothschild PR, Pagnoux C, Seror R, Brézin AP, Delair E, Guillevin L. Ophthalmologic manifestations of systemic necrotizing vasculitides at diagnosis: a retrospective study of 1286 patients and review of the literature. *Semin Arthritis Rheum.* 2013;42(5):507–514.

Treatment and prognosis

Mortality secondary to renal failure or mesenteric, cerebral, or cardiac infarction is common in PAN. In patients with untreated PAN, the 5-year survival rate is 13%; however, with treatment, the rate improves to 80%. Treatment usually includes systemic corticosteroids and IMT, typically cyclophosphamide. PAN should be considered in the differential diagnosis of ANCA-negative retinal vasculitis because appropriate diagnosis and management can be lifesaving.

Gayraud M, Guillevin L, le Toumelin P, et al; French Vasculitis Study Group. Long-term follow-up of polyarteritis nodosa, microscopic polyangiitis, and Churg-Strauss syndrome: analysis of four prospective trials including 278 patients. *Arthritis Rheum.* 2001;44(3):666–675.

Pagnoux C, Mendel A. Treatment of systemic necrotizing vasculitides: recent advances and important clinical considerations. *Expert Rev Clin Immunol.* 2019;15(9):939–949.

Granulomatosis With Polyangiitis and Microscopic Polyangiitis

Granulomatosis with polyangiitis (GPA) is a multisystem inflammatory disorder that features the following classic triad:

- necrotizing granulomatous vasculitis of the upper and lower respiratory tract
- focal segmental glomerulonephritis
- necrotizing vasculitis of small arteries and veins

Paranasal sinus involvement is the most characteristic clinical feature of GPA, followed by pulmonary and renal disease. Glomerulonephritis eventually develops in 85% of patients and is a high risk for mortality, so early disease detection is important.

Like GPA, *microscopic polyangiitis (MPA)* is an ANCA-associated vasculitis. MPA and GPA may have similar clinical features, but biopsy specimens from patients with MPA lack granulomatous findings. In addition, MPA is associated with ANCA directed against myeloperoxidase (MPO; see the section "Diagnosis"), whereas GPA is usually associated with an elevated level of ANCA directed against proteinase 3 (PR3). Ophthalmic involvement is also less common in MPA than in GPA.

Manifestations

Patients with GPA may present with sinusitis featuring bloody nasal discharge, pulmonary symptoms, and arthritis. Dermatologic manifestations, including purpura (often in the lower extremities), ulcers, and subcutaneous nodules, occur in 50% of patients. Neurologic findings such as mononeuritis multiplex (most common), cranial neuropathies, seizures, stroke syndromes, and cerebral vasculitis are reported in one-third of patients.

Fifteen percent of patients with GPA have ocular or orbital involvement at presentation, and in up to 50% of patients with GPA, ocular involvement occurs over time. Orbital involvement may be due to contiguous spread of the granulomatous inflammatory process from the paranasal sinuses into the orbit. Orbital pseudotumor, distinct from the sinus inflammation, may also occur. Inflamed nasal and paranasal sinus mucosa may become secondarily infected and may progress to orbital cellulitis and/or dacryocystitis. Orbital disease can cause compressive ischemic optic neuropathy.

Up to 40% of individuals with GPA have scleritis of any type, particularly diffuse anterior or necrotizing disease, with or without peripheral ulcerative keratitis. Approximately 10% of patients with ophthalmic GPA have nonspecific unilateral or bilateral anterior, intermediate, or posterior uveitis, with varying degrees of vitritis. Retinal disease, while uncommon, may include cotton-wool spots, intraretinal hemorrhage, artery or vein occlusion, or retinitis. Complications such as retinal neovascularization (Fig 10-5),

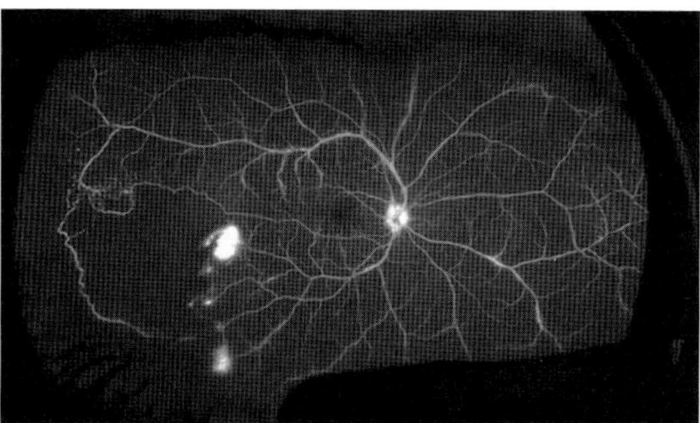

Figure 10-5 Granulomatosis with polyangiitis. FA shows peripheral nonperfusion and retinal neovascularization. *(Reproduced with permission from Huvard MJ, Pecen PE, Palestine AG. The clinical characteristics of noninfectious occlusive retinal vasculitis.* Ophthalmol Retina. *2022;6(1):43–48.)*

vitreous hemorrhage, and neovascular glaucoma may also arise. Vision loss occurs in up to 40% of patients with GPA, especially among those with long-standing or inadequately treated disease.

Kitching AR, Anders HJ, Basu N, et al. ANCA-associated vasculitis. *Nat Rev Dis Primers.* 2020;6(1):71.

Kubal AA, Perez VL. Ocular manifestations of ANCA-associated vasculitis. *Rheum Dis Clin North Am.* 2010;36(3):573–586.

Diagnosis

ANCAs are specific markers for a group of systemic vasculitides that include GPA, MPA, eosinophilic GPA (Churg-Strauss syndrome), renal-limited vasculitis, and pauci-immune glomerulonephritis. These antibodies are directed against cytoplasmic azurophilic granules within neutrophils and monocytes. Immunofluorescence staining patterns suggest 2 main classes of ANCAs:

- The cytoplasmic ANCA, or c-ANCA, pattern is both sensitive and specific for GPA and is present in up to 95% of affected patients. PR3 is the most common target antigen.
- The perinuclear ANCA, or p-ANCA, pattern is associated with MPA, renal-limited vasculitis, and pauci-immune glomerulonephritis. MPO is the most common antigenic target.

Two assays are available for these antibodies, and ideally, both assays are used for diagnosis:

- indirect immunofluorescence for c- and p-ANCA (more sensitive)
- enzyme-linked immunosorbent assay (ELISA) testing for the autoantibodies PR3-ANCA and MPO-ANCA (more specific)

Laboratory evaluation may also reveal proteinuria or hematuria and elevated erythrocyte sedimentation rate (ESR) and C-reactive protein (CRP) values. Chest radiography may show nodular, diffuse, or cavitary lesions. A tissue biopsy specimen showing necrotizing or granulomatous inflammation can establish a histologic diagnosis.

Treatment

Without treatment of GPA, the 1-year mortality rate is 80%. Therefore, the condition is usually treated aggressively with systemic corticosteroids and IMT, such as rituximab or cyclophosphamide. The ophthalmologist's role in recognizing GPA-associated eye disease is critical, as timely diagnosis and treatment may prevent not only ocular morbidity but also patient mortality.

Susac Syndrome

Initially reported by Susac and colleagues in 1979, Susac syndrome (also referred to as *SICRET syndrome,* for *s*mall *i*nfarctions of *c*ochlear, *r*etinal, and *e*ncephalic *t*issue) is an immune-mediated, occlusive microvascular endotheliopathy. Patient age at onset is typically 20–40 years (range, 7–70 years), and women are more likely than men to be affected by a 3:1 ratio.

Manifestations

The clinical triad of Susac syndrome consists of

- encephalopathy
- low- to mid-frequency sensorineural hearing loss and/or tinnitus
- branch retinal artery occlusions

Most patients do *not* display the complete triad at disease onset, rendering diagnosis a challenge. The differential diagnosis includes multiple sclerosis, herpetic encephalitis, acute disseminated encephalomyelitis, sarcoidosis, and Behçet disease.

In patients with Susac syndrome, fundus examination may reveal yellow arteriolar wall deposits ("Gass plaques") that may represent an immunologic reaction in the arteriolar wall. Unlike cholesterol or Hollenhorst plaques, these deposits usually occur away from arteriolar bifurcations and may be transient. Retinal arteries may be diffusely or locally narrowed with a "boxcar" segmentation of the blood column at the level of peripheral retinal arteries (Fig 10-6A). Vitreous haze or cells are minimal or absent. In active disease, angiography shows focal, nonperfused retinal arterioles with arterial wall hyperfluorescence (Fig 10-6B). Embolic material or inflammatory reactions are not seen around the vessels. In magnetic resonance imaging, multifocal supratentorial white matter lesions involving the central corpus callosum are highly suggestive of Susac syndrome. When a diagnosis of Susac syndrome is being considered, formal audiology testing can be performed to assess for sensorineural hearing loss.

Treatment

Therapy for Susac syndrome often features a combination of high-dose corticosteroids, intravenous immunoglobulin, cyclophosphamide, antimetabolite therapy, and rituximab. The disease course varies, and patients may need long-term therapy. Serial fluorescein angiography helps monitor for ophthalmic disease recurrence.

Heng LZ, Bailey C, Lee R, Dick A, Ross A. A review and update on the ophthalmic implications of Susac syndrome. *Surv Ophthalmol.* 2019;64(4):477–485.

Rennebohm RM, Asdaghi N, Srivastava S, Gertner E. Guidelines for treatment of Susac syndrome – an update. *Int J Stroke.* 2020;15(5):484–494.

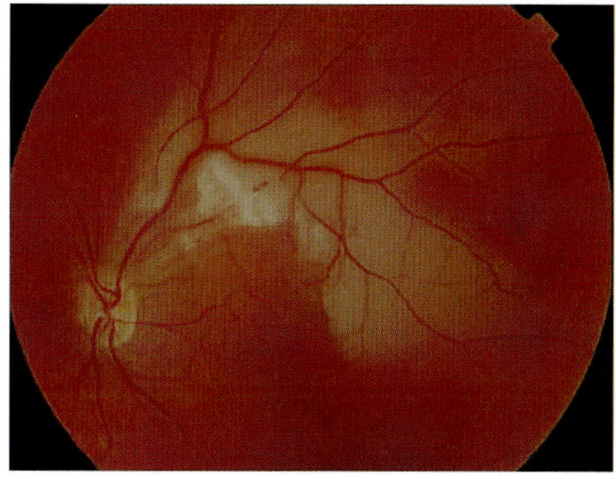

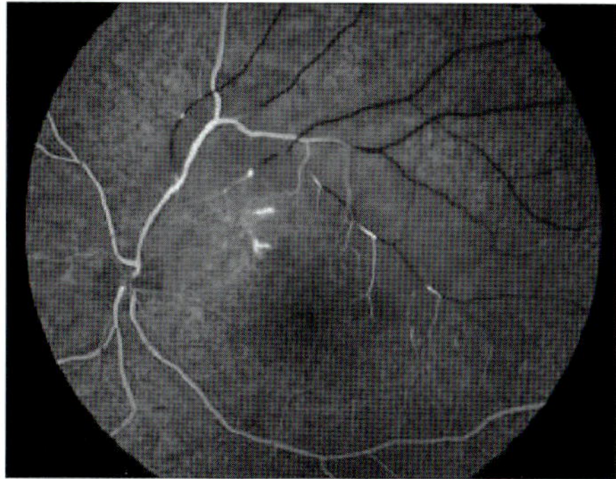

Figure 10-6 Susac syndrome. **A,** Color fundus photograph revealing an area of intraretinal whitening corresponding to a superotemporal branch artery occlusion in the left eye. **B,** FA showing a superotemporal branch artery occlusion with multiple areas of segmental staining well away from sites of bifurcation. *(Courtesy of Albert T. Vitale, MD.)*

Panuveitis With Possible Systemic Manifestations

Sarcoidosis

Sarcoidosis is a multisystem inflammatory disease of unknown etiology with a wide range of systemic and ocular manifestations. In patients with sarcoidosis, the lungs are most commonly affected (90% of cases); followed by the liver, spleen, or lymph nodes (25%–35%); the eyes (12%–50%); the skin (12%–25%); the joints (10%); and the CNS (5%–10%). Cardiac sarcoidosis is probably underdiagnosed; while 5% of patients with sarcoidosis may have clinically detectable cardiac disease, autopsy studies suggest cardiac involvement in 20%–30% of affected patients. The most common cause of sarcoidosis-related death is pulmonary disease, followed by cardiac disease. Overall, the sarcoidosis mortality rate is approximately 5%.

Sarcoidosis affects all ethnic groups worldwide; the highest prevalence is in northern European countries (40 per 100,000). In the United States, the disease is more common in Black patients than in White patients: the prevalence is 36 cases per 100,000 Black individuals versus 11 cases per 100,000 White individuals, and the cumulative lifetime risks are 2.4% versus 0.85%, respectively. No single etiologic agent or genetic locus has been definitively identified in the pathogenesis of sarcoidosis, although environmental exposures (ie, agricultural, infectious) likely play a role in directly triggering inflammation in those with a susceptible genetic background. Familial clustering also suggests a genetic predisposition; siblings of patients with sarcoidosis have a fivefold-increased risk of acquiring the disease. In the United States, lower socioeconomic status is associated with increased severity of disease and higher morbidity and mortality from sarcoidosis. Factors contributing to worse outcomes likely include limited access to medical care and physician implicit bias. See BCSC Section 1, *Update on General Medicine,* for further discussion of social determinants of health.

Although the age at onset for sarcoidosis is usually between 20 and 50 years, the disorder should be investigated as the cause of uveitis in patients of all ages; for example, epidemiologic studies suggest a second sarcoidosis peak between 50 and 65 years of age. Patients with late-onset sarcoidosis are more likely than younger patients to have uveitis, and they are less likely to have asymptomatic abnormalities on chest radiography.

Pediatric cases of sarcoidosis are rare. When children younger than 5 years are affected, they are less likely than adults to have pulmonary disease and more likely to have cutaneous and joint involvement. In this age group, pediatric sarcoidosis, JIA-associated anterior uveitis, and familial juvenile systemic granulomatosis may also overlap in terms of ocular and articular involvement. See Chapter 8 for a discussion of JIA-associated anterior uveitis.

In young patients, acute systemic sarcoidosis may present and spontaneously remit within 2 years. One form of acute sarcoidosis, *Löfgren syndrome,* is characterized by erythema nodosum, febrile arthropathy, bilateral hilar lymphadenopathy, and acute iritis. This syndrome responds well to systemic corticosteroids and has a good long-term prognosis. *Heerfordt syndrome* (uveoparotid fever), another form of acute sarcoidosis, is characterized by uveitis, parotitis, fever, and facial nerve palsy. In contrast, chronic sarcoidosis presents insidiously, persists longer than 2 years, and often involves lung disease and chronic uveitis.

Uveitis, along with granulomatous dermatitis and arthritis, is also observed in patients with *familial juvenile systemic granulomatosis* (ie, *Blau syndrome*), an autosomal dominant disease caused by mutations in the *NOD2* gene. The ophthalmic presentation is similar to that of ocular sarcoidosis and should be suspected when there is a family history of granulomatous disease.

Hena KM. Sarcoidosis epidemiology: race matters. *Front Immunol.* 2020;11:537382. doi:10.3389/fimmu.2020.537382

Moller DR, Rybicki BA, Hamzeh NY, et al. Genetic, immunologic, and environmental basis of sarcoidosis. *Ann Am Thorac Soc.* 2017;14(suppl 6):S429–S436.

Yee AM. Sarcoidosis: rheumatology perspective. *Best Pract Res Clin Rheumatol.* 2016;30(2):334–356.

Manifestations

The characteristic lesion of sarcoidosis is a noncaseating granuloma without histologic evidence of infection or foreign body (Fig 10-7). See BCSC Section 4, *Ophthalmic Pathology and Intraocular Tumors,* for additional details on histologic findings of sarcoidosis.

Ocular sarcoidosis can affect any ocular tissue, including the orbit and adnexa. Common findings include cutaneous lesions (Fig 10-8) as well as granulomas in the orbit and eyelids. Palpebral and bulbar conjunctival nodules can be easily biopsied to provide histologic confirmation of the diagnosis (Fig 10-9). Infiltration of the lacrimal gland, meanwhile, may cause dacryoadenitis and keratoconjunctivitis sicca.

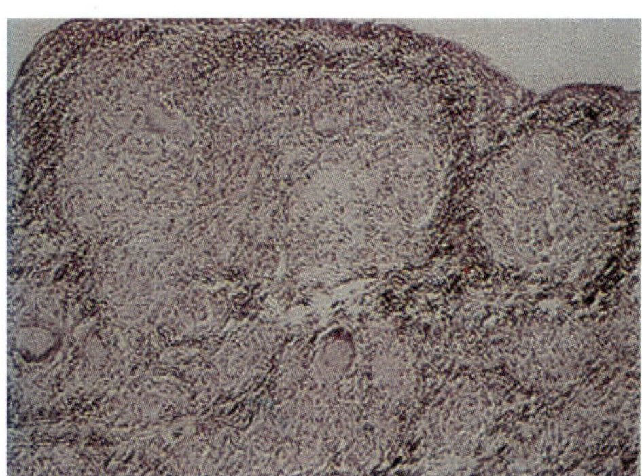

Figure 10-7 Sarcoidosis. Histologic view of conjunctival biopsy. Note the giant cells and granulomatous inflammation.

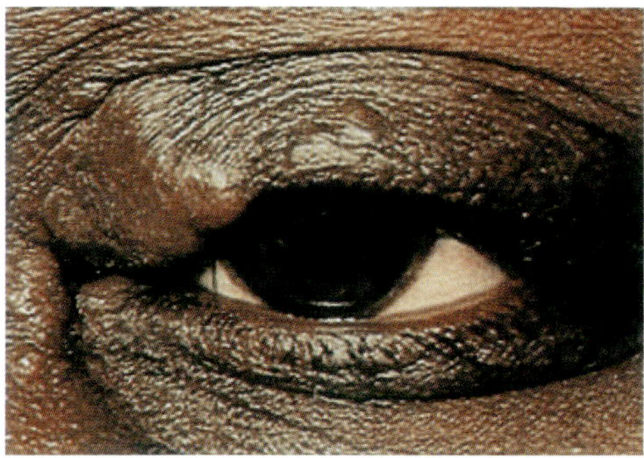

Figure 10-8 Sarcoidosis. Skin lesions.

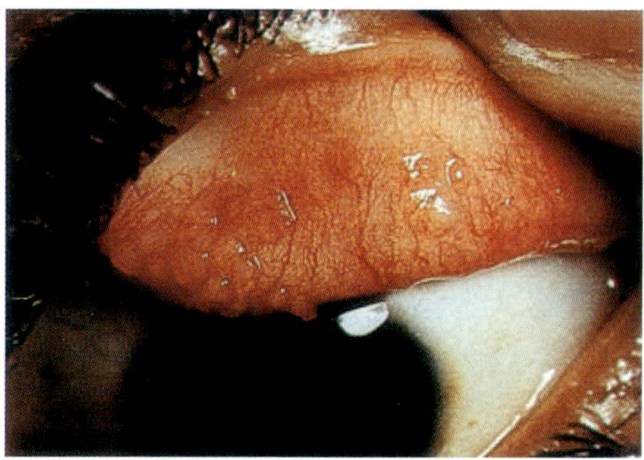

Figure 10-9 Sarcoidosis. Conjunctival nodules.

Uveitis is the most common manifestation of ocular sarcoidosis, occurring in 61% of patients. Overall, sarcoidosis accounts for 5%–10% of uveitis cases in tertiary care centers in the United States. Most sarcoidosis-associated uveitis cases (71%) are anterior. Presenting symptoms include acute onset of eye pain, redness, and photophobia. Alternatively, chronic granulomatous anterior uveitis may be more insidious, with the gradual development of blurred vision, floaters, and mild periorbital aching. Clinical findings of granulomatous anterior uveitis include *mutton-fat keratic precipitates (KPs)* (Fig 10-10), *Koeppe* (pupillary margin) and *Busacca* (iris stroma) iris nodules (Fig 10-11), and white clumps of cells in the anterior vitreous. The cornea is infrequently involved, but nummular infiltrates and inferior endothelial opacification have been observed. Band keratopathy may occur as a result of chronic uveitis or hypercalcemia. The formation of posterior synechiae and peripheral anterior synechiae

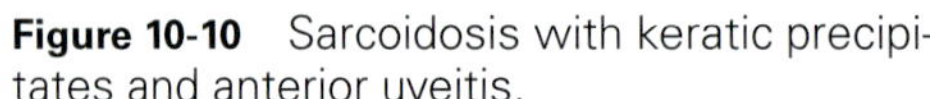

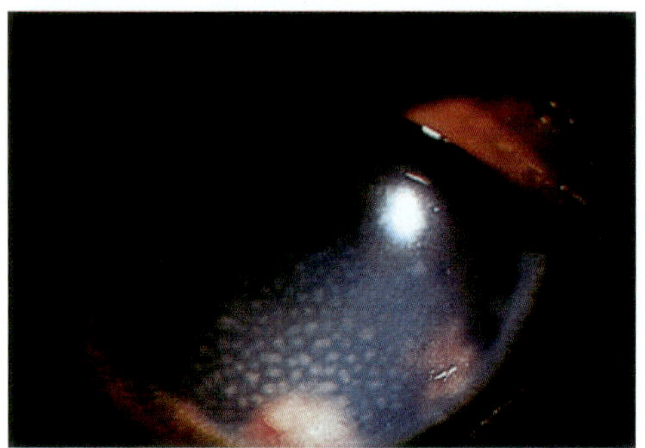

Figure 10-10 Sarcoidosis with keratic precipitates and anterior uveitis.

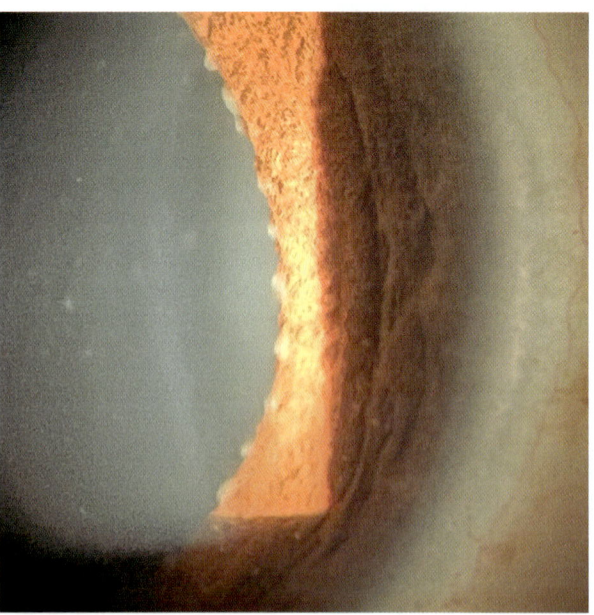

Figure 10-11 Koeppe nodules. *(Courtesy of Sam S. Dahr, MD, MS.)*

can be extensive, leading to iris bombé and secondary angle closure; glaucoma due to sarcoid uveitis complications is a poor prognostic sign associated with severe vision loss.

Posterior segment manifestations occur in up to 20% of patients with ocular sarcoidosis. Vitreous involvement includes cellular-proteinaceous clumps *(snowballs)* with or without vitreous inflammatory cell infiltrate. Vitreous cells may also form semi-linear strands or "string of pearls." Vitreous inflammation may be the primary site of involvement (ie, intermediate uveitis) or accompany sarcoidosis-associated panuveitis. Acute chorioretinal disease can present as multiple small yellow choroidal granulomas (Fig 10-12) that can evolve into hypopigmented atrophic spots, sometimes with a rim of pigment hyperplasia. Large choroidal granulomas may cause exudative retinal detachment. Granulomas also may involve the retina or optic nerve. *Dalen-Fuchs nodules,* a mixture of lymphocytes and epithelioid histiocytes located between the RPE and Bruch membrane, can occur. Linear or segmental venous sheathing or periphlebitis is common, and retinal macroaneurysms may also develop. *Candlewax drippings,* or *taches de bougie* (Fig 10-13), are irregular nodular granulomas along venules. Retinovascular involvement may also manifest as branch or central retinal vein occlusion and peripheral retinal capillary nonperfusion.

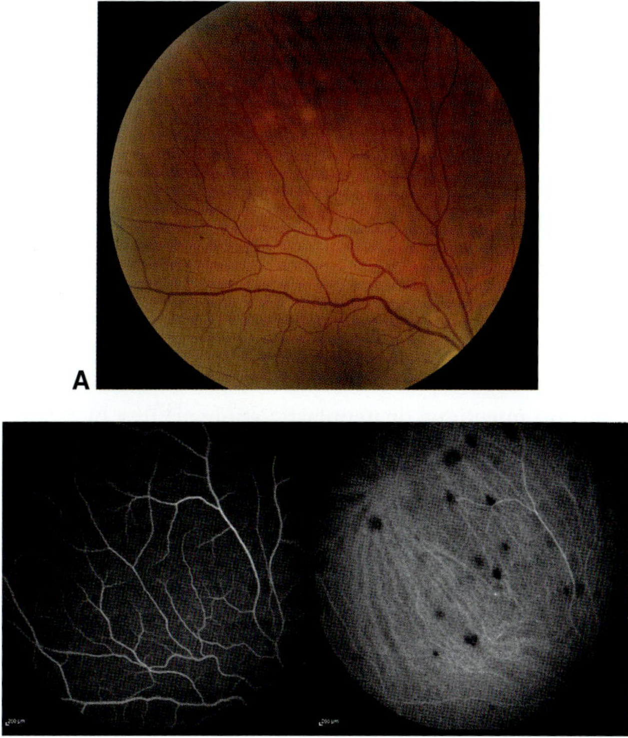

Figure 10-12 Sarcoidosis. **A,** Color fundus photograph of small, deep yellow lesions. **B,** FA *(left)* shows no hyperfluorescence associated with clinically seen lesions. Indocyanine green imaging *(right)* shows multiple small hypocyanescent lesions more numerous than appreciated clinically. *(Courtesy of Wendy M. Smith, MD.)*

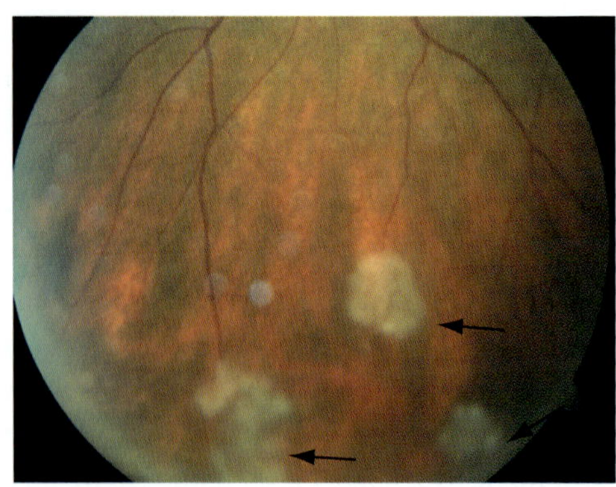

Figure 10-13 Sarcoidosis. Color fundus photograph of taches de bougie, or candlewax drippings *(arrows)*. *(Courtesy of Sam S. Dahr, MD, MS.)*

Complications of posterior segment inflammation include macular edema, retinal neovascularization and vitreous hemorrhage, and choroidal neovascularization (CNV) associated with choroidal lesions. Papillitis secondary to uveitis can develop, although more prominent optic disc swelling from papilledema may occur with neurosarcoidosis. Sarcoidosis can also cause an inflammatory optic neuropathy without uveitis.

Acharya NR, Browne EN, Rao N, Mochizuki M; International Ocular Sarcoidosis Working Group. Distinguishing features of ocular sarcoidosis in an international cohort of uveitis patients. *Ophthalmology*. 2018;125(1):119–126.

Kidd DP, Burton BJ, Graham EM, Plant FT. Optic neuropathy associated with systemic sarcoidosis. *Neurol Neuroimmunol Neuroinflamm*. 2016;3(5):e270.

Standardization of Uveitis Nomenclature (SUN) Working Group. Classification criteria for sarcoidosis-associated uveitis. *Am J Ophthalmol*. 2021;228:220–230.

Diagnosis

The diagnosis of sarcoidosis is based on cumulative evidence obtained from clinical observations, laboratory testing, radiologic studies, and tissue biopsy. As noted previously, definitive diagnosis requires the presence of characteristic histologic findings (noncaseating granuloma with no infectious or neoplastic etiology) in a biopsy specimen; in some cases, however, the diagnosis may be considered probable because of clinical and radiologic evidence, as long as other causes such as tuberculosis (TB) and syphilis have been ruled out.

For the ophthalmologist who is investigating suspected ocular sarcoidosis, a starting point could be a chest x-ray, as abnormalities are present at some point in up to 90% of patients with the disorder. Bilateral hilar with or without mediastinal lymphadenopathy is strongly suggestive of sarcoidosis. However, pulmonary pathology may not persist throughout the disease course, or it may not be detectable by chest radiography. When clinical suspicion for sarcoidosis is high, high-resolution chest computed tomography (CT) is more sensitive than chest x-ray for confirmation. However, the potential clinical utility of the CT scan (ie, the likelihood of changing management of the ocular disease when there are no other signs or symptoms of extraocular sarcoidosis) must be weighed against the risk of increased radiation and the higher cost of the test. If the chest image is abnormal, pulmonary function testing and a pulmonology consultation may be considered. Bronchoscopy with bronchoalveolar lavage and/or endobronchial ultrasound-guided transbronchial needle aspiration may provide histologic proof of sarcoidosis. The characteristic finding from lavage is mononuclear alveolitis with increased $CD4^+$ lymphocytes.

Laboratory testing may include serum levels of angiotensin-converting enzyme (ACE) and lysozyme. If the patient is taking a systemic ACE inhibitor, the ACE level is unlikely to be significantly elevated; however, the lysozyme value may still be informative. A series of biopsy-proven or probable cases of ocular sarcoidosis reported a combined sensitivity of 61% and specificity of 88% for elevated levels of ACE, lysozyme, or both. It is important to note that lysozyme levels can be elevated in patients with chronic renal failure, especially end-stage disease. Other serum test results such as calcium and liver enzyme levels may be abnormal in patients with sarcoidosis, but they are not very useful for diagnosis.

The review of systems should be the guide for additional evaluations of sarcoidosis because other disease sites may have substantial associated morbidity. Signs and symptoms of neurologic involvement may include new-onset headaches, seizures, bowel/bladder dysfunction, gait disturbance, and paresthesias. A patient with suspected ocular sarcoidosis should be asked about symptoms of cardiac arrhythmia (ie, unexplained fainting) or heart failure. Cardiac sarcoidosis is rare, but it can be asymptomatic as well as a cause of sudden cardiac arrest; therefore, some advocate obtaining a screening electrocardiogram in all patients with suspected ocular sarcoidosis, as definitive proof of sarcoidosis could be lifesaving for patients with cardiac disease. Fluorine-18-fluorodeoxyglucose positron emission tomography may be used to identify occult sarcoidosis disease activity and potential sites for biopsy. However, this imaging modality is expensive and involves extensive radiation exposure, so it should be reserved for scenarios in which the correct diagnosis would truly change management (ie, differentiating between neoplastic, inflammatory, and infectious diseases.)

Han YS, Rivera-Grana E, Salek S, Rosenbaum JT. Distinguishing uveitis secondary to sarcoidosis from idiopathic disease: cardiac implications. *JAMA Ophthalmol.* 2018; 136(2):109–115.

McKay KM, Lim LL, Van Gelder RN. Rational laboratory testing in uveitis: a Bayesian analysis. *Surv Ophthalmol.* 2021;66(5):802–825.

Mochizuki M, Smith JR, Takase H, Kaburaki T, Acharya NR, Rao NA; International Workshop on Ocular Sarcoidosis Study Group. Revised criteria of International Workshop on Ocular Sarcoidosis (IWOS) for the diagnosis of ocular sarcoidosis. *Br J Ophthalmol.* 2019;103(10):1418–1422.

Treatment

Local and systemic corticosteroids are appropriate for initial treatment and short-term control of ocular sarcoidosis. Topical cycloplegia should be utilized to prevent synechiae formation until anterior segment inflammation is well controlled. Posterior segment disease usually requires systemic corticosteroids; for sarcoid uveitis, intravitreal corticosteroids, including implants, can be adjunctive or primary treatment, but systemic disease will be untreated.

Systemic IMT should be used when there is persistent or recurrent vision-threatening ocular sarcoidosis despite administration of corticosteroids or when complications arise with their use. Repeated short courses of systemic corticosteroids or monotherapy with serial intravitreal corticosteroids can lead to cumulative damage from waxing and waning ocular inflammation. Options for systemic IMT include methotrexate, mycophenolate mofetil, azathioprine, cyclosporine, tacrolimus, and leflunomide. The tumor necrosis factor (TNF) inhibitors adalimumab and infliximab have been shown to be effective in treating sarcoid uveitis. Paradoxically, a sarcoid-like syndrome is a rare adverse effect of etanercept, another TNF inhibitor.

Factors associated with vision loss from ocular sarcoidosis include chronic intermediate or posterior uveitis, glaucoma, and delayed involvement of a uveitis specialist.

Takase H, Acharya NR, Babu K, et al. Recommendations for the management of ocular sarcoidosis from the International Workshop on Ocular Sarcoidosis. *Br J Ophthalmol.* 2021;105(11):1515–1519.

Sympathetic Ophthalmia

Sympathetic ophthalmia (SO) is a rare, bilateral granulomatous panuveitis that develops after surgical or accidental trauma to one eye (the *exciting eye*). After a latent period ranging from months to years, uveitis develops in the uninjured fellow eye (the *sympathizing eye*). In a recent series, one-third of patients developed SO within 3 months of ocular injury or surgery, and less than one-half did so within 1 year of the event. Earlier studies found that SO was more likely to occur after accidental penetrating ocular trauma than after ocular surgery; however, owing to improved access to emergency surgical care after ocular trauma (particularly in combat situations), SO is now more commonly associated with ocular surgery such as pars plana vitrectomy. In rare cases, SO may develop after nonpenetrating ocular surgery, such as transscleral ciliary body laser, panretinal photocoagulation, and radioactive plaque therapy.

The precise etiology of SO is unknown, but it is hypothesized to be an autoimmune reaction to previously sequestered ocular antigens from the RPE or choroid that reach conjunctival lymphatic channels and initiate an immunopathologic T-lymphocyte response. There may be a genetic predisposition to SO, as affected patients are more likely to express human leukocyte antigen (HLA)-DR4, HLA-DRw53, and HLA-DQw3 haplotypes compared with the general population. Of note, SO and VKH syndrome have nearly identical immunogenetics and share many of the same pathologic ophthalmic features.

Anikina E, Wagner S, Liyanage S, Sullivan P, Pavesio C, Okhravi N. The risk of sympathetic ophthalmia after vitreoretinal surgery. *Ophthalmol Retina.* 2022;6(5):347–360.

Chu XK, Chan CC. Sympathetic ophthalmia: to the twenty-first century and beyond. *J Ophthalmic Inflamm Infect.* 2013;3(1):49.

Fromal OV, Swaminathan V, Soares RR, Ho AC. Recent advances in diagnosis and management of sympathetic ophthalmia. *Curr Opin Ophthalmol.* 2021;32(6):555–560.

He B, Tanya SM, Wang C, Kezouh A, Torun N, Ing E. The incidence of sympathetic ophthalmia after trauma: a meta-analysis. *Am J Ophthalmol.* 2022;234:117–125.

Manifestations

As mentioned previously, in SO the injured/postsurgical eye is the exciting eye and the fellow eye is the sympathizing eye. Patients with SO typically present with asymmetric bilateral panuveitis, in which the exciting eye exhibits more severe inflammation than the sympathizing eye, at least initially. However, prior enucleation, phthisis, or corneal opacity may preclude observation of inflammation in the exciting eye. Early SO symptoms may also include near vision loss (secondary to ciliary body edema), photosensitivity, pain, floaters, photopsia, and metamorphopsia. In rare cases, there may be extraocular signs and symptoms similar to those observed in VKH syndrome (ie, cerebral spinal fluid pleocytosis, sensory neural hearing disturbance, alopecia, poliosis, and vitiligo).

Anterior segment findings include granulomatous KPs, thickening of the iris from lymphocytic infiltration, and posterior synechiae. Intraocular pressure (IOP) may be elevated because of trabeculitis, or it may be low as a result of ciliary body hyposecretion. Moderate to severe vitritis is usually present. Fundus examination typically shows multiple serous retinal detachments and yellow-white midperipheral lesions known as *Dalen-Fuchs nodules* (Fig 10-14). With time, these lesions can coalesce into areas of chorioretinal atrophy. Optic nerve edema followed by optic atrophy, chronic macular edema, CNV, and cataract may also develop.

Two fluorescein angiography (FA) patterns may be seen in acute SO, sometimes concurrently: (1) multiple areas of early pinpoint hyperfluorescence (Fig 10-15) with late pooling corresponding to areas of serous retinal detachments; and (2) early hypofluorescence and late staining of chorioretinal lesions. Indocyanine green angiography (ICGA) shows numerous hypocyanescent foci (Fig 10-16), whereas fundus autofluorescence (FAF)

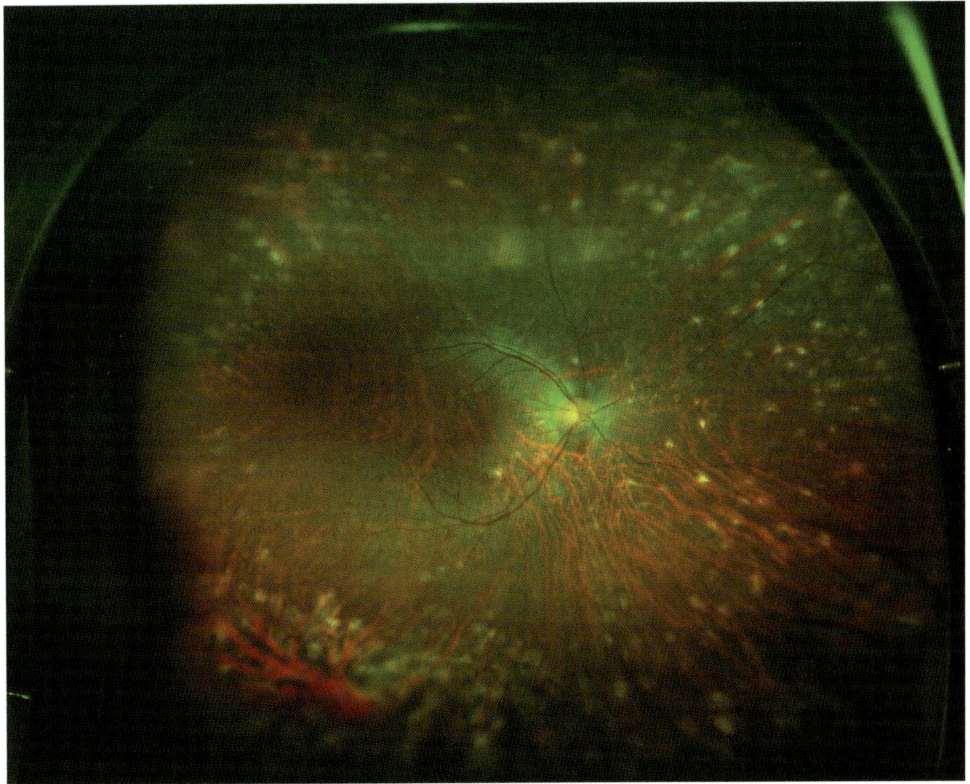

Figure 10-14 Sympathetic ophthalmia. Wide-field fundus photograph shows multiple yellow-white lesions known as *Dalen-Fuchs nodules.* *(Courtesy of Emilio M. Dodds, MD.)*

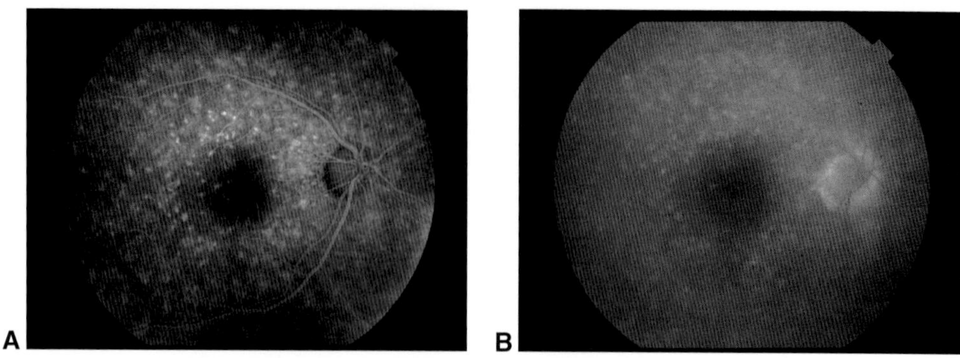

Figure 10-15 Sympathetic ophthalmia. **A,** Early FA demonstrates pinpoint hyperfluorescence. **B,** Late FA shows staining. *(Courtesy of Emilio M. Dodds, MD.)*

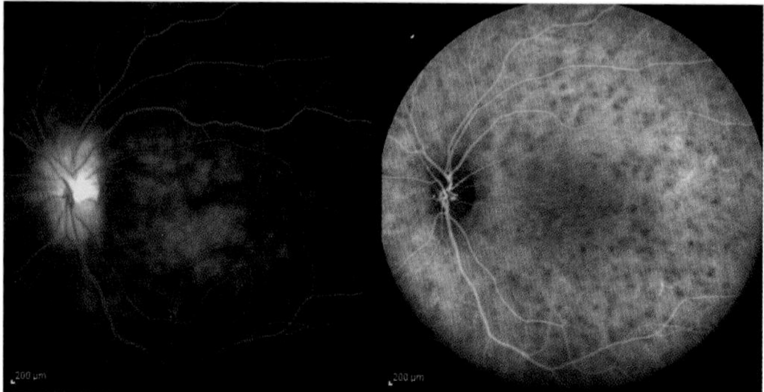

Figure 10-16 Sympathetic ophthalmia. *Left,* FA shows substantial late disc leakage with moderate late central macular leakage. *Right,* Indocyanine green angiography demonstrates multiple hypocyanescent lesions that are more numerous than lesions found on clinical examination or FA. *(Courtesy of Wendy M. Smith, MD.)*

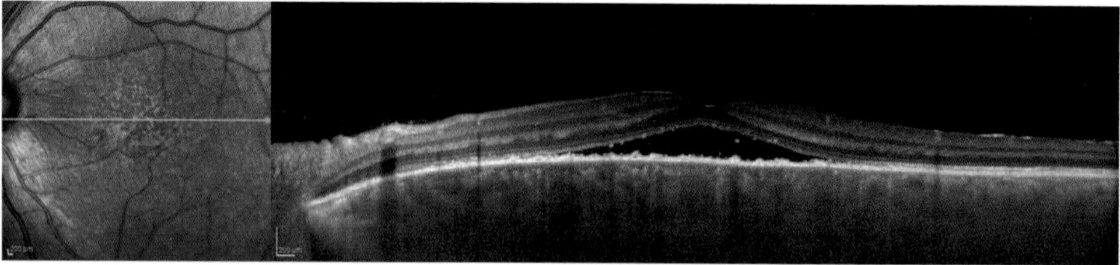

Figure 10-17 Sympathetic ophthalmia. Enhanced depth imaging (EDI)-OCT of the same patient as in Figure 10-16 shows subfoveal fluid with massive, diffuse choroidal thickening. *(Courtesy of Wendy M. Smith, MD.)*

shows hypoautofluorescence secondary to blockage by nodules or atrophy. Optical coherence tomography (OCT) may show choroidal folds and thickening, retinal edema, and/or subretinal fluid (Fig 10-17). Choroidal thickening may also be demonstrated by B-scan ultrasonography.

The histologic features of SO are similar for both the exciting and sympathizing eyes. The entire uveal tract is infiltrated by a diffuse granulomatous, nonnecrotizing inflammatory response that is composed primarily of lymphocytes plus epithelioid cells and a few giant cells. In the choroid, the choriocapillaris is classically spared, at least in the early stage. Dalen-Fuchs nodules, also found in sarcoidosis and VKH, are composed of lymphocytes and epithelioid histiocytes and are located between the RPE and Bruch membrane (see BCSC Section 4, *Ophthalmic Pathology and Intraocular Tumors*).

Mahajan S, Invernizzi A, Agrawal R, Biswas J, Rao NA, Gupta V. Multimodal imaging in sympathetic ophthalmia. *Ocul Immunol Inflamm.* 2017;25(2):152–159.

Diagnosis

The diagnosis of SO is clinical and should be suspected in any patient with bilateral uveitis after ocular trauma or surgery. The differential diagnosis includes TB, sarcoidosis, syphilis, traumatic or postoperative endophthalmitis, and endogenous fungal endophthalmitis. SO and lens-associated uveitis (phacoantigenic) may occur concurrently and share similar clinical features; in the absence of SO, lens-associated uveitis can be differentiated by the absence of choroidal thickening. SO and VKH can also have very similar clinical presentations; however, by definition patients with VKH have no history of ocular injury.

Treatment

In primary penetrating ocular trauma, every effort should be made to salvage eyes with a reasonable prognosis for useful vision, as SO is rare and treatable. When the globe is grossly disorganized with no discernible visual potential, enucleation within 2 weeks of injury may be considered to reduce the risk of SO. Although controversial, enucleation may still be preferred to evisceration, because it removes all residual uveal tissue that may predispose patients to the development of SO. See BCSC Section 7, *Oculofacial Plastic and Orbital Surgery,* for further discussion of enucleation versus evisceration. Regardless of visual potential, once SO has developed, enucleation of the exciting eye does not appear to reduce inflammation in the sympathizing eye. In fact, the exciting eye may eventually become the better-seeing eye.

Treatment of SO usually involves local and/or systemic corticosteroids combined with systemic IMT. Long-term therapy is necessary in most patients, and if the inflammation is severe and vision threatening, alkylating agents should be used. With prompt and aggressive systemic therapy, the visual prognosis of SO is good; 60% of patients achieve a final visual acuity of 20/40, although up to 25% decline to 20/200 or worse in the sympathizing eye.

Lubin JR, Albert DM, Weinstein M. Sixty-five years of sympathetic ophthalmia: a clinicopathologic review of 105 cases (1913–1978). *Ophthalmology.* 1980;87(2):109–121.

Vogt-Koyanagi-Harada Syndrome

Vogt-Koyanagi-Harada (VKH) syndrome is a multisystem disease characterized by bilateral granulomatous posterior uveitis or panuveitis that is usually accompanied by auditory, neurologic, and integumentary manifestations. Ethnic groups affected by VKH include individuals of East Asian, South Asian, Middle Eastern, Hispanic, and Native American ancestry. Accordingly, the incidence of VKH varies geographically: in tertiary referral centers for uveitis, VKH accounts for 6%–8% of cases in Asia, 1.2% in the Middle East, 1%–4% in North America, and 2%–4% in Brazil.

The precise pathogenesis of VKH is unknown, but current evidence implicates a T-cell–mediated process directed against melanin-containing cells in the eyes, ears, skin, and meninges. A genetic predisposition for VKH is supported by a strong association with HLA-DR4 among Japanese patients and with HLA-DR1 or HLA-DR4 among Hispanic patients in Southern California.

Abu El-Asrar AM, Van Damme J, Struyf S, Opdenakker G. New perspectives on the immunopathogenesis and treatment of uveitis associated with Vogt-Koyanagi-Harada disease. *Front Med (Lausanne).* 2021;8:705796. doi:10.3389/fmed.2021.705796

Rao NA. Pathology of Vogt-Koyanagi-Harada disease. *Int Ophthalmol.* 2007;27(2–3):81–85.

Sakata VM, da Silva FT, Hirata CE, de Carvalho JF, Yamamoto JH. Diagnosis and classification of Vogt-Koyanagi-Harada disease. *Autoimmun Rev.* 2014;13(4-5):550–555.

Manifestations

Prodrome Before the onset of ocular symptoms, patients with VKH may experience headache, nausea, meningismus, dysacusia, tinnitus, fever, orbital pain, photophobia, and hypersensitivity of the skin to touch. Focal neurologic signs are rare but may include cranial neuropathies, hemiparesis, aphasia, transverse myelitis, and ganglionitis. Cerebrospinal fluid analysis reveals lymphocytic pleocytosis with normal levels of glucose in more than 80% of patients. Central dysacusia of the higher frequencies occurs in approximately 30% of patients early in the disease course, usually improving within 2–3 months.

Previous investigators described 4 stages of VKH uveitis, but multimodal imaging suggests VKH is a continuum from early- to late-stage disease.

Early stage The early stage of VKH is characterized by bilateral granulomatous anterior uveitis, a variable degree of vitritis, thickening of the choroid, optic nerve edema, and multiple serous retinal detachments (Fig 10-18A). Rare cases may be unilateral. The focal serous retinal detachments are often small and shallow, forming a cloverleaf pattern around the posterior pole, but they may coalesce and evolve into bullous exudative detachments. The posterior pole exudative retinal detachments may be associated with substantial vision loss. Other findings include granulomatous KPs and pupillary margin nodules. IOP may be elevated with shallowing of the anterior chamber because of ciliary body edema or annular choroidal detachment. Alternatively, ciliary body shutdown may result in low IOP.

Late stage In late-stage VKH, there may be features of a smoldering panuveitis including anterior chamber inflammation, vitritis, and choroiditis/choroidal thickening. Repeated bouts of granulomatous anterior uveitis may occur, but recurrent serous retinal detachment is uncommon in late-stage disease. Additional sequelae of chronic inflammation include posterior subcapsular cataract, glaucoma, CNV, and subretinal fibrosis.

The orange-red "sunset-glow" fundus of VKH evolves as a result of depigmentation of the choroid, and juxtapupillary depigmentation may also occur. Small, round, discrete, depigmented, atrophic chorioretinal spots may develop in the peripheral fundus (Fig 10-18B). Perilimbal vitiligo (Sugiura sign) is present in up to 85% of Japanese patients with VKH but is rarely observed among White patients with the disease (Fig 10-19). In up to 30% of patients, integumentary changes such as vitiligo, alopecia, and poliosis develop (Fig 10-20), which can coincide with fundus depigmentation as a later finding. Among Hispanic patients, the incidence of cutaneous and other extraocular manifestations is relatively low.

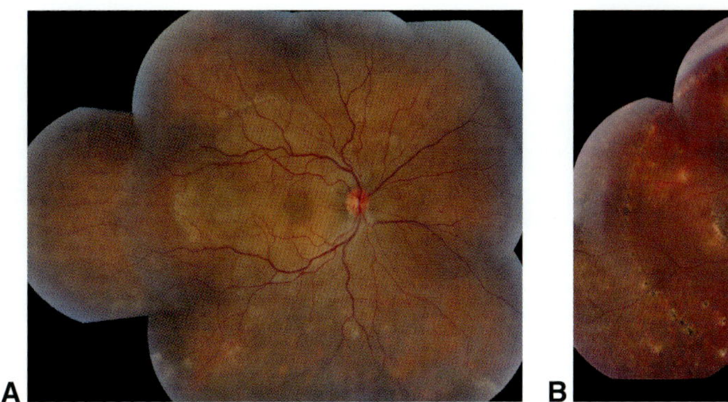

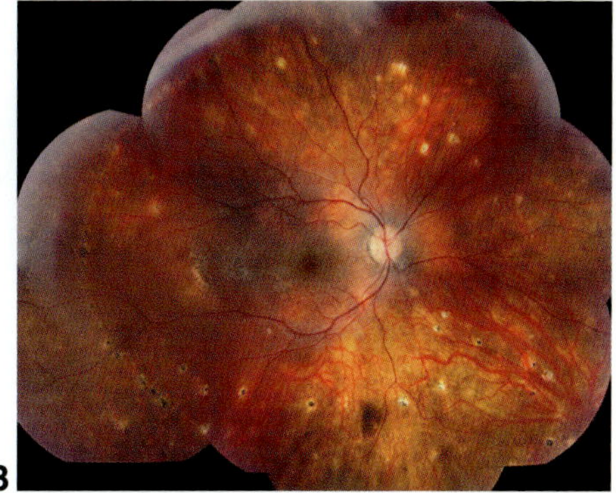

Figure 10-18 Vogt-Koyanagi-Harada syndrome. **A,** Color fundus photograph montage from initial presentation shows exudative retinal detachments. **B,** After treatment, residual depigmented deep lesions in the periphery and diffuse sunset-glow fundus changes are seen. *(Courtesy of Jared E. Knickelbein, MD, PhD, and Nida Sen, MD/National Eye Institute.)*

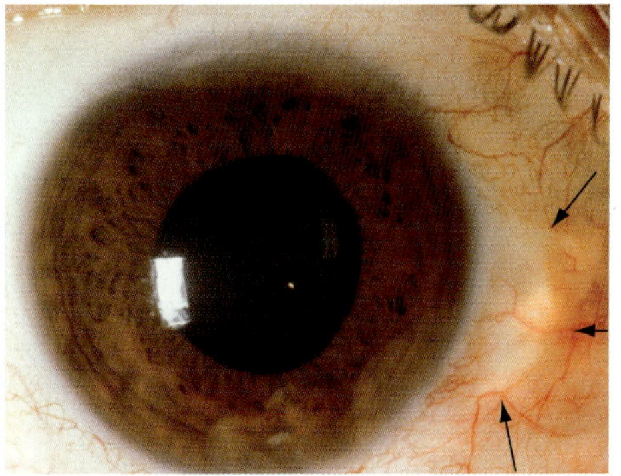

Figure 10-19 Perilimbal vitiligo (Sugiura sign) *(arrows). (Courtesy of Albert T. Vitale, MD.)*

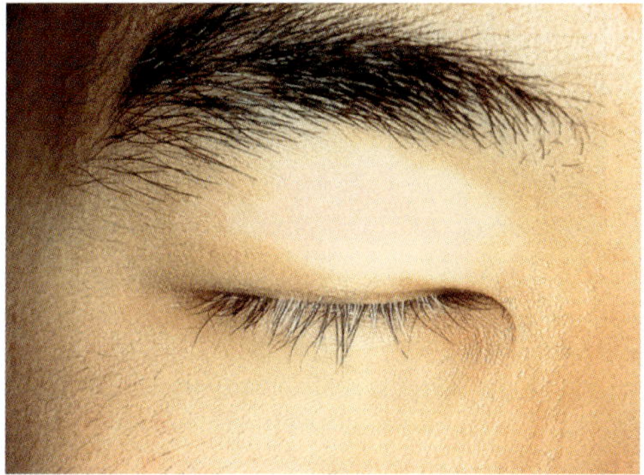

Figure 10-20 Vogt-Koyanagi-Harada syndrome. Vitiligo of the upper eyelid and marked poliosis in the late stage. *(Courtesy of Ramana S. Moorthy, MD.)*

Imaging findings

In the early stage of VKH, FA reveals punctate hyperfluorescent foci followed by pooling in areas of neurosensory detachment (Fig 10-21). Optic disc leakage occurs in most cases, but macular edema and retinovascular leakage are less common. In late-stage disease, alternating areas of hyperfluorescent window defects (from RPE loss) and hypofluorescence (from chorioretinal atrophy and pigment migration) are seen.

ICGA in early-stage VKH shows initial choroidal perfusion delay and subsequent segmental or diffuse choroidal vessel hypercyanescence indicating inflammatory vasculopathy. Hypocyanescent dark dots, likely corresponding to choroidal granulomas, are also seen. These hypocyanescent dark dots are often more widespread than clinical examination findings, and thus ICGA can be used to detect and monitor subclinical choroidal inflammation.

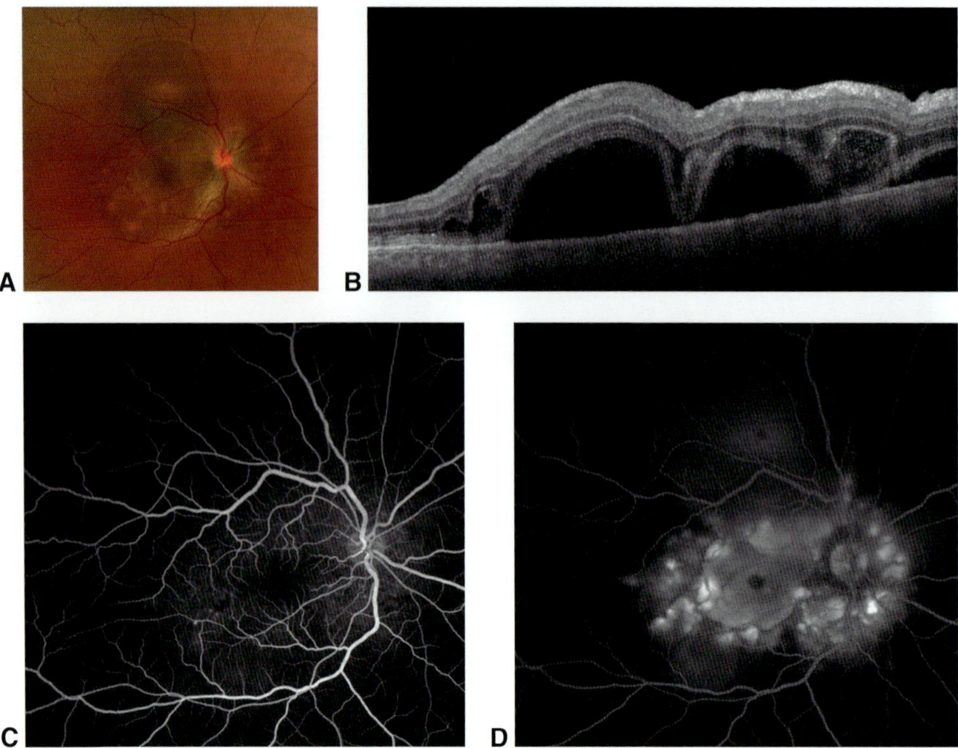

Figure 10-21 Vogt-Koyanagi-Harada syndrome. **A,** Color photograph shows multiple serous retinal detachments. **B,** OCT scan reveals characteristic loculated spaces of subretinal fluid with fibrinous septa extending from the outer retina to the retinal pigment epithelium. **C,** FA shows early pinpoint hyperfluorescence. **D,** Late-phase FA shows leakage and pooling within multiple serous detachments. *(Courtesy of Karen R. Armbrust, MD, PhD.)*

Ultrasonography may display low to medium reflective thickening of the posterior choroid, exudative retinal detachment, vitreous opacities, and posterior thickening of the sclera and/or episclera.

OCT is useful for monitoring serous macular detachments, macular edema, and choroidal neovascular membranes. In the presence of multiple serous detachments, OCT may show loculated areas of subretinal fluid with fibrinous septa extending from the retina to the RPE (see Fig 10-21B). Enhanced depth imaging OCT displays massive choroidal thickening in the early stage that decreases with treatment (Fig 10-22). Recurrent choroidal thickening may precede the appearance of anterior chamber cells if VKH activity increases. FAF may show hyperautofluorescence in early-stage disease (early damage to RPE from inflammation) with areas of hypoautofluorescence corresponding to serous detachments. Later, hypoautofluorescent spots may develop as a result of RPE loss and chorioretinal atrophy.

Histologic findings

In early-stage VKH there is a diffuse, nonnecrotizing, granulomatous inflammation that is virtually identical to the pattern seen in SO. The uveal inflammation consists of

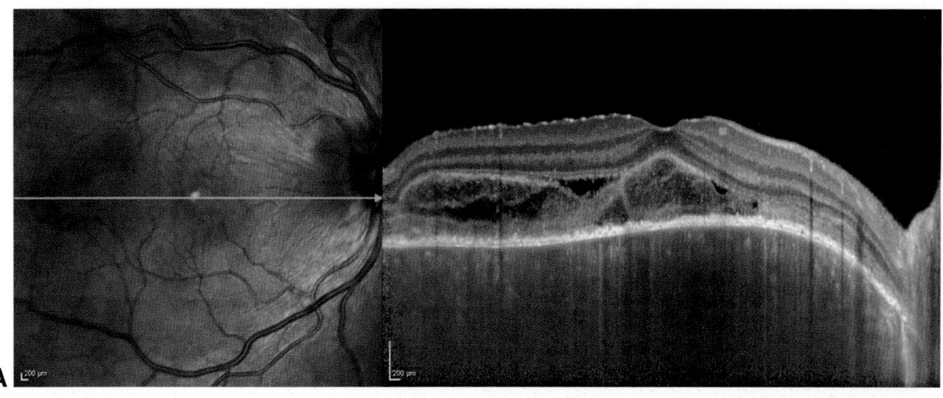

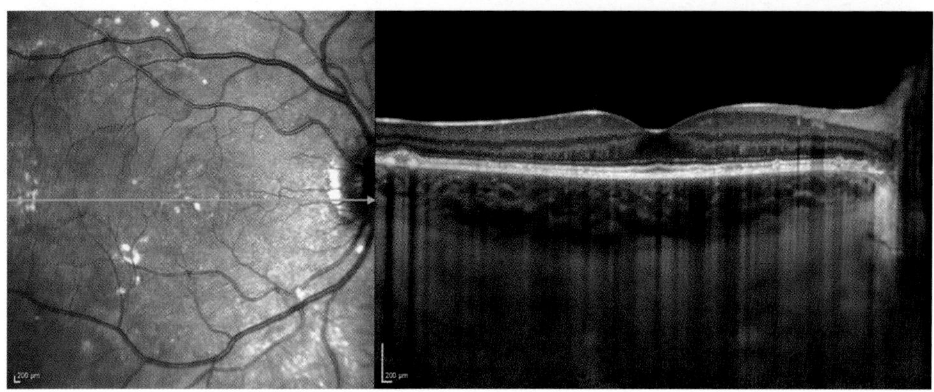

Figure 10-22 Vogt-Koyanagi-Harada syndrome. **A,** EDI-OCT shows turbid subretinal fluid and massive choroid thickening. **B,** After treatment, the subretinal fluid and choroidal thickening resolved. *(Courtesy of Jared R. Knickelbein, MD, PhD, and Nida Sen, MD/National Eye Institute.)*

lymphocytes, macrophages, and epithelioid and multinucleated giant cells with preservation of the choriocapillaris. The peripapillary choroid is the predominant site of inflammation, but the ciliary body and iris may also be involved.

In late-stage VKH, the choriocapillaris is damaged and sometimes obliterated. The number of choroidal melanocytes decreases with loss of melanin pigment (corresponding to the sunset-glow fundus).

Diagnosis

Vogt-Koyanagi-Harada syndrome is a clinical diagnosis; no confirmatory diagnostic tests exist. The 2001 International Committee Revised Diagnostic Criteria included categories of "complete," "incomplete," and "probable" VKH. More recently, the Standardization of Uveitis Nomenclature (SUN) Working Group sought to minimize misclassification by dividing cases into early-stage (Table 10-1) and late-stage (Table 10-2) diseases. Patients may have overlap of early- and late-stage diseases.

The differential diagnosis of VKH includes SO, uveal effusion syndrome, posterior scleritis, vitreoretinal lymphoma, choroidal lymphoma, acute posterior multifocal placoid

Table 10-1 Classification Criteria for Early-Stage Vogt-Koyanagi-Harada Syndrome

Criteria: require #1 or #2 below

1. Evidence of Vogt-Koyanagi-Harada syndrome (posterior uveitis with serous detachment) and no history of penetrating trauma or vitreoretinal surgery prior to disease onset
   a. Serous (exudative) retinal detachment AND
   b. Multiloculated appearance on fluorescein angiogram or septa on optical coherence tomography

OR

2. Panuveitis[a] with ≥2 of the following within 4 weeks and no history of penetrating trauma or vitreoretinal surgery prior to disease onset:
   a. Headache OR
   b. Tinnitus OR
   c. Dysacusis OR
   d. Meningismus OR
   e. Cerebrospinal fluid pleocytosis

Exclusions

1. Positive serology for syphilis using a treponemal test
2. Evidence for sarcoidosis (either bilateral hilar adenopathy on chest imaging or tissue biopsy demonstrating noncaseating granulomas)

[a]Patients with uveitis should have evidence of choroidal involvement on clinical examination, fluorescein angiography, indocyanine green angiography, or optical coherence tomography.

Adapted with permission from SUN Working Group. Classification criteria for Vogt-Koyanagi-Harada disease. *Am J Ophthalmol.* 2021;228:205–211.

Table 10-2 Classification Criteria for Late-Stage Vogt-Koyanagi-Harada Syndrome

Criteria: history of early-stage Vogt-Koyanagi-Harada syndrome plus #1 or #2 below

1. Sunset-glow fundus

OR

2. Uveitis[a] AND at least 1 of the following: vitiligo, poliosis, or alopecia

Exclusions

1. Positive serology for syphilis using a treponemal test
2. Evidence for sarcoidosis (either bilateral hilar adenopathy on chest imaging or tissue biopsy demonstrating noncaseating granulomas)

[a]Uveitis may be (1) chronic anterior uveitis, (2) anterior and intermediate uveitis, or (3) panuveitis with multifocal choroiditis (Dalen-Fuchs–like nodules).

Adapted with permission from SUN Working Group. Classification criteria for Vogt-Koyanagi-Harada disease. *Am J Ophthalmol.* 2021;228:205–211.

pigment epitheliopathy, bilateral diffuse uveal melanocytic proliferation, TB-associated uveitis, and sarcoidosis.

Abouammoh MA, Gupta V, Hemachandran S, Herbort CP, Abu El-Asrar AM. Indocyanine green angiographic findings in initial-onset acute Vogt-Koyanagi-Harada disease. *Acta Ophthalmol.* 2016;94(6):573–578.

Jap A, Chee SP. Imaging in the diagnosis and management of Vogt-Koyanagi-Harada disease. *Int Ophthalmol Clin.* 2012;52(4):163–172.

Jap A, Chee SP. The role of enhanced depth imaging optical coherence tomography in chronic Vogt-Koyanagi-Harada disease. *Br J Ophthalmol.* 2017;101(2):186–189.

Treatment and prognosis

Aggressive therapy for VKH can produce good visual outcomes, especially when used early in the disease course. Initial treatment is high-dose systemic corticosteroids followed by a taper. Within 3 months, oral corticosteroids are tapered to 10 mg or less daily and then decreased very slowly (often at a rate of 1 mg per month) over the subsequent 6–12 months to prevent late-stage VKH. Local steroid injections should be used with caution, as patients with VKH may have an increased risk of developing elevated IOP.

Most practitioners also initiate systemic IMT at the onset of VKH to reduce the risk of chronic inflammation with subsequent pigment loss, chorioretinal atrophy, and loss of visual function. Systemic treatment with corticosteroids or IMT reduces the risk of vision loss and the development of structural complications such as CNV and subretinal fibrosis.

Greco A, Fusconi M, Gallo A, et al. Vogt-Koyanagi-Harada syndrome. *Autoimmun Rev.* 2013;12(11):1033–1038.

Herbort CP Jr, Abu El Asrar AM, Takeuchi M, et al. Catching the therapeutic window of opportunity in early initial-onset Vogt-Koyanagi-Harada uveitis can cure the disease. *Int Ophthalmol.* 2019;39(6):1419–1425.

Behçet Disease

Behçet disease (BD) is a chronic, relapsing, multisystem vasculitis known for the triad of (1) painful oral ulcers, (2) genital lesions, and (3) recurrent (often high-grade) uveitis. BD may also affect the joints, skin, heart, gastrointestinal system, and CNS. No environmental or infectious factors have been definitely linked to BD. The disorder is clinically and experimentally unlike other autoimmune diseases.

The disease has been described for more than 2,500 years; in the early 20th century, it was formally characterized by Adamantiades and Behçet. Affected patients often have ancestry derived from the ancient Silk Road, extending from Greece and Turkey in the eastern Mediterranean to China, Korea, and Japan along the eastern rim of Asia.

The prevalence of BD varies from as high as 20–421 cases per 100,000 inhabitants in Turkey to 13.5–30 cases per 100,000 people in Asia. The estimated prevalence in the United States is 5.2 cases per 100,000 people. Onset typically occurs in the third and fourth decades, but the disease can also present in childhood or after age 50 years. Both sexes are affected equally, but BD may have a more severe course in males. Uveitis may be especially severe in young males aged 15–25 years, and diagnosis of BD is often delayed in this demographic. Although some familial cases exist, most are sporadic.

Hammam N, Li J, Evans M, et al. Epidemiology and treatment of Behçet's disease in the USA: insights from the Rheumatology Informatics System for Effectiveness (RISE) Registry with a comparison with other published cohorts from endemic regions. *Arthritis Res Ther.* 2021;23(1):224.

Yazici H, Seyahi E, Hatemi G, Yazici Y. Behçet syndrome: a contemporary view. *Nat Rev Rheumatol.* 2018;14(2):107–119.

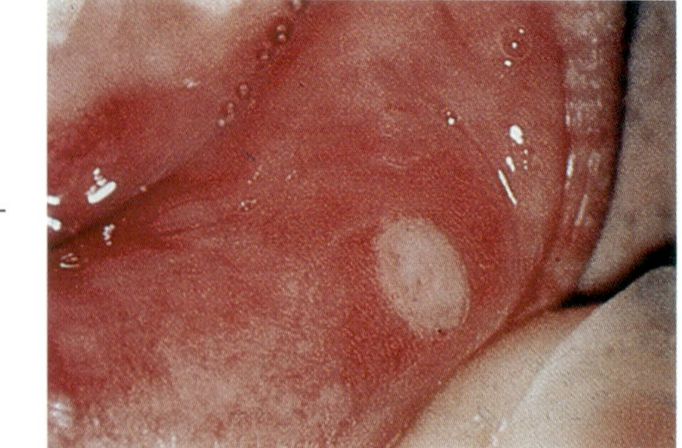

Figure 10-23 Behçet disease. Mucous membrane ulcers (oral aphthae).

Nonocular manifestations

In patients with BD, painful oral aphthae can occur on the lips, gums, palate, tongue, uvula, and posterior pharynx (Fig 10-23). These discrete, round lesions are white with red rims, vary in size from 2 to 15 mm, and last 7–10 days until healing with zero to minimal scarring. Genital ulcers, which occur on the scrotum or penis in men and on the vulva and vaginal mucosa in women, are deeper and larger and heal with more scarring.

Skin lesions include painful or recurrent erythema nodosum, often over extensor surfaces such as the tibia, but also on the face, neck, and buttocks. Pustular acnelike spots called *pseudofolliculitis* may occur on the upper thorax and face. Skin lesions may resolve with minimal or no scarring. Nearly 40% of patients with BD exhibit cutaneous pathergy: the development of a sterile pustule at the site of a venipuncture or an injection; however, this is not pathognomonic.

Systemic vasculitis affecting any size artery or vein in the body occurs in up to 25% of patients with BD. Examples include arterial occlusions and aneurysms and superficial or deep venous thrombosis and varices. Cardiac involvement can manifest as granulomatous endocarditis, myocarditis, endomyocardial fibrosis, coronary arteritis, or pericarditis. Gastrointestinal lesions, such as ulcers involving the esophagus, stomach, and intestines, are seen in more than 50% of Japanese patients with BD, for whom it is a major cause of morbidity. Lung involvement is mainly pulmonary arteritis with aneurysmal dilatation of the pulmonary artery. Moreover, 50% of patients with BD develop arthritis, commonly of the knee, elbow, hand, or ankle.

Thirty percent of patients with ocular BD have neurologic involvement, and 10% of patients with *neuro-BD* have ocular disease. Brain or brainstem white matter lesions may cause motor dysfunction, stroke, and cognitive/behavioral changes. CNS vasculitis or meningeal inflammation may provoke headaches and aseptic meningitis, respectively. Neuro-ophthalmic involvement may also include cranial nerve palsies, papillitis, and papilledema from venous sinus thrombosis.

Ocular manifestations

Up to 70% of patients with BD have ocular manifestations; however, ocular involvement is not usually an initial presenting symptom or sign, and it may develop years after involvement of other organs. In addition, ocular BD usually does not cause chronic inflammation; it is typically an acute and explosive inflammation that spontaneously resolves in a few weeks, potentially with substantial vision loss when there is retinal ischemia from vaso-occlusive disease.

When uveitis occurs in patients with BD, it is most often bilateral and nongranulomatous and can occur in all potential anatomical sites. However, the most common forms of ocular BD are posterior uveitis and panuveitis (50%–80% of cases), which may be profoundly sight threatening as well as more severe in men. A characteristic finding is occlusive retinal vasculitis affecting arteries and veins, which may manifest as multifocal chalky white retinitis, often with surrounding retinal hemorrhage (Figs 10-24, 10-25). Other posterior manifestations of ocular BD include vitritis with or without dense haze, retinal artery and vein occlusions, macular edema, and macular atrophy. Repeated occlusions cause whitening and sclerosis of retinal vessels. Retinal ischemia can stimulate retinal and iris neovascularization. The optic nerve is affected in 25% of patients with ocular BD. Vasculitis affecting the posterior ciliary vessels may cause optic papillitis and subsequent optic atrophy.

In a minority of cases, anterior uveitis may be the only ocular manifestation of BD. Although BD is associated with hypopyon, this is not a common occurrence. A classic description is a sudden-onset hypopyon that shifts with patient head position or disperses with head shaking. The eye may appear relatively quiet despite the hypopyon, or the patient may experience symptoms of acute anterior uveitis (ie, redness, photophobia, and pain). In addition, relapses of anterior uveitis can lead to posterior synechiae, iris bombé, and

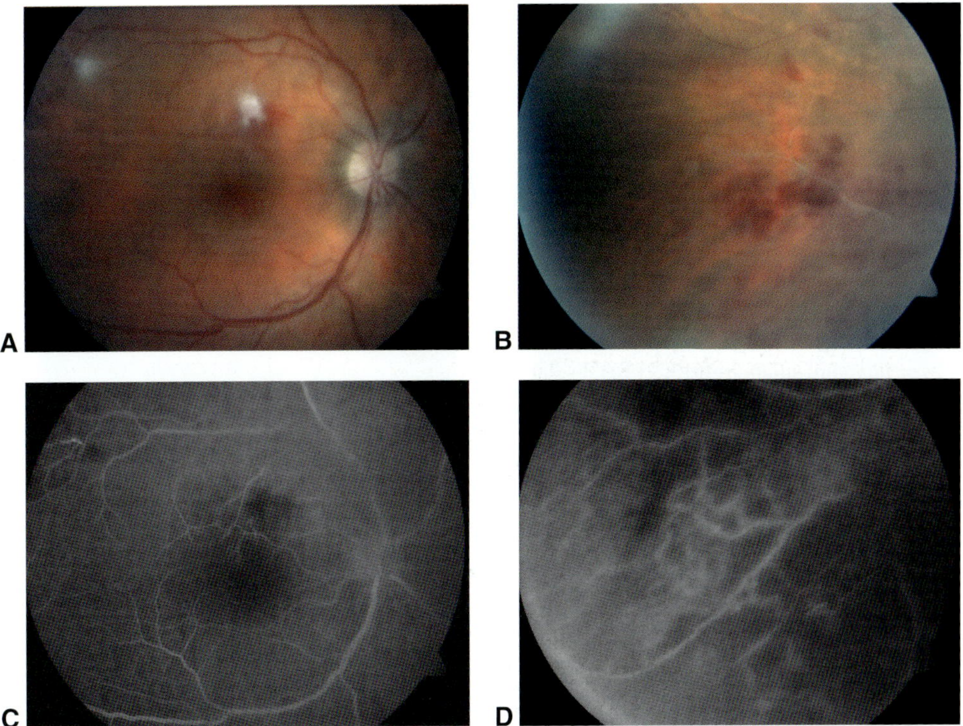

Figure 10-24 Behçet disease with retinitis and vasculitis in a 17-year-old male. **A,** Fundus photograph shows retinitis and hemorrhage in the macula. **B,** Fundus photograph shows retinitis, hemorrhage, and vascular occlusion in the midzone. **C,** Mid-phase FA of the macula. **D,** Peripheral FA shows nonperfusion and vessel staining. *(Courtesy of Sam S. Dahr, MD, MS.)*

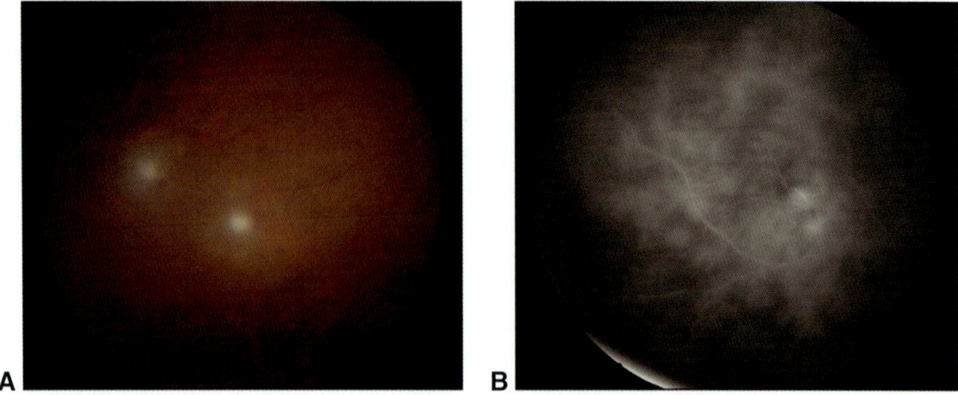

Figure 10-25 Behçet disease. **A,** Fundus photograph of retinitis. **B,** FA shows a ferning pattern of small vessel leakage and focal areas of more intense hyperfluorescence. *(Courtesy of Sam S. Dahr, MD, MS.)*

angle-closure glaucoma. Less common anterior segment features include episcleritis, scleritis, conjunctival ulcers, and corneal immune ring opacities.

In cases of acute ocular BD, FA may show islands of hyperfluorescence corresponding to capillaritis in the posterior and midzones of the retina (see Fig 10-25B). These islands may or may not correspond to clinically visible retinitis and are important indicators of active or impending inflammation. Larger vessels as well as the optic nerve may leak and/or stain. When early signs of inflammation are observed on FA, treatment may prevent an explosive attack. Later sequelae on FA include foveal capillary pruning, islands of capillary nonperfusion, telangiectasias and remodeling, and neovascularization (see Fig 10-24C, D). OCT can show inflammatory retinal edema as well as later macular atrophy.

Kaçmaz RO, Kempen JH, Newcomb C, et al; Systemic Immunosuppressive Therapy for Eye Diseases Cohort Study Group. Ocular inflammation in Behçet disease: incidence of ocular complications and of loss of visual acuity. *Am J Ophthalmol.* 2008;146(6):828–836.

Tugal-Tutkun I, Gupta V, Cunningham ET. Differential diagnosis of Behçet uveitis. *Ocul Immunol Inflamm.* 2013;21(5):337–350.

Tugal-Tutkun I, Ozdal P, Oray M, Onal S. Review for diagnostics of the year: multimodal imaging in Behçet uveitis. *Ocul Immunol Inflamm.* 2017;25(1):7–19.

Pathogenesis

Histologically, neutrophils, T lymphocytes, macrophages, and plasma cells accumulate around the vasa vasorum and perivascular area, generating immunoglobulin and complement-containing immune complexes (Fig 10-26). Necrotizing, neutrophilic, obliterative perivasculitis with or without fibrinoid necrosis develops in capillaries, arteries, and veins of all sizes. Local aggregates of B lymphocytes and plasma cells may be present, contributing to immune complex deposition. The vascular endothelium, meanwhile, shows upregulated expression of adhesion molecules.

Diagnosis

The differential diagnosis of BD includes HLA-B27–associated anterior uveitis, reactive arthritis, JIA, inflammatory bowel disease–associated uveitis, sarcoidosis, and Susac

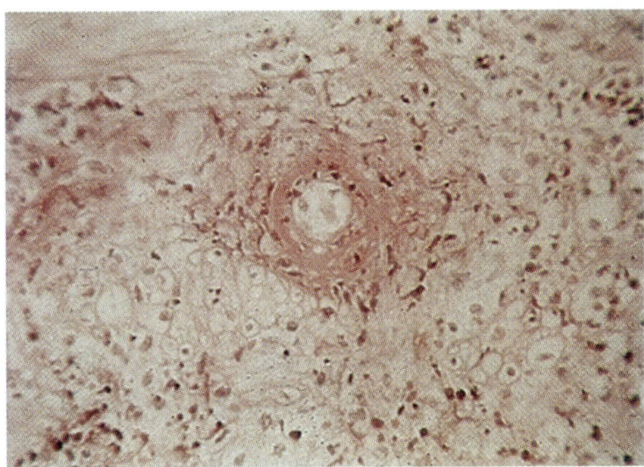

Figure 10-26 Behçet disease. Histologic view of perivascular inflammation.

Table 10-3 International Study Group Criteria for the Diagnosis of Behçet Disease

Recurrent oral aphthous ulcers (at least 3 times per year) plus 2 of the following criteria:
1. Recurrent genital ulcers
2. Ocular inflammation
3. Skin lesions
4. Positive cutaneous pathergy test result

Adapted from International Study Group for Behçet's Disease. Criteria for diagnosis of Behçet's disease. *Lancet.* 1990;335(8697):1078–1080.

syndrome. Systemic vasculitides such as SLE, PAN, and GPA are also included in the differential. In addition, infections such as acute retinal necrosis, toxoplasmosis, and syphilis and masquerade syndromes such as lymphoma may cause a retinitis that mimics BD.

BD is a clinical diagnosis (Table 10-3). Although HLA typing, cutaneous pathergy testing, and blood tests such as ESR and CRP can provide supportive evidence for BD, none definitively establishes the diagnosis. Of note, although the HLA-B51 allele is strongly associated with BD, it is not one of the diagnostic criteria. This association—much like the association between mucocutaneous BD and HLA-B12—is not reproducible in all populations, and testing lacks the sensitivity and specificity necessary to support routine diagnostic use.

Yazici Y, Hatemi G, Bodaghi B, et al. Behçet syndrome. *Nat Rev Dis Primers.* 2021;7(1):67.

Treatment of ocular Behçet disease

The goals of ocular BD treatment are twofold: (1) quickly control acute inflammation to minimize damage; and (2) treat chronic inflammation and reduce the frequency and severity of future attacks. Close collaboration with other specialists, such as rheumatologists, dermatologists, neurologists, and gastroenterologists, is often indicated to treat this multisystem disease.

Systemic corticosteroids are usually necessary to control acute inflammation. Periocular and intravitreal corticosteroids may be a useful adjunct in select patients. Corticosteroid monotherapy should be avoided in sight-threatening ocular BD because of the risk of severe rebound attacks during tapering.

Posterior segment ocular BD is an absolute indication for prompt initiation of systemic IMT. An American expert panel recommended TNF inhibitor therapy with infliximab or adalimumab as first- or second-line IMT for ocular BD. In contrast, a European League Against Rheumatism panel recommended using azathioprine (with corticosteroids) as first-line IMT for ocular BD and cyclosporine or infliximab as second-line treatment. Studies have demonstrated the long-term efficacy and relative safety of infliximab for severe refractory ocular BD. Rapid and complete control of disease may be achieved with decreased retinovascular leakage on FA, preservation of vision, and decreased recurrences. Adalimumab has been studied to a lesser extent, but the data are promising.

Other antimetabolites (mycophenolate mofetil and methotrexate) and T-cell inhibitors (eg, tacrolimus) may also be used to treat ocular BD. Alkylating agents such as chlorambucil and oral or pulsed intravenous cyclophosphamide can be effective, but they are used less frequently because of serious adverse effects. Colchicine is used for orogenital disease and anterior uveitis, but it is not effective in patients with BD and posterior uveitis.

Interferon alfa-2a is a recombinant interferon with antiviral, antitumor, and immunomodulatory properties. Thanks to its low cost and compatibility with concomitant latent TB infection, it is often used (principally outside the United States) as first-line treatment for ocular BD. Potential adverse effects include associated flulike syndrome, depression, suicidal ideation, neutropenia, alopecia, and liver enzyme abnormalities.

Many patients require combination therapy for ocular BD. Potential combinations include an antimetabolite plus a TNF inhibitor, an antimetabolite plus a T-cell inhibitor, or a T-cell inhibitor plus a TNF inhibitor.

Hatemi G, Christensen R, Bang D, et al. 2018 update of the EULAR recommendations for the management of Behçet's syndrome. *Ann Rheum Dis.* 2018;77(6):808–818.

Keino H, Okada AA, Watanabe T, Nakayama M, Nakamura T. Efficacy of infliximab for early remission induction in refractory uveoretinitis associated with Behçet disease: a 2-year follow-up study. *Ocul Immunol Inflamm.* 2017;25(1):46–51.

Levy-Clarke G, Jabs DA, Read RW, Rosenbaum JT, Vitale A, Van Gelder RN. Expert panel recommendations for the use of anti–tumor necrosis factor biologic agents in patients with ocular inflammatory disorders. *Ophthalmology.* 2014;121(3):785–796.

Zierhut M, Abu El-Asrar AM, Bodaghi B, Tugal-Tutkun I. Therapy of ocular Behçet disease. *Ocul Immunol Inflamm.* 2014;22(1):64–76.

Prognosis

Worldwide, visual prognosis is guarded in patients with ocular BD. Nearly 25% of those with chronic ocular BD have vision loss due to macular edema, occlusive retinal vasculitis, optic atrophy, and glaucoma. In general, adult males tend to have worse visual outcomes than females. The presence of posterior synechiae, persistent inflammation, elevated IOP, and hypotony are predictive factors for vision loss. Owing to the chronic relapsing nature of BD, exacerbations may occur after long periods of remission. However, visual prognosis can be improved with early and aggressive use of systemic IMT.

CHAPTER 11

Infectious Uveitis: Bacterial Causes

This chapter includes a related video. Go to www.aao.org/bcscvideo_section09 or scan the QR code in the text to access this content.

Highlights

- Bacterial uveitis most commonly presents as posterior uveitis. Causative organisms include *Treponema pallidum, Mycobacterium tuberculosis,* and less frequently, *Borrelia burgdorferi* and *Bartonella* species.
- Syphilis is reemerging globally and should be considered in the differential diagnosis of any intraocular inflammatory disease.
- Tuberculosis-associated uveitis can arise in the absence of detectable active systemic disease, and the diagnosis is presumptive in most cases.
- Ocular involvement occurs in 5%–10% of individuals with cat-scratch disease (bartonellosis) and may manifest as neuroretinitis, focal/multifocal retinitis, and less frequently, Parinaud oculoglandular syndrome.

Syphilis

Syphilis is a reemerging multisystem, chronic bacterial infection caused by the spirochete *Treponema pallidum.* Transmission occurs most often through sexual contact, but transplacental infection of the fetus is also possible, mainly after the 10th week of pregnancy. In the United States, the infection reached an all-time low in 2000; since then, however, the incidence rates of all stages of syphilis have been increasing among men (particularly those who have sex with men), as well as among women. This rise is associated with an almost twofold increase in the incidence of congenital syphilis in the United States (from 9.4 to 15.7 per 100,000 live births).

Ocular manifestations of both the congenital and acquired forms of syphilis are numerous. Although syphilis is thought to be responsible for less than 2% of all uveitis cases, it is one of the great masqueraders in medicine and should always be considered in the differential diagnosis of any intraocular inflammatory disease. Also, syphilitic uveitis is one of the few forms of uveitis that can be cured with appropriate antimicrobial therapy, even in patients with HIV coinfection. Delay in the diagnosis of syphilitic uveitis may lead to permanent vision loss as well as substantial neurologic and cardiac morbidity, which early treatment may prevent. See BCSC Section 1, *Update on General Medicine,* for additional discussion of the systemic aspects of syphilis.

Centers for Disease Control and Prevention. *Sexually Transmitted Disease Surveillance, 2020.* US Dept of Health and Human Services. Accessed September 15, 2022. https://www.cdc.gov/std/statistics/2020/

Congenital Syphilis

The prevalence of congenital syphilis is increasing in the United States in parallel with higher rates of infection in young women. The increased prevalence is associated with limited, late, or no prenatal care, without serologic screening for the infection. Maternal primary or secondary syphilis is more likely to be transmitted to the fetus than latent syphilis (see the section Acquired Syphilis for discussion of the stages of syphilis); maternal-fetal transmission becomes less likely as the duration of maternal infection increases. See BCSC Section 6, *Pediatric Ophthalmology and Strabismus,* for additional information on congenital syphilis.

Ocular signs of congenital syphilis may present at birth or decades later. Manifestations include congenital cataract, uveitis, interstitial keratitis, optic neuritis, and glaucoma. In early congenital infection, the most frequent form of uveitis is multifocal chorioretinitis followed by retinal vasculitis. Both may result in a bilateral salt-and-pepper retinopathy that can affect the peripheral retina, posterior pole, or even a single quadrant. The retinopathy is not progressive, and the patient may have normal visual acuity. Less often, there may be a bilateral secondary degeneration of the retinal pigment epithelium (RPE) that can mimic retinitis pigmentosa, with narrowing of the retinal and choroidal vessels, optic disc pallor with sharp margins, and variable deposits of pigment.

The most common ocular sign of untreated late congenital syphilis is nonulcerative stromal interstitial keratitis, which occurs in up to 50% of cases, most commonly in girls (Fig 11-1). The constellation of interstitial keratitis, cranial nerve VIII deafness, and Hutchinson teeth is called the *Hutchinson triad.* Interstitial keratitis may also be accompanied by anterior uveitis that occurs in response to *T pallidum* in the cornea (keratouveitis). Symptoms include intense pain and photophobia. Blood vessels can invade the cornea, and late stages show deep "ghost" (nonperfused) stromal vessels and corneal opacities. If untreated, the corneal inflammation may resolve, but residual focal or diffuse corneal opacification or scarring can cause severe vision loss. Anterior uveitis accompanying interstitial keratitis may be difficult to visualize because of corneal haze. Glaucoma may also occur. For further discussion of interstitial keratitis, see BCSC Section 8, *External Disease and Cornea.*

Acquired Syphilis

Primary syphilis

Primary syphilis follows an incubation period of approximately 3 weeks and is characterized by a *chancre,* a painless, solitary lesion that originates at the site of inoculation. The chancre heals spontaneously, and signs of dissemination appear after a variable quiescent period of several weeks to months. The central nervous system (CNS) may be seeded with treponemes during this period, often in the absence of neurologic findings.

Secondary syphilis

Secondary syphilis occurs 6–8 weeks after resolution of the chancre and is heralded by the appearance of lymphadenopathy and a generalized maculopapular rash (Fig 11-2) that may be prominent on the palms and soles. Uveitis occurs in approximately 10% of cases. This stage is followed by a latent period, occurring within 1 year of infection (early latency) to decades later (late latency).

Tertiary syphilis

Approximately one-third of untreated patients develop tertiary syphilis, which may be further subcategorized as *benign tertiary syphilis* (the characteristic lesion is a gumma, most frequently found on the skin and mucous membranes but also in the choroid and iris), *cardiovascular syphilis,* and *neurosyphilis.* Although uveitis may occur in up to 5% of patients whose disease has progressed to tertiary syphilis, it can occur at any stage of infection, including primary

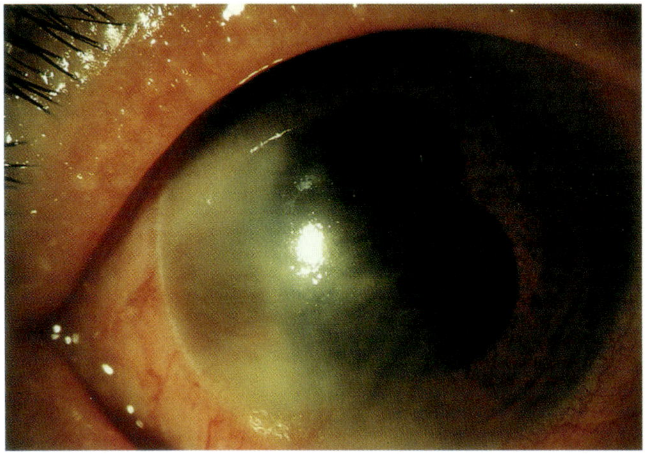

Figure 11-1 Ocular syphilis. Active syphilitic interstitial keratitis.

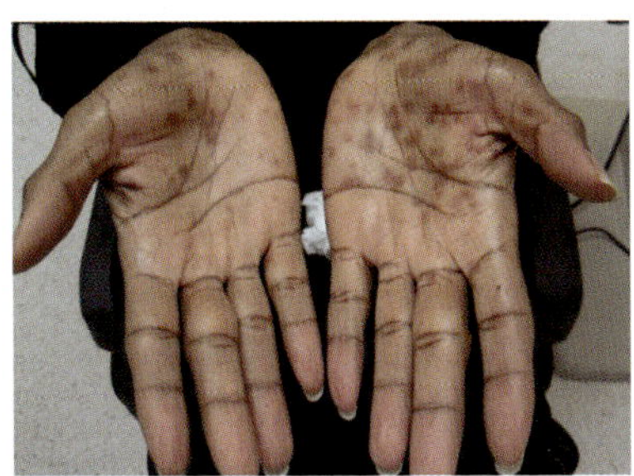

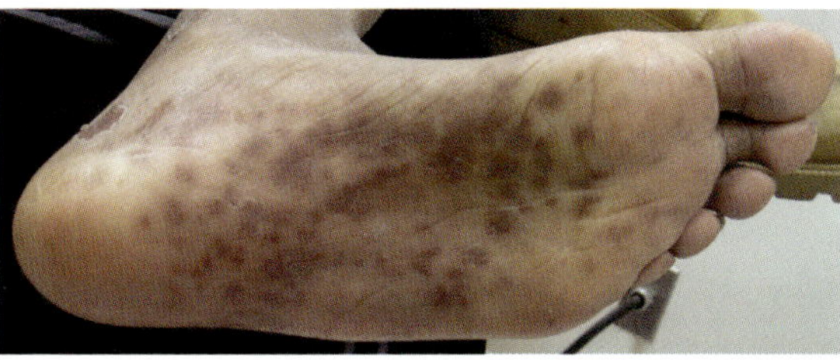

Figure 11-2 Syphilis. A characteristic maculopapular rash on the palms and soles of a patient diagnosed with syphilis. *(Courtesy of Wendy M. Smith, MD/National Eye Institute.)*

disease. Because the eye is an extension of the CNS, ocular syphilis is considered a manifestation of neurosyphilis, a concept that has important diagnostic and therapeutic implications.

Ocular involvement

Ocular manifestations of acquired syphilis are protean, and any structure of the eye (including conjunctiva, sclera, cornea, lens, uvea, retina, and optic nerve), as well as the cranial nerves and pupillomotor pathways, can be involved. Patients may present with pain, redness, photophobia, blurred vision, and floaters. Intraocular inflammation may be granulomatous or nongranulomatous, unilateral or bilateral, and it may affect anterior or posterior segment structures. Anterior segment findings can include iris roseola, vascularized papules (iris papulosa), large red nodules (iris nodosa), and gummata. Interstitial keratitis, posterior synechiae, lens dislocation, and iris atrophy may also occur.

Posterior segment findings of acquired syphilis include vitritis, chorioretinitis, focal or multifocal retinitis, necrotizing retinochoroiditis, retinal vasculitis, exudative retinal detachment, isolated papillitis, and neuroretinitis. The most common manifestation is focal or multifocal chorioretinitis, usually associated with a variable degree of vitritis (Fig 11-3). Typically, the lesions are small and grayish yellow and are located in the postequatorial fundus; however, they may become confluent. Retinal vasculitis, optic disc edema, and serous retinal detachment, with exudates appearing around the disc and the retinal arterioles, may accompany the chorioretinitis.

The clinical appearance and angiographic characteristics of syphilitic posterior placoid chorioretinitis are essentially pathognomonic for secondary syphilis (Fig 11-4, Video 11-1). Findings include placoid, yellowish-gray lesions at the level of the RPE, often with accompanying vitritis. The lesions may be solitary or multifocal, macular or papillary. Characteristics of posterior placoid chorioretinitis on multimodal imaging include the following:

- *Fundus autofluorescence (FAF).* The lesions are hyperautofluorescent.
- *Fluorescein angiography (FA).* Lesions show early hypofluorescence and late staining, with retinal perivenous staining.
- *Indocyanine green angiography (ICGA).* Lesions are hypofluorescent.
- *Optical coherence tomography (OCT).* Images show irregularities at the level of the RPE, disorganization, and loss of outer retinal layers.

VIDEO 11-1 SD-OCT of syphilitic posterior placoid chorioretinitis.
Courtesy of Daniel V. Vasconcelos-Santos, MD, PhD.

Less common posterior segment findings include focal retinitis, periphlebitis, and, infrequently, exudative retinal detachment. Syphilis may present as a focal retinitis or as a peripheral necrotizing retinochoroiditis that may resemble acute retinal necrosis or progressive outer retinal necrosis (Fig 11-5). Although the foci of retinitis may become confluent and are frequently associated with retinal vasculitis, syphilitic retinitis progresses more slowly than retinitis in acute retinal necrosis and responds dramatically to therapy with intravenous penicillin, often with a good visual outcome. Distinctive punctate inner retinal infiltrates have also been observed (Fig 11-6). Isolated retinal vasculitis that affects the retinal arterioles, capillaries, and larger arteries or veins (or both) is another feature of syphilitic

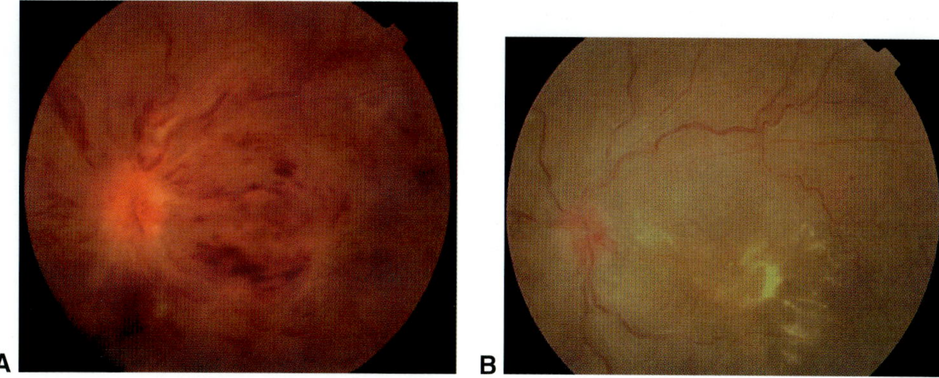

Figure 11-3 Syphilitic chorioretinitis. **A,** Fundus photograph of acute syphilitic chorioretinitis. Note the extensive involvement of the optic disc, retina, and choroid in the posterior pole. **B,** Fundus photograph showing chorioretinitis after 2 weeks of intravenous penicillin therapy. Note the subretinal hard exudate that is organizing, as well as the reduction in disc edema and choroidal inflammation. *(Courtesy of Ramana S. Moorthy, MD.)*

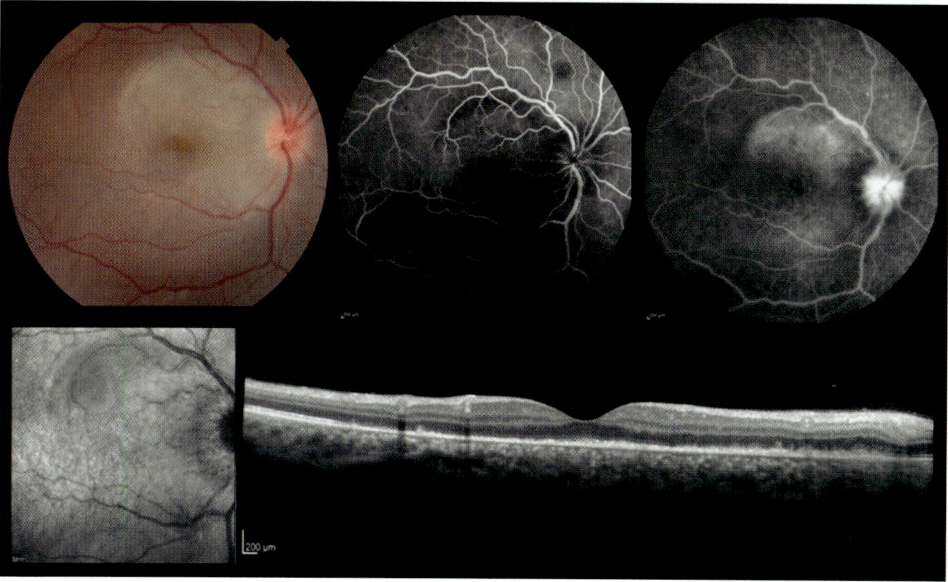

Figure 11-4 Features of syphilitic posterior placoid chorioretinitis on multimodal imaging. Fundus photograph *(top left),* fluorescein angiography (FA; *top middle and top right*), and spectral-domain optical coherence tomography (SD-OCT; *bottom*). Progressive placoid hyperfluorescence is seen on FA *(top right),* corresponding to the yellowish geographic infiltrate in the posterior pole *(top left).* SD-OCT reveals deep granular changes, with disruption of outer retinal layers and underlying homogeneous hyperreflectivity of the inner choroid. *(Courtesy of Daniel V. Vasconcelos-Santos, MD, PhD.)*

intraocular inflammation and may best be appreciated on FA. Focal retinal vasculitis may masquerade as a branch retinal vein and/or arterial occlusion.

Neuro-ophthalmic manifestations of syphilis, including the Argyll Robertson pupil, ocular motor nerve palsies, optic neuropathy, and retrobulbar optic neuritis, appear most frequently

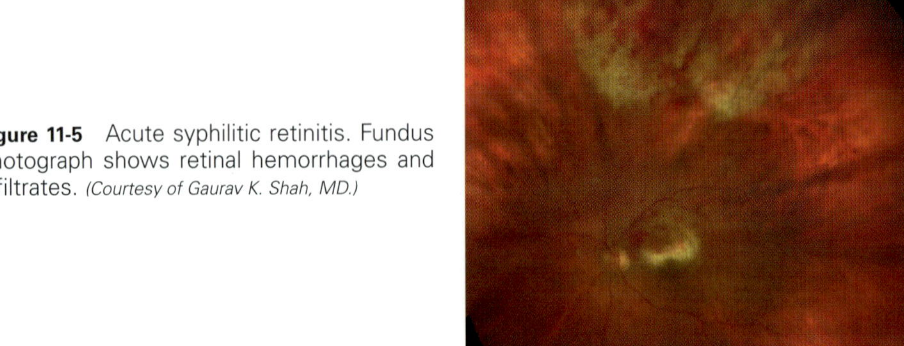

Figure 11-5 Acute syphilitic retinitis. Fundus photograph shows retinal hemorrhages and infiltrates. *(Courtesy of Gaurav K. Shah, MD.)*

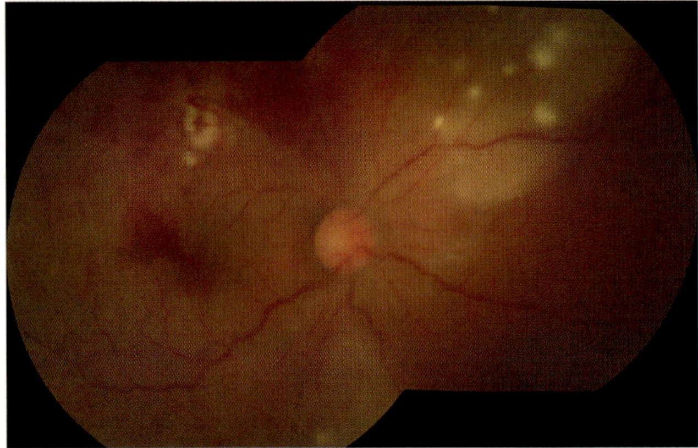

Figure 11-6 Syphilitic posterior uveitis. Fundus photograph reveals punctate inner retinal infiltrates overlying an area of retinal edema superonasally. *(Courtesy of Daniel V. Vasconcelos-Santos, MD, PhD.)*

in patients with tertiary syphilis or neurosyphilis. Syphilis is an important entity to consider in the differential diagnosis of patients with neuroretinitis and papillitis who present with macular star formation. See BCSC Section 5, *Neuro-Ophthalmology,* for further discussion.

Immunocompromised patients with syphilis may present with atypical ocular disease patterns. Optic neuritis and neuroretinitis are more common as the initial presentation in these patients, and disease recurrences may be noted even after appropriate antibacterial therapy.

Eandi CM, Neri P, Adelman RA, Yannuzzi LA, Cunningham ET Jr; International Syphilis Study Group. Acute syphilitic posterior placoid chorioretinitis: report of a case series and comprehensive review of the literature. *Retina.* 2012;32(9):1915–1941.

Furtado JM, Simões M, Vasconcelos-Santos D, et al. Ocular syphilis. *Surv Ophthalmol.* 2022;67(2):440–462.

Jumper JM, Randhawa S. Imaging syphilis uveitis. *Int Ophthalmol Clin.* 2012;52(4):121–129.

Rasoldier V, Gueudry J, Chapuzet C, et al. Early symptomatic neurosyphilis and ocular syphilis: a comparative study between HIV-positive and HIV-negative patients. *Infect Dis Now.* 2021;51(4):351–356.

Diagnosis

The diagnosis of syphilitic uveitis is supported by the history and clinical presentation and confirmed by results of serologic testing. Recently, the Standardization of Uveitis Nomenclature (SUN) Working Group defined diagnostic criteria for ocular syphilis that incorporate characteristic ocular findings with serologic evidence.

According to the US Centers for Disease Control and Prevention (CDC), newly diagnosed syphilis cases should be reported to public health authorities according to local regulations. Public health departments can help identify sexual contacts of the patient who are at risk for acquiring and transmitting the disease. All patients diagnosed with syphilis should receive HIV testing because there is a high frequency of coinfection.

Standardization of Uveitis Nomenclature (SUN) Working Group. Classification criteria for syphilitic uveitis. *Am J Ophthalmol.* 2021;228:182–191.

Van Gelder RN. Diagnostic testing in uveitis. *Focal Points: Clinical Modules for Ophthalmologists.* American Academy of Ophthalmology; 2013, module 4.

Nontreponemal and treponemal antigen tests

There are 2 types of serologic tests for syphilis: nontreponemal and treponemal (Table 11-1). Nontreponemal tests (eg, rapid plasma reagin [RPR], VDRL) detect antibodies against host and bacterial lipoidal antigens released during infection. Treponemal tests (eg, fluorescent treponemal antibody absorption [FTA-ABS], syphilis immunoglobulin [Ig] G) detect antibodies against proteins specific to *T pallidum.* The traditional testing sequence starts with a nontreponemal test followed by confirmatory treponemal tests. Recently, treponemal immunoassays have become the preferred initial test because of their improved speed and automated testing and their ability to detect disease in early or latent stages. This testing strategy is called the *reverse sequence syphilis screening algorithm.* Treponemal tests have a higher positive predictive value in patients with uveitis and should be used in conjunction with nontreponemal tests to diagnose ocular syphilis. Treponemal IgG kits are available commercially for home use in the United States.

Nontreponemal antibody titers (eg, RPR, VDRL test) correlate with disease activity, generally increasing during primary or secondary syphilis and decreasing with spirochete inactivity, such as during latent syphilis or after adequate antibiotic treatment. They are useful barometers for monitoring therapy for both systemic and ocular disease. Results of treponemal tests (eg, FTA-ABS, syphilis IgG) become positive during the secondary stage of syphilis

Table 11-1 Types of Serologic Testing for Syphilis

Nontreponemal
Venereal Disease Research Laboratory (VDRL)
Rapid plasma reagin (RPR)
Treponemal
Treponema pallidum antibodies via enzyme immunoassays (EIAs) or chemiluminescence immunoassays (CIAs)
Microhemagglutination assay for *T pallidum* antibodies (MHA-TP)
Fluorescent treponemal antibody absorption (FTA-ABS) assay

and remain positive throughout the patient's life; as such, they are not useful in assessing therapeutic response.

As a result of passive transfer of IgG across the placenta, VDRL and FTA-ABS IgG test results are positive among infants born to mothers with syphilis. For this reason, serodiagnosis of congenital syphilis is made using the FTA-ABS IgM test, the results of which can indicate acute infection in an infant.

False-positive and false-negative results may occur with both types of tests. False-positive nontreponemal tests occur in various conditions, including the following:

- systemic lupus erythematosus and other autoimmune diseases
- pregnancy, vaccinations, advanced age, intravenous drug use
- infectious diseases such as leprosy, bacterial endocarditis, tuberculosis, infectious mononucleosis, HIV, atypical pneumonia, and malaria
- spirochetal infections (eg, rickettsial infections, Lyme disease, leptospirosis)
- other treponemal infections (yaws, pinta, and bejel)

False-positive treponemal test results are rare (1%–2%) and may be associated with similar conditions. False-negative nontreponemal testing may occur in primary or secondary syphilis when high antibody titers prevent formation of antibody/antigen complexes (the "prozone" effect), or in late-stage syphilis when spirochetes are inactive. Both treponemal and nontreponemal test results become positive approximately 2–4 weeks after infection, so false-negative tests may occur in asymptomatic patients with recent exposure. Both the false-positive and false-negative rates of serologic testing may be greater in HIV-infected patients.

Patients with syphilitic uveitis may require a lumbar puncture with examination of cerebrospinal fluid (CSF), especially if they have neurologic symptoms. A positive CSF-VDRL result and/or pleocytosis is diagnostic for neurosyphilis, as the CSF-VDRL can be nonreactive in some cases of active CNS involvement. In patients with neurosyphilis and abnormal CSF findings, spinal fluid examinations must be repeated every 6 months until the cell count and protein level return to normal and the VDRL is nonreactive.

Cantor AG, Pappas M, Daeges M, Nelson HD. Screening for Syphilis: Updated Evidence Report and Systematic Review for the US Preventive Services Task Force. *JAMA.* 2016; 315(21):2328–2337.

Other diagnostic techniques

Primary syphilis can be diagnosed by direct visualization of spirochetes with dark-field microscopy and by direct fluorescent antibody tests of lesion exudates or tissue. Polymerase chain reaction (PCR)-based DNA amplification techniques may be used on intraocular fluids, CSF fluids, or fluid taken from swabs of mucosal sites or ulcerative lesions.

Treatment

For all stages of syphilis, parenteral penicillin G is the preferred treatment. Regardless of immune status, patients with syphilitic uveitis should be treated with the regimen used for neurosyphilis: intravenous aqueous penicillin G for 10–14 days. Penicillin is the first choice for neurosyphilis, congenital infection, or infection in people who are pregnant or coinfected with HIV. Patients with penicillin allergy may require desensitization. For penicillin-allergic patients who do not have neurosyphilis or HIV coinfection, alternatives include doxycycline or tetracycline. For penicillin-allergic patients with ocular syphilis, ceftriaxone and chloramphenicol have been reported to be effective alternatives.

In the first 24 hours of treatment, patients should be monitored for the development of the *Jarisch-Herxheimer reaction,* a hypersensitivity response of the host to treponemal antigens released in large numbers as spirochetes are killed. Patients can have constitutional symptoms such as fever, chills, hypotension, tachycardia, and malaise, and they may also experience concomitant worsening of intraocular inflammation that may require local and/or systemic corticosteroids. In most cases, supportive care and observation are sufficient.

Topical, periocular, and/or systemic corticosteroids, with concurrent antibiotic treatment, may be useful adjuncts for treating the intraocular inflammation associated with syphilitic uveitis. Use of systemic, periocular, or intravitreal corticosteroids in patients with undiagnosed syphilis can worsen the disease and may result in irreversible vision loss. When the diagnosis of ocular syphilis is significantly delayed, patients may develop chronic uveitis that requires ongoing anti-inflammatory treatment after the antibiotic course is completed.

Centers for Disease Control and Prevention. *Sexually Transmitted Infections Treatment Guidelines, 2021.* US Dept of Health and Human Services. Accessed September 15, 2022. https://www.cdc.gov/std/treatment-guidelines/

Queiroz RP, Smit DP, Peters RPH, Vasconcelos-Santos DV. Double trouble: challenges in the diagnosis and management of ocular syphilis in HIV-infected individuals. *Ocul Immunol Inflamm.* 2020;28(7):1040–1048.

Tuberculosis

Tuberculosis (TB) is a rare cause of ocular disease in the United States. The TB incidence rate in the United States has decreased from 52.6 cases per 100,000 persons in 1953 to 2.2 cases per 100,000 in 2020. Worldwide, however, TB remains an important systemic infectious disease, with more than 10.4 million new cases and 1.7 million deaths reported annually. Nearly one-third of the world's population is infected, and 95% of cases occur in resource-limited countries. In the United States, the incidence of uveitis attributable to TB at tertiary care clinics is less than 1%, whereas at referral centers in India, the incidence is up to 10%.

The most important risk factor for TB infection in the United States is country of birth, with 71.5% of infections occurring in persons born outside the United States. Additional risk factors include medical conditions such as diabetes and HIV infection and social and occupational factors such as homelessness, substance use, and employment or residence in a congregate setting (eg, a correctional facility or long-term care facility).

Mycobacterium tuberculosis, the etiologic agent of TB, is an acid-fast–staining obligate aerobe most commonly transmitted in aerosolized droplets. The organism has an affinity for highly oxygenated tissues, so tubercular lesions are commonly found in the apices of the lungs as well as in the choroid. While primary infection may occur due to recent exposure to *M tuberculosis,* the majority of cases (up to 90%) develop as a result of reactivation of latent infection in immunocompromised patients. Immunocompromised patients are also at risk for widespread hematogenous dissemination of *M tuberculosis,* known as *miliary TB.*

Testing for TB exposure is typically completed in patients who are starting systemic immunosuppressive medication, especially tumor necrosis factor (TNF) inhibitors.

In approximately 80% of infected patients, pulmonary TB develops. Among the 20% with extrapulmonary disease, 50% have a normal chest radiograph, and up to 20% have a negative purified protein derivative (PPD) skin test. Patients coinfected with HIV are more likely to have extrapulmonary disease, especially with deteriorating immune function. The classic presentation of symptomatic disease—fever, night sweats, and weight loss—can occur in both pulmonary and extrapulmonary infection.

Alli HD, Ally N, Mayet I, Dangor Z, Madhi SA. Global prevalence and clinical outcomes of tubercular uveitis: a systematic review and meta-analysis. *Surv Ophthalmol.* 2022;67(3): 770–792.

Centers for Disease Control and Prevention. *Reported Tuberculosis in the United States, 2020.* US Dept of Health and Human Services; 2020. Accessed November 10, 2022. https://www.cdc.gov/tb/statistics/reports/2020/

Ocular Involvement

Most patients with TB-associated ocular inflammatory disease have no active TB infection elsewhere in the body. The ocular manifestations may result from either active ocular infection or an immunologic reaction to extraocular organism. External ocular findings include scleritis (especially necrotizing), phlyctenulosis, interstitial keratitis, and corneal infiltrates. Tubercular uveitis is typically a chronic granulomatous disease that may affect the anterior or posterior segment or both. While granulomatous anterior uveitis can be an isolated finding, it is more likely to occur with posterior segment disease. Anterior segment manifestations may include mutton-fat keratic precipitates, iris nodules, posterior synechiae, and secondary glaucoma (Fig 11-7), although nongranulomatous uveitis may also occur. Patients may experience a waxing and waning course, with the development of macular edema (Fig 11-8). Neuroretinitis can also occur.

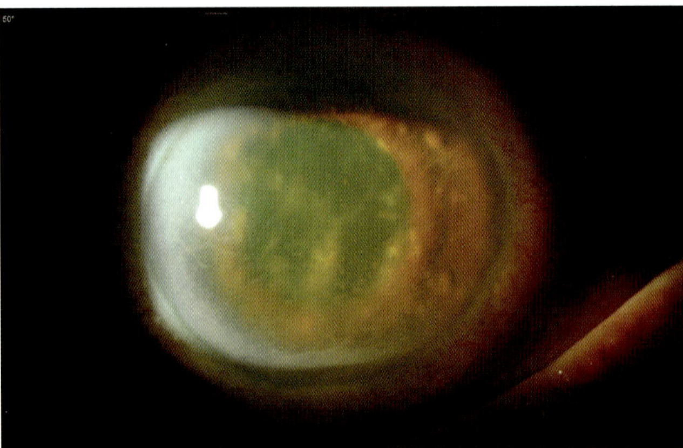

Figure 11-7 Ocular tuberculosis. Anterior segment photograph shows severe fibrinous inflammation and large iris nodules. Polymerase chain reaction testing of aqueous fluid was positive for *Mycobacterium tuberculosis.* *(Courtesy of H. Nida Sen, MD/National Eye Institute.)*

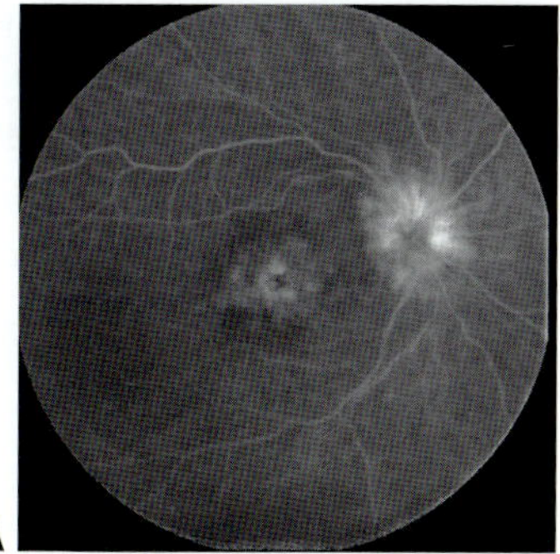
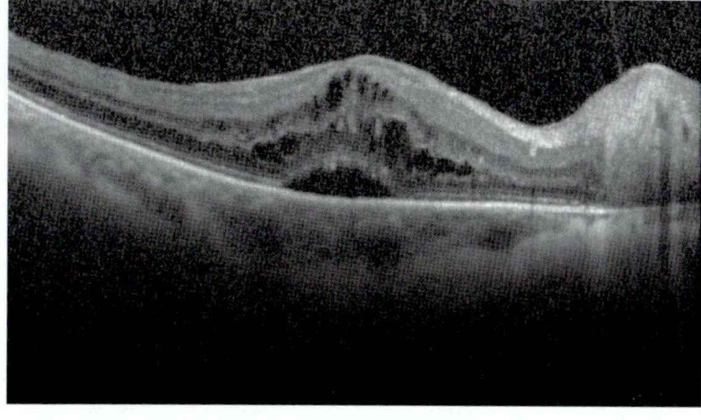

Figure 11-8 Chronic tuberculosis-associated uveitis. **A,** FA shows disc and macular leakage. **B,** SD-OCT confirms macular edema. *(Courtesy of Daniel V. Vasconcelos-Santos, MD, PhD.)*

CLINICAL PEARL

Possible ocular manifestations of TB include necrotizing scleritis, choroidal granuloma (tuberculoma), serpiginous-like choroiditis, and retinal vasculitis (often occlusive).

Choroidal involvement

The most common presentation is disseminated choroiditis that is characterized by multiple (from 5 to hundreds) deep, discrete, yellowish lesions (tubercles) between 0.5 mm and 3.0 mm in diameter (Fig 11-9). These lesions are located predominantly in the posterior pole and may be accompanied by granulomatous anterior uveitis, vitritis, disc edema, and nerve fiber layer hemorrhages. Alternatively, there can be a single, focal, large (4–14-mm), elevated choroidal mass (tuberculoma) that may be accompanied by neurosensory retinal detachment and macular star formation (Fig 11-10). Choroidal tubercles may be one of the earliest signs of disseminated disease and are more common in immunocompromised hosts. On FA, active choroidal lesions display early hypofluorescence and hyperfluorescence with late leakage, and cicatricial lesions show early blocked fluorescence with late staining. ICGA reveals early- and late-stage hypofluorescence corresponding to the choroidal lesions, which are frequently more numerous than those seen on clinical examination or FA. Other manifestations include multifocal choroiditis, frequently with a serpiginoid pattern termed *serpiginous-like choroiditis* (also called *multifocal serpiginoid choroiditis*) (Fig 11-11). In patients with HIV infection/AIDS, tubercular choroiditis may progress despite effective antituberculosis therapy.

Retinal involvement

Retinal involvement in TB is usually secondary to extension of the choroidal disease or an immunologic response to mycobacteria and should be differentiated from *Eales disease,* a peripheral retinal vasculitis that presents in otherwise healthy young men aged 20–40 years with recurrent, unilateral retinal and vitreous hemorrhage and subsequent involvement of the fellow eye. The disease may be associated with tuberculin hypersensitivity. Interestingly, a few studies employing PCR-based assays have detected *M tuberculosis* DNA in aqueous,

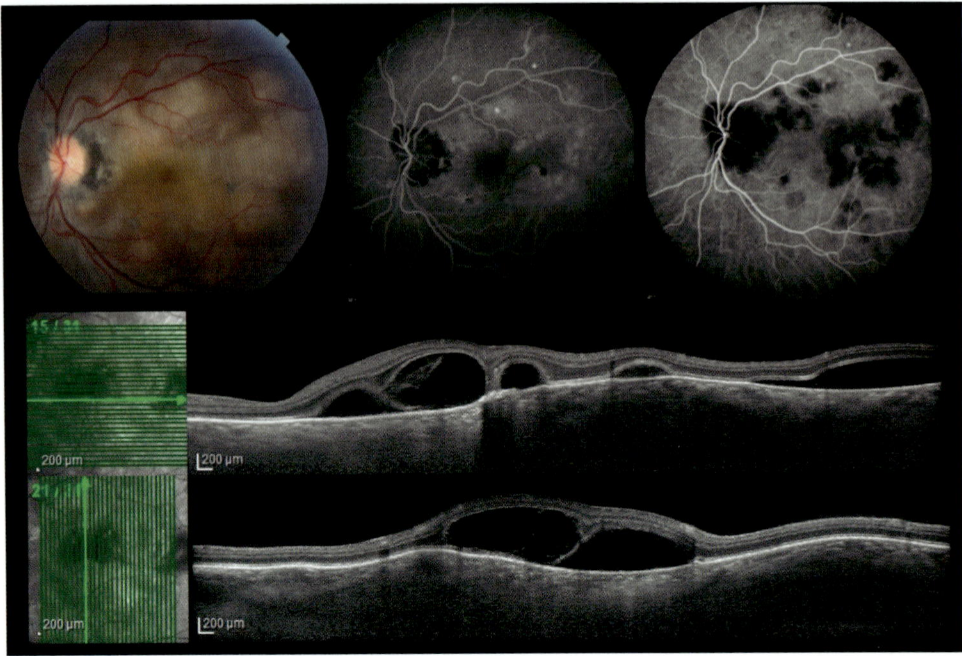

Figure 11-9 Tubercular multifocal choroiditis. Fundus photography *(top left)* shows multiple pockets of subretinal fluid overlying choroidal tubercles. FA *(top middle)* reveals multifocal leakage, and indocyanine green angiography *(top right)* delineates hypocyanescence, presumably corresponding to areas of choroidal inflammatory infiltration. SD-OCT *(bottom)* shows choroidal nodules (tubercles) with overlying bacillary detachments. *(Courtesy of Daniel V. Vasconcelos-Santos, MD, PhD.)*

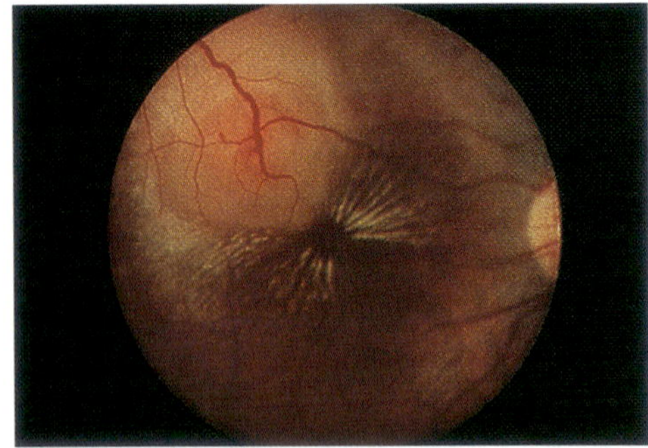

Figure 11-10 Ocular tuberculosis. Fundus photograph demonstrates a choroidal tubercle (tuberculoma) with a macular star formation).

vitreous, and epiretinal membranes from patients with Eales disease. Periphlebitis is commonly seen in patients with Eales disease and may be accompanied by venous occlusion, peripheral nonperfusion, neovascularization (Fig 11-12), and eventual development of tractional retinal detachment in some cases. See BCSC Section 12, *Retina and Vitreous,* for additional discussion of Eales disease.

Other posterior segment findings of TB include subretinal abscess, choroidal neovascularization, optic neuritis, and panophthalmitis.

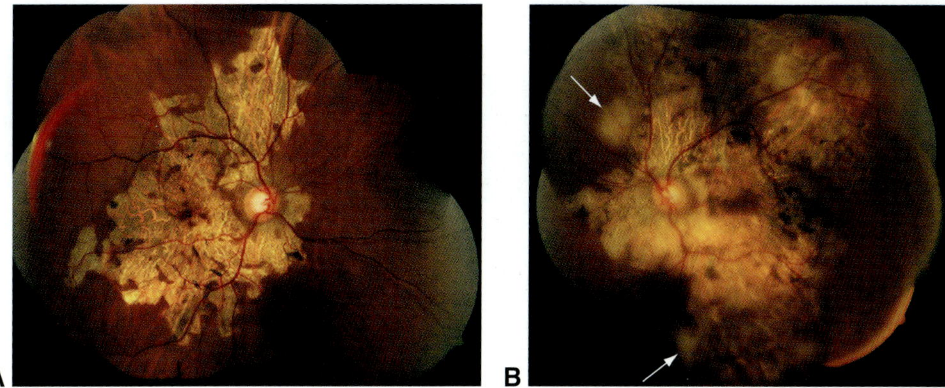

Figure 11-11 Ocular tuberculosis. Fundus photographs showing tubercular choroiditis masquerading as atypical serpiginous-like choroiditis. **A,** The right eye shows inactive disease. **B,** The left eye (from same patient as in part A) shows areas of new activity *(arrows)* as well as areas of scarring. *(Reproduced with permission from Leveque TK, Van Gelder RN. Uveitis. In: Stein HA, Stein RM, Freeman MI, Stein RL, eds.* The Ophthalmic Assistant: A Text for Allied and Associated Ophthalmic Personnel. *11th ed. Elsevier; 2022:484.)*

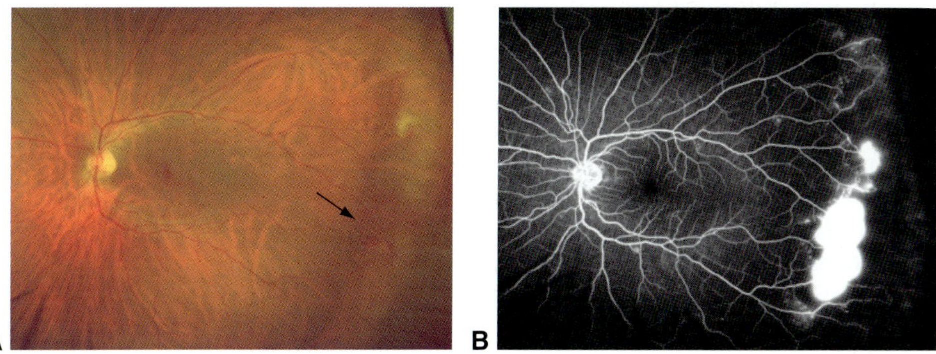

Figure 11-12 Eales disease. **A,** Wide-angle fundus photograph of Eales disease with retinal hemorrhage with neovascularization *(arrow).* **B,** Angiographic image shows peripheral retinal nonperfusion and neovascularization (temporally), in addition to perivenular hyperfluorescence (periphlebitis). *(Courtesy of Emilio M. Dodds, MD.)*

Diagnosis

Definitive diagnosis of TB requires direct evidence of mycobacteria in bodily fluids or tissues. A history of recent exposure to TB or a positive TB test result warrants a concerted search for systemic infection using chest imaging, and/or microbiologic analysis of specimens from other body sites. However, failure to demonstrate systemic disease does not exclude the possibility of ocular involvement. In many cases of ocular TB, the diagnosis is presumptive and based on the presence of TB exposure risk factors, clinical findings of ocular disease consistent with TB (eg, choroidal granuloma, serpiginous-like choroiditis), and positive TB screening tests.

A positive result on the tuberculin skin test using PPD (purified protein derivative of *Mycobacterium bovis*) or the serum interferon-gamma release assay (IGRA) can indicate previous exposure to TB, but it does not provide proof of active systemic or ocular infection. The IGRA blood test is useful when the patient has been immunized with the BCG vaccine; a positive IGRA result suggests exposure to TB, whereas an immune reaction to the PPD usually occurs in BCG-vaccinated patients and thus does not necessarily indicate TB infection. Antibodies against purified cord factor, the most antigenic and abundant cell wall component of tubercle bacilli, have been detected by enzyme-linked immunosorbent assay (ELISA) and may be useful for rapid serodiagnosis of pulmonary TB, in addition to providing supportive data for the diagnosis of ocular infection.

In cases of suspected ocular TB with no evidence of systemic infection, ocular fluid or tissue testing can be attempted. Nucleic acid amplification techniques, with either transcription-mediated amplification of 16S ribosomal RNA or PCR amplification of unique DNA sequences of *M tuberculosis,* can be used to detect intraocular TB. However, the yield from ocular fluids may be low because *M tuberculosis* has a thick cell wall and the organism is less likely to be present in aqueous or vitreous. In atypical or vision-threatening cases where it is important to rule out masquerade syndromes, chorioretinal biopsy in conjunction with PCR testing and routine histologic examination may be necessary.

Agarwal A, Agrawal R, Gunasekaran DV, et al. The Collaborative Ocular Tuberculosis Study (COTS)-1 Report 3: Polymerase Chain Reaction in the Diagnosis and Management of Tubercular Uveitis: Global Trends. *Ocul Immunol Inflamm.* 2019;27(3):465–473.

Betzler BK, Gupta V, Agrawal R. Clinics of ocular tuberculosis: a review. *Clin Exp Ophthalmol.* 2021;49(2):146–160.

Lewinsohn DM, Leonard MK, LoBue PA, et al. Official American Thoracic Society/Infectious Diseases Society of America/Centers for Disease Control and Prevention Clinical Practice Guidelines: Diagnosis of Tuberculosis in Adults and Children. *Clin Infect Dis.* 2017;64(2):111–115.

Testi I, Agrawal R, Mahajan S, et al. Tubercular uveitis: nuggets from Collaborative Ocular Tuberculosis Study (COTS)-1. *Ocul Immunol Inflamm.* 2020;28(sup1):8–16.

CLINICAL PEARL

In patients with uveitis, possible indications for TB testing include

- ocular findings suggestive of TB (ie, choroidal granuloma, serpiginous-like choroiditis, necrotizing scleritis)
- high pretest probability of TB because of risk factors for TB exposure and/or systemic symptoms that are concerning for TB infection
- screening before initiation of systemic immunosuppressive medication

Treatment

In brief, TB treatment entails an initial 2-month induction course of isoniazid, rifampin, pyrazinamide, and ethambutol (quadruple drug therapy), followed by 2-drug therapy for 4–7 months. More than 95% of immunocompetent patients may be successfully treated with a full course of therapy, provided they adhere to the regimen. Treatment protocols have been standardized and are available from the CDC. Comanagement with an infectious diseases specialist and the local health department is usually recommended.

Because ocular TB can be a difficult diagnosis to definitively confirm, the treatment approach varies depending on the features of ocular disease and the likelihood of extraocular TB infection. Recently, the Collaborative Ocular Tuberculosis Study Consensus Group developed new guidelines for the management of tubercular uveitis that are based on multiple factors, such as the type of uveitis.

Indications to treat tubercular uveitis with quadruple drug therapy include (1) recent conversion to a positive TB test; (2) chest radiograph findings consistent with TB; (3) positive mycobacterial culture or *M tuberculosis* PCR. If a patient with suspected tubercular uveitis has a positive TB test and a normal chest radiograph, quadruple drug therapy may be indicated when the ocular inflammation is strongly suggestive of TB or the uveitis has been recalcitrant to systemic immunomodulatory therapy (IMT).

After quadruple drug therapy is started, tubercular uveitis may paradoxically worsen, requiring concurrent treatment with corticosteroids (topical and/or systemic) for the inflammatory component of the disease. Delayed diagnosis may lead to chronic tubercular uveitis; after at least one month of quadruple drug therapy, cautious initiation of systemic immunosuppressive medication may be considered with the agreement of the infectious diseases specialist.

As mentioned previously, because there is a risk of reactivation of latent infection, all patients should be screened for TB exposure before starting systemic IMT, especially TNF inhibitors. Patients with latent TB may be treated for 6–12 months with isoniazid with or without rifapentine or rifampin.

Agrawal R, Gunasekeran DV, Grant R, et al; Collaborative Ocular Tuberculosis Study (COTS)-1 Study Group. Clinical features and outcomes of patients with tubercular uveitis treated with antitubercular therapy in the Collaborative Ocular Tuberculosis Study (COTS)-1. *JAMA Ophthalmol.* 2017;135(12):1318–1327.

Agrawal R, Testi I, Bodaghi B, et al; Collaborative Ocular Tuberculosis Study Consensus Group. Collaborative Ocular Tuberculosis Study Consensus Guidelines on the Management of Tubercular Uveitis—Report 2: Guidelines for Initiating Antitubercular Therapy in Anterior Uveitis, Intermediate Uveitis, Panuveitis, and Retinal Vasculitis. *Ophthalmology.* 2021;128(2):277–287.

Agrawal R, Testi I, Mahajan S, et al; Collaborative Ocular Tuberculosis Study Consensus Group. Collaborative Ocular Tuberculosis Study Consensus Guidelines on the Management of Tubercular Uveitis—Report 1: Guidelines for Initiating Antitubercular Therapy in Tubercular Choroiditis. *Ophthalmology.* 2021;128(2):266–276.

Lyme Disease

Lyme disease (LD) is the most common tick-borne illness in the United States, where it is caused by the spirochete *Borrelia burgdorferi.* Outside the United States, LD is caused by different *Borrelia* species, including *Borrelia afzelii* and *Borrelia garinii.* Animal reservoirs include deer, horses, cows, rodents, birds, cats, and dogs. The spirochete is transmitted to humans through the bite of an infected tick, *Ixodes scapularis* in the northeast, mid-Atlantic, and midwestern United States and *Ixodes pacificus* in the western United States. The disease affects men (53% of cases) slightly more often than women, and it has a bimodal age distribution, with peaks in children aged 5–14 years and in adults aged 50–59 years. There is a seasonal variation, with most cases occurring between May and August. Prevention strategies include avoiding tick-infested habitats, using tick repellents, wearing protective outer garments, removing ticks promptly, and reducing tick populations.

Clinical Features

The 3 stages of LD have protean systemic manifestations. Intraocular inflammation is very rare. See BCSC Section 1, *Update on General Medicine,* for more information about LD.

Stage 1

The most characteristic feature of stage 1, or *localized* disease, is a macular rash known as *erythema chronicum migrans* at the site of the tick bite (Fig 11-13). It appears within 2–28 days of the bite in at least 70% of patients, often appearing as a "bull's-eye" lesion with central clearing. Constitutional symptoms appear at this stage and include fever, malaise, fatigue, myalgias, and arthralgias.

Stage 2

Stage 2, or *early disseminated* disease, occurs days to weeks after exposure. Spirochetes spread hematogenously to the skin, CNS, joints, heart, and eyes. A secondary erythema chronicum migrans rash may appear at sites remote from the tick bite. If LD is left untreated, up to 80% of patients with erythema chronicum migrans develop joint manifestations, most commonly monoarthritis or oligoarthritis involving the large joints, typically the knee.

Neurologic involvement, which occurs in up to 15% of untreated patients with LD, can develop in stage 2 or 3. Lyme neuroborreliosis may include meningitis, encephalitis, painful radiculitis, or unilateral or bilateral Bell palsy. In endemic areas, as many as 25% of new-onset cranial nerve VII palsies may be attributed to *B burgdorferi* infection.

Stage 3

Stage 3, or *late disseminated* disease, occurs more than 5 months after the initial infection. The most frequent systemic manifestation is episodic arthritis that may become chronic and is associated with human leukocyte antigen (HLA)-DR4 and -DR2 haplotypes in North

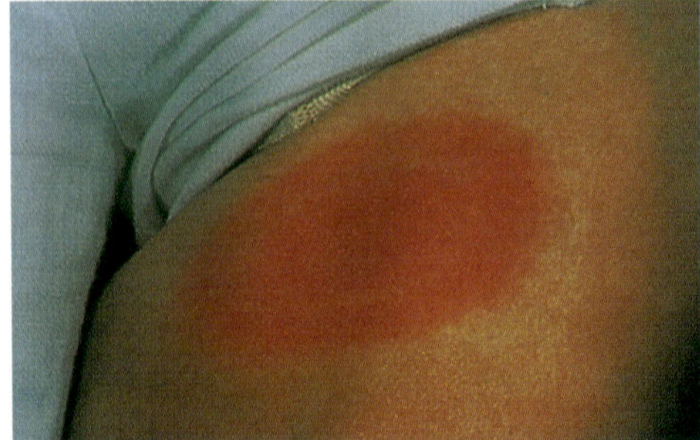

Figure 11-13 Lyme disease. External photograph shows a single dense erythematous lesion consistent with erythema chronicum migrans in a patient with Lyme disease. *(Courtesy of Alan B. MacDonald, MD.)*

America. Chronic systemic findings include acrodermatitis chronica atrophicans, neuropsychiatric disease, radiculopathy, chronic fatigue, peripheral neuropathy, and memory loss.

Steere AC, Strle F, Wormser GP, et al. Lyme borreliosis. *Nat Rev Dis Primers.* 2016;2:16090. doi:10.1038/nrdp.2016.90

Ocular Involvement

The spectrum of ocular findings in patients with LD varies with disease stage.

In early stage 1 disease, the most common ocular finding, occurring in approximately 11% of patients, is a follicular conjunctivitis. Episcleritis is a less frequent manifestation.

Intraocular inflammation is a rare manifestation of LD. It has been reported in stage 2 and, rarely, in stage 3 disease. All forms of uveitis have been described, with intermediate uveitis being the most common. Vitritis may be severe and accompanied by a granulomatous anterior chamber reaction. Other findings include choroiditis, retinal vasculitis, and exudative retinal detachment. A type of peripheral multifocal choroiditis has been described in patients with LD and is characterized by multiple small, round, punched-out lesions associated with vitritis, similar to those present in sarcoidosis. Choroidal involvement may lead to pigment epithelial clumping resembling the inflammatory changes that occur with syphilis or rubella. Retinal vasculitis, found in association with peripheral multifocal choroiditis or vasculitic branch retinal vein occlusion, may be more common than previously known.

Neuro-ophthalmic manifestations of LD occur more frequently than uveitis. In stage 2, multiple cranial neuropathies can occur, unilaterally or bilaterally, either sequentially or simultaneously. Optic nerve findings include papillitis (most common), neuroretinitis, optic neuritis, and papilledema associated with meningitis. Horner syndrome has also been reported.

The most common ocular manifestation of stage 3 disease is presumed immune-mediated keratitis. In rare cases, episcleritis may occur. Both may present months to years after the onset of infection. Typically, infiltrates are bilateral, patchy, focal, and stromal. Subepithelial infiltrates with indistinct borders, peripheral keratitis with stromal edema, and corneal neovascularization can also occur.

Bernard A, Seve P, Abukhashabh A, et al. Lyme-associated uveitis: clinical spectrum and review of literature. *Eur J Ophthalmol.* 2020;30(5):874–885.

Sathiamoorthi S, Smith WM. The eye and tick-borne disease in the United States. *Curr Opin Ophthalmol.* 2016;27(6):530–537.

Diagnosis

It should be emphasized that intraocular inflammation is not a common manifestation of LD. In a patient with no risk factors for tick bite and no signs or symptoms of systemic inflammatory disease, it is very unlikely that new-onset uveitis is related to LD. Therefore, serologic screening for LD does not need to be part of a standard workup for new-onset uveitis.

The diagnosis of early LD can be made on the basis of the history and clinical presentation. For example, if a patient in a Lyme-endemic area presents with a bull's-eye rash after a tick bite, a primary care provider may opt to treat with a course of antibiotics for presumed LD. Otherwise, for the diagnosis of active LD or previous infection, the CDC recommends serum ELISA testing for Lyme IgM and IgG, followed by confirmatory Western immunoblot testing. False-positive results can occur in patients with syphilis or other infections, as well as in various rheumatologic diseases. Similar to the approach used for patients with syphilitic uveitis, investigations for CNS disease may be warranted for patients with uveitis and LD.

Caplash S, Gangaputra S, Kesav N, et al. Usefulness of routine Lyme screening in patients with uveitis. *Ophthalmology.* 2019;126(12):1726–1728.

Rifkin LM, Vadboncoeur J, Minkus CC, et al. The utility of Lyme testing in the workup of ocular inflammation. *Ocul Immunol Inflamm.* 2021;29(1):149–153.

Schwartz AM, Hinckley AF, Mead PS, Hook SA, Kugeler KJ. Surveillance for Lyme disease—United States, 2008–2015. *MMWR Surveill Summ.* 2017;66(22):1–12.

Treatment

Treatment for LD is based on the stage of infection. Oral antibiotic regimens include amoxicillin, 500 mg 3 times/day; doxycycline, 100 mg 2 times/day; or cefuroxime axetil, 500 mg 2 times/day. For patients with ocular involvement, the route of administration and duration of antibiotic treatment have not been established. Those with severe posterior segment involvement may be treated with intravenous (IV) antibiotics according to dosing regimens for neurologic LD (ie, ceftriaxone 2 g IV daily, cefotaxime 2 g IV every 8 hours, or penicillin G 18–24 million units/day IV divided every 4 hours). As with syphilis, the Jarisch-Herxheimer reaction may complicate antibiotic therapy.

After appropriate antibiotic therapy is initiated, anterior segment inflammation may be treated with topical corticosteroids and mydriatics. The use of systemic corticosteroids has been described as part of the management of LD; however, the routine use of corticosteroids is controversial, as it has been associated with an increase in antibiotic treatment failures.

Lantos PM, Rumbaugh J, Bockenstedt LK, et al. Clinical Practice Guidelines by the Infectious Diseases Society of America (IDSA), American Academy of Neurology (AAN), and American College of Rheumatology (ACR): 2020 Guidelines for the Prevention, Diagnosis, and Treatment of Lyme Disease. *Arthritis Care Res (Hoboken).* 2021;73(1):1–9.

Leptospirosis

Leptospirosis is a zoonotic infection with a worldwide distribution. It occurs most frequently in tropical and subtropical regions and is caused by the gram-negative spirochete *Leptospira interrogans.* The natural reservoirs for *Leptospira* organisms include livestock, horses, dogs, and rodents, which excrete the organism in their urine. Humans contract the disease upon exposure to contaminated soil or water; thus, groups at risk include agricultural workers, sewer workers, veterinarians, fishery and slaughterhouse workers, and military personnel, as well as swimmers, triathletes, and whitewater rafters. The disease is not known to spread from person to person, but maternal–fetal transmission might occur infrequently. Leptospirosis is very rare in the United States, with 100–150 cases identified annually, half of them in Puerto Rico. Globally, 1 million people are estimated to be infected each year, with almost 60,000 deaths. Since 2013, leptospirosis has been reinstated as a nationally notifiable disease in the United States.

Leptospirosis is frequently a biphasic disease. The initial, or *leptospiremic,* phase follows an incubation period of 2–4 weeks and is heralded by the abrupt onset of fever, chills, headache, myalgias, vomiting, and diarrhea. Approximately 10% of infected individuals will develop severe septicemic leptospirosis or *Weil disease,* which is characterized by renal and hepatocellular dysfunction and is fatal in 30% of cases. Leptospires may be isolated from the blood and CSF but are cleared rapidly as the disease progresses to the second, or *immune,* phase, which is characterized by meningitis, leptospiruria, cranial nerve palsies, myelitis, and uveitis. The organism may persist for longer periods in immunologically privileged sites, such as the brain and the eye.

Centers for Disease Control and Prevention. *Leptospirosis: Healthcare Workers.* US Dept of Health and Human Services; 2018. Accessed November 28, 2022. http://www.cdc.gov/leptospirosis/health_care_workers/index.html

Ocular Involvement

Ocular involvement can occur in both the leptospiremic and immune phases, but frequently there is a prolonged interval between systemic and ocular disease. The earliest and most common sign of ocular leptospirosis is circumcorneal conjunctival hyperemia. The development of intraocular inflammation (in 10%–44% of patients) can manifest as mild anterior uveitis, neuroretinitis, or panuveitis with retinal vasculitis and is the more serious, potentially vision-threatening complication.

Sivakumar RR. Ocular leptospirosis: lack of awareness among ophthalmologists and challenges in diagnosis. *Curr Opin Ophthalmol.* 2022;33(6):532–542.

Diagnosis

The differential diagnosis of leptospiral uveitis includes HLA-B27–associated uveitis, idiopathic pars planitis, Behçet disease, Eales disease, sarcoidosis-associated uveitis, and tubercular and syphilitic uveitis. Appropriate history and laboratory evaluation help distinguish these entities from leptospiral uveitis. A definitive diagnosis requires isolation of the organism from bodily fluids. A presumptive diagnosis is made on the basis of serologic assays. Rapid serologic assays such as ELISA and complement-fixation tests for the detection of IgM antibodies against leptospiral antigens are highly sensitive and specific; PCR-based assays are under evaluation. Leptospirosis may cause a false-positive result on the RPR or FTA-ABS test.

Treatment

For mild or moderate cases, penicillin G (1.5 million units IV every 6 hours) or oral doxycycline (100 mg twice daily for 1 week) may be used. It is not known whether systemic antibiotic treatment can prevent long-term complications such as uveitis. However, systemic antibiotic treatment should be considered for ocular disease that occurs even months after onset of the acute systemic disease. In addition, topical, periocular, or systemic corticosteroids, together with mydriatic and cycloplegic drugs, are routinely used to treat intraocular inflammation and complications. The visual prognosis for patients with leptospiral uveitis is quite favorable despite severe panuveitis.

Nocardiosis

Nocardia asteroides is a gram-positive rod with partially acid-fast beaded branching filaments—a bacterium that acts like a fungus. The organism is commonly found in soil, and initial infection occurs by ingestion or inhalation, causing an insidious inflammation. Immunocompromised individuals are more likely to be infected than immunocompetent persons. *N asteroides* causes a potentially lethal disease characterized by pneumonia and disseminated abscesses. Ocular involvement is rare, but it may be the presenting problem.

Garg P. Fungal, mycobacterial, and *Nocardia* infections and the eye: an update. *Eye (Lond).* 2012;26(2):245–251.

Ocular Involvement

Ocular involvement occurs by hematogenous spread of the bacteria, and essentially any ocular structure can be affected, including periorbital tissue and the adnexa. Symptoms vary from the mild pain and redness of anterior uveitis to severe pain and decreased vision from panophthalmitis. Findings may include keratitis; necrotizing scleritis; or an isolated, unilateral choroidal or subretinal mass or abscess (Fig 11-14) with minimal vitritis. Panuveitis may also develop, with anterior chamber cell and flare, vitritis, and multiple choroidal abscesses with overlying retinal detachments mimicking fungal endophthalmitis.

Diagnosis

Diagnosis can be established with a culture of the organism taken from tissue or fluid, by vitreous aspiration for Gram stain and culture, or occasionally by enucleation and microscopic identification of *N asteroides*. Where available, molecular techniques such as panbacterial 16S ribosomal RNA PCR or PCR for *Nocardia* species may be used.

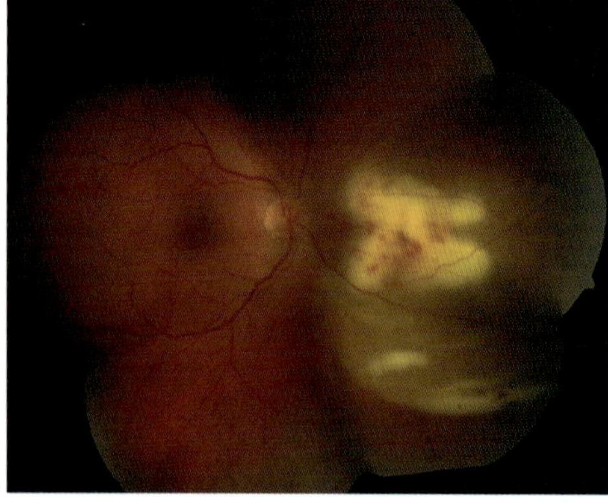

Figure 11-14 Ocular nocardiosis. Fundus photograph reveals a subretinal abscess in the nasal retina. *(Courtesy of Gaurav K. Shah, MD.)*

Treatment

Treatment of *N asteroides* infection with systemic sulfonamide (trimethoprim-sulfamethoxazole) may be required for protracted periods. Combination therapy with additional antibiotics may be necessary.

Bartonellosis

Bartonella henselae is a small, fastidious gram-negative rod that was initially isolated from the tissue of patients with bacillary angiomatosis of AIDS. It is known to be the principal etiologic agent of cat-scratch disease (CSD), a feline-associated zoonotic disease. CSD is found worldwide, with an estimated annual incidence rate in the United States of 9.3 cases per 100,000 persons. The highest age-specific incidence is among children younger than 10 years. Cats are the primary mammalian reservoir of *B henselae* and other species that can cause CSD, such as *Bartonella quintana.* The cat flea is an important vector for the transmission of these organisms among cats. CSD is transmitted to humans by the scratches, licks, and bites of domestic cats, particularly kittens. The disease follows a seasonal pattern, occurring predominantly in the fall and winter, and is most prevalent in the southern states, California, and Hawaii.

Systemic manifestations of CSD include a mild to moderate flulike illness associated with regional adenopathy that usually precedes the ocular manifestations of the disease. An erythematous papule, vesicle, or pustule usually forms at the primary site of cutaneous injury 3–10 days after primary inoculation and 1–2 weeks before the onset of lymphadenopathy and constitutional symptoms. Less commonly, more severe and disseminated disease may develop that is associated with encephalopathy, aseptic meningitis, osteomyelitis, hepatosplenic disease, pneumonia, and pleural and pericardial effusions.

Biancardi AL, Curi AL. Cat-scratch disease. *Ocul Immunol Inflamm.* 2014;22(2):148–154.

Ocular Involvement

Ocular involvement occurs in 5%–10% of patients with CSD and includes Parinaud oculoglandular syndrome (unilateral granulomatous conjunctivitis and regional lymphadenopathy) in approximately 5% of patients. The differential diagnosis of Parinaud oculoglandular syndrome includes tularemia, TB, syphilis, sporotrichosis, and acute *Chlamydia trachomatis* infection. See BCSC Section 8, *External Disease and Cornea,* for further discussion.

Ocular bartonellosis has a wide array of posterior segment and neuro-ophthalmic findings. Although the most common finding in *B henselae* infection is a small focal area of retinitis, the best-known posterior segment manifestation is neuroretinitis, which occurs in 1%–2% of patients with CSD and follows the onset of constitutional symptoms by 2–3 weeks. It is characterized by abrupt vision loss, unilateral optic disc edema, and macular star formation with or without focal or multifocal retinitis. Visual acuity ranges from 20/25 to 20/200 or worse. Although the presentation is most often unilateral, bilateral cases of neuroretinitis have been reported and are frequently asymmetric. Optic disc edema, associated with peripapillary serous retinal detachment, has been observed 2–4 weeks before the appearance of the macular star and may be a sign of systemic *B henselae* infection. The development of the macular star is variable (Fig 11-15) and may be partial or incomplete, usually resolving in approximately 8–12 weeks. Table 11-2 lists other entities that may cause neuroretinitis.

Patients with *Bartonella*-associated neuroretinitis may exhibit some degree of anterior chamber inflammation and vitritis. Discrete, focal, or multifocal retinal and/or choroidal

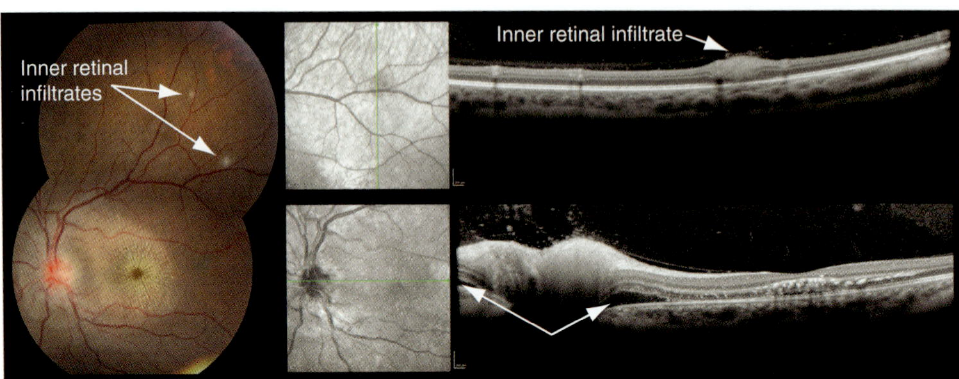

Figure 11-15 Ocular bartonellosis. *Left,* Color fundus photograph of the left eye of a patient with cat-scratch disease shows neuroretinitis with optic disc involvement associated with a macular star. Punctate retinal infiltrates (retinitis) are also visible superiorly *(arrows). Upper right,* SD-OCT scan delineates the inner retinal infiltrate *(arrow). Lower right,* The scan reveals subretinal fluid (peripapillary serous retinal detachments, *arrows*), intraretinal exudates, vitreous inflammatory infiltration, and optic disc and macular edema. *(Courtesy of Daniel V. Vasconcelos-Santos, MD, PhD.)*

Table 11-2 Differential Diagnosis of Neuroretinitis

Infectious conditions	
Bartonellosis *(Bartonella henselae)*	Mumps
Diffuse unilateral subacute neuroretinitis *(Ancylostoma caninum, Baylisascaris procyonis)*	Rocky Mountain spotted fever
	Salmonella
	Syphilis
	Toxocariasis
Ehrlichiosis	Toxoplasmosis
Herpes simplex	Tuberculosis
Leptospirosis	Varicella
Lyme disease	
Noninfectious conditions	
Acute systemic hypertension	Idiopathic intracranial hypertension
Anterior ischemic optic neuropathy	Leukemic infiltration of the optic nerve
Diabetes	Sarcoidosis
Idiopathic condition	
Recurrent idiopathic neuroretinitis	

lesions measuring 50–300 μm are common posterior segment findings. Both arterial and venous occlusive disease, as well as localized neurosensory macular detachments, have been described in association with focal retinitis. Other posterior segment ocular complications include epiretinal membranes, inflammatory mass of the optic nerve head, peripapillary angiomatosis, intermediate uveitis, retinal white dot syndromes, orbital abscess, isolated optic disc edema, and panuveitis. Immunosuppressed individuals may display a retinal vasoproliferative response, leading to single or multiple angiomatoid lesions involving retina and/or choroid.

Amer R, Tugal-Tutkun I. Ophthalmic manifestations of bartonella infection. *Curr Opin Ophthalmol.* 2017;28(6):607–612.

Chi SL, Stinnett S, Eggenberger E, et al. Clinical characteristics in 53 patients with cat scratch optic neuropathy. *Ophthalmology.* 2012;119(1):183–187.

Johnson A. Ocular complications of cat scratch disease. *Br J Ophthalmol.* 2020;104(12): 1640–1646.

Diagnosis

A diagnosis of CSD is made on the basis of characteristic clinical features together with confirmatory serologic testing. Serum anti–*B henselae* antibodies can be detected with indirect fluorescent antibody assay, enzyme immunoassays, or Western blot analysis; all methodologies have good sensitivity and specificity. A single positive indirect fluorescent antibody or enzyme immunoassay titer for IgG or IgM is sufficient to confirm the diagnosis of CSD. Other diagnostic approaches include bacterial cultures that may require several weeks for colonies to become apparent; skin testing, which has a sensitivity of up to 100% and a specificity of up to 98%; and PCR-based techniques that target the bacterial 16S ribosomal RNA gene or *B henselae* DNA.

Suhler ED, Lauer AK, Rosenbaum JT. Prevalence of serologic evidence of cat scratch disease in patients with neuroretinitis. *Ophthalmology.* 2000;107(5):871–876.

Treatment

Definitive treatment guidelines have not emerged for CSD because in many cases it is a self-limiting illness with an overall excellent systemic prognosis. Visual outcomes vary, depending on the location and severity of intraocular inflammation. A variety of antibiotics, including doxycycline, ciprofloxacin, erythromycin, rifampin, trimethoprim-sulfamethoxazole, and gentamicin, have been used in the treatment of more severe systemic or ocular manifestations, even though their efficacy has not been demonstrated conclusively. A typical regimen for immunocompetent patients older than 8 years consists of doxycycline, 100 mg orally twice daily for 4–6 weeks. For more severe infections, doxycycline may be given intravenously or used in combination with rifampin, 300 mg orally twice daily; in immunocompromised individuals, this treatment is extended for 4 months. Children with CSD may be treated with azithromycin. The effectiveness of oral corticosteroids on the course of systemic and ocular disease is unknown, even though these agents are frequently used in cases in which the optic nerve/macula is threatened.

Whipple Disease

Whipple disease is a rare multisystem disease caused by the *Tropheryma whipplei* bacterium. It is most common in middle-aged White men. Migratory arthritis occurs in 80% of cases, and gastrointestinal symptoms, including diarrhea, steatorrhea, and malabsorption, occur in 75%. Intestinal loss of protein results in pitting edema and weight loss. Cardiomyopathy and valvular disease can also occur. CNS involvement occurs in 10% of cases and causes seizures, dementia, and coma. Neuro-ophthalmic signs can include cranial nerve palsies, nystagmus, and ophthalmoplegia. Some patients develop a progressive supranuclear palsy–like condition. See also BCSC Section 5, *Neuro-Ophthalmology,* for discussion of the neuro-ophthalmic manifestations of Whipple disease.

Ocular Involvement

Intraocular involvement is rare, occurring in less than 5% of cases. Patients can present with bilateral panuveitis and retinal vasculitis, as well as with multifocal chorioretinitis (Fig 11-16). Both anterior uveitis and moderate vitritis are present. Diffuse chorioretinal inflammation and diffuse retinal vasculitis in the perifoveal and midperipheral regions may occur. Retinal vascular occlusions and retinal hemorrhages may result from the vasculitis. Optic disc edema and, later, optic atrophy may occur. Unusual granular, crystalline deposits on the iris, capsular bag, and intraocular lens have also been reported.

Touitou V, Fenollar F, Cassoux N, et al. Ocular Whipple's disease: therapeutic strategy and long-term follow-up. *Ophthalmology.* 2012;119(7):1465–1469.

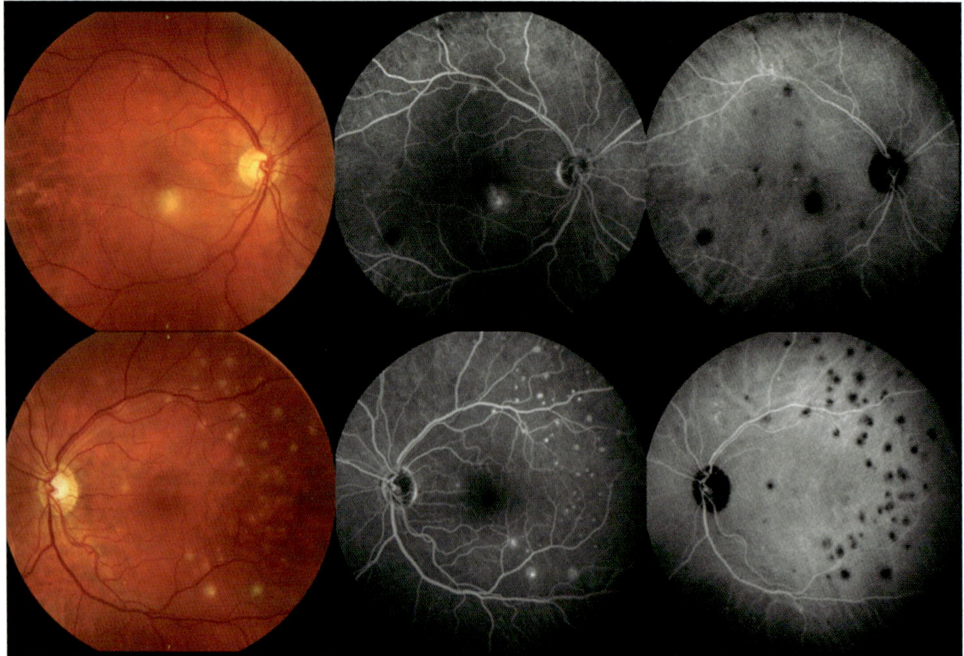

Figure 11-16 Whipple disease. Fundus photography *(left),* FA *(middle),* and indocyanine green angiography *(right)* demonstrate bilateral multifocal chorioretinitis. *(Courtesy of Wendy M. Smith, MD.)*

Diagnosis

The gold standard for diagnosis of Whipple disease is a duodenal biopsy that demonstrates a periodic acid–Schiff-positive bacillus in macrophages within intestinal villi. A PCR analysis of peripheral blood and vitreous may show *T whipplei* DNA and confirm the diagnosis. Culturing of *T whipplei* is difficult but possible. The differential diagnosis of uveitis associated with Whipple disease includes diseases that can cause retinal vasculitis with multisystem involvement, including sarcoidosis, systemic lupus erythematosus, polyarteritis nodosa, and Behçet disease. Vitreoretinal lymphoma should also be considered in older adults with substantial vitreal infiltration.

Boumaza A, Ben Azzouz E, Arrindell J, Lepidi H, Mezouar S, Desnues B. Whipple's disease and *Tropheryma whipplei* infections: from bench to bedside. *Lancet Infect Dis.* 2022;22(10):e280–e291. doi:10.1016/S1473-3099(22)00128-1

Treatment

Comanagement with an infectious diseases specialist is warranted. The preferred treatment is systemic trimethoprim-sulfamethoxazole. Patients allergic to sulfonamides may be treated with ceftriaxone, tetracycline, or chloramphenicol. Treatment duration may vary from 1 to 3 months, but relapses occur in 30% of cases, necessitating prolonged (up to 1 year) treatment. Retinal vasculitis can resolve with treatment, but neurologic deficits become permanent. Untreated, Whipple disease can be fatal.

CHAPTER 12

Infectious Uveitis: Nonbacterial Causes

This chapter includes a related video. Go to www.aao.org/bcscvideo_section09 or scan the QR code in the text to access this content.

Highlights

- Viruses, fungi, protozoa, helminths, and bacteria can cause infectious uveitis, and any part of the uveal tract can be involved. This chapter on nonbacterial pathogens is organized according to the causative organism and subcategorized by the anatomical location of inflammation.
- Herpes simplex, varicella-zoster, and cytomegalovirus may cause an isolated anterior uveitis or retinitis. In all patients with suspected viral infection, the eyes should be dilated to look for possible posterior segment disease.
- The viral retinopathies include acute retinal necrosis, progressive outer retinal necrosis, and cytomegalovirus retinitis. Diagnosis is principally clinical, although polymerase chain reaction testing can be utilized to identify the causative pathogen.
- In humans, *Toxoplasma gondii* infection is either acquired or congenital. Recently acquired disease may present as a focal retinochoroiditis in the absence of a retinochoroidal scar.
- Ophthalmic presentations of ocular toxocariasis include a chronic endophthalmitis (25% of cases), a posterior pole granuloma (25% of cases), or a peripheral granuloma (50% of cases).

Viral Uveitis

Herpesviridae Family

The herpesviruses, which include some of the most common human viruses, are double-stranded DNA microorganisms. Members of the family Herpesviridae discussed in this chapter are herpes simplex virus (HSV), varicella-zoster virus (VZV), cytomegalovirus (CMV), and Epstein-Barr virus. For a discussion of Herpesviridae member *Human herpesvirus 8,* which is associated with Kaposi sarcoma, see Chapter 13. For additional information, see BCSC Section 1, *Update on General Medicine.*

The uveitic entities associated with herpesvirus infection include isolated anterior uveitis and posterior uveitis or panuveitis. The following section is organized by anatomical involvement.

Herpes simplex virus, varicella-zoster virus, and cytomegalovirus

Anterior uveitis In immunocompetent patients, HSV, VZV, or CMV may cause an isolated acute or chronic anterior uveitis with or without keratitis. Dermatitis, rash, conjunctivitis, episcleritis, and scleritis may accompany HSV- and VZV-associated anterior uveitis but typically not anterior uveitis associated with CMV. Although bilateral cases of herpetic anterior uveitis have been reported, the disorder is classically unilateral.

FEATURES AND DIAGNOSIS Primary infection with VZV causes varicella (chickenpox), characterized by a full-body vesicular rash. Up to 40% of patients with primary VZV infection develop a *bilateral acute nongranulomatous anterior uveitis* that is asymptomatic, mild, and self-limiting. Reactivation of VZV within V_1 (ophthalmic division of cranial nerve V) causes herpes zoster ophthalmicus (HZO), a painful vesicular rash in the associated dermatome. Cutaneous vesicles at the tip of the nose (ie, Hutchinson sign) indicate nasociliary nerve involvement and an increased likelihood of ocular involvement (Fig 12-1). In patients with HZO, care should be taken to identify other ophthalmic manifestations of the disease, such as keratitis, anterior uveitis, conjunctivitis, episcleritis, scleritis, acute retinal necrosis, nonnecrotizing retinitis, and cranial nerve palsy.

Infection with VZV may be considered in the differential diagnosis of chronic unilateral anterior uveitis, even when the cutaneous component of the infection occurred in the past or was minimal when present. However, patients may also develop VZV-associated anterior uveitis without ever experiencing a cutaneous component (ie, varicella-zoster

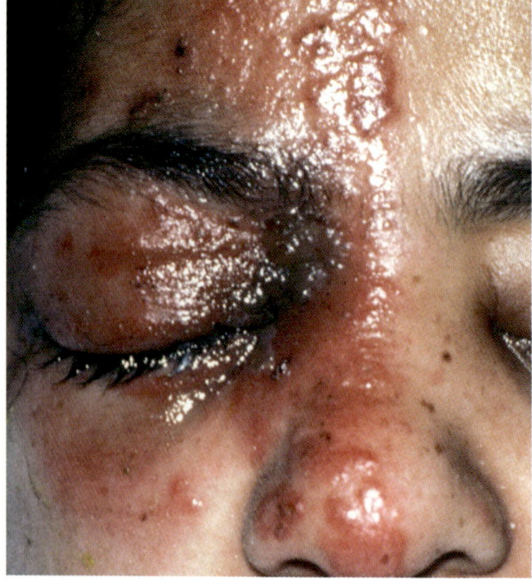

Figure 12-1 Herpes zoster ophthalmicus. Painful, dermatomal vesicular rash. *(Courtesy of Debra A. Goldstein, MD.)*

sine herpete). Primary infection or reactivation of *HSV-associated* anterior uveitis may also occur with or without blepharoconjunctivitis and periocular vesicles. See BCSC Section 8, *External Disease and Cornea,* for additional information about HSV, VZV, and CMV infections of the anterior segment.

Acute anterior chamber inflammation with ocular hypertension can be a helpful diagnostic hallmark of herpetic anterior uveitis. Although most inflammatory syndromes are associated with *decreased* intraocular pressure (IOP) as a result of ciliary body inflammation-related hyposecretion, herpetic anterior uveitis may cause trabeculitis that results in *very high IOP* (ie, 50–60 mm Hg). Elevated IOP can also be caused by inflammatory cells obstructing the trabecular meshwork. Of note, CMV has been associated with glaucomatocyclitic crisis and Fuchs uveitis syndrome, entities that may present acutely with elevated IOP (see Chapter 8).

Keratic precipitates (KPs) caused by HSV and VZV may be granulomatous or nongranulomatous and sometimes occur with associated pigmentation, especially in chronic uveitis. Diffuse, stellate KPs can occur with all three types of herpetic anterior uveitis, while ring-shaped clusters or scant, small, white-domed KPs are pathognomonic for CMV. Anterior uveitis may be accompanied by corneal endotheliitis and edema with all three viruses, but only HSV and VZV are associated with dendritiform epithelial involvement, reduced corneal sensation, and neurotrophic keratitis. Stromal keratitis is more typical of HSV and VZV than of CMV. Similarly, hyphema, hypopyon, and posterior synechia may be seen with HSV and VZV, but they do not routinely occur with CMV-associated anterior uveitis. Iris atrophy is a later characteristic of herpetic inflammation that is not typically present in the first few days to weeks of the initial episode of uveitis. The atrophy may be patchy or sectorial (Fig 12-2A) and is visualized as transillumination defects upon retroillumination at the slit lamp (Figs 12-2B, 12-3).

Distinguishing between HSV, VZV, and CMV can have implications for treatment and prognosis of anterior uveitis. When diagnostic uncertainty could change treatment, anterior chamber paracentesis may be performed to distinguish HSV and VZV from CMV (see the following section). In addition, all patients with suspected viral anterior uveitis should have a careful dilated examination of both eyes to assess for posterior segment disease, as a missed or delayed diagnosis could lead to blindness.

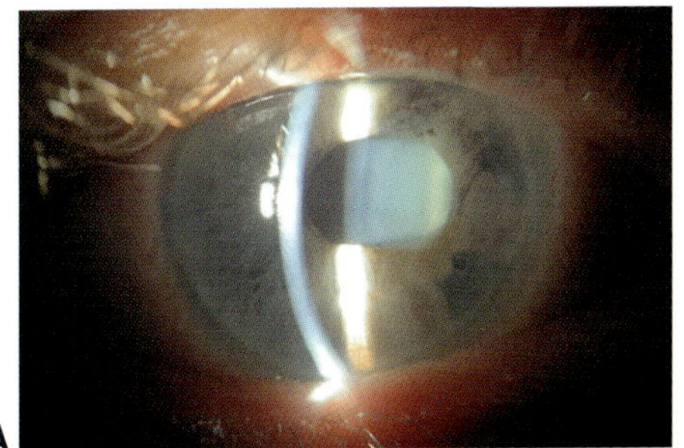

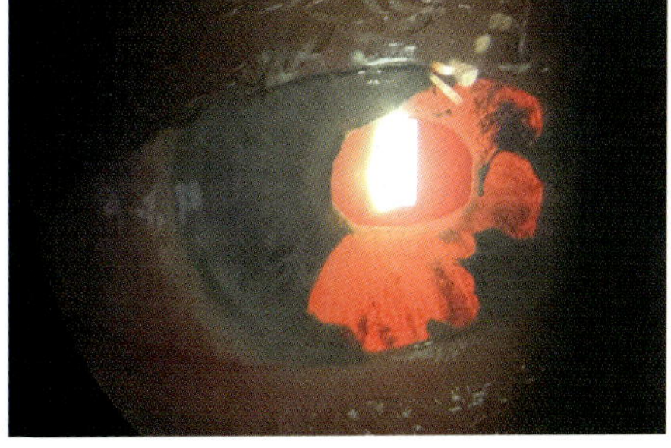

Figure 12-2 Iris stromal atrophy in a patient with herpes simplex virus anterior uveitis. **A,** Anterior segment photograph. **B,** Visualized as transillumination defects with retroillumination at the slit lamp. *(Courtesy of Sam S. Dahr, MD, MS.)*

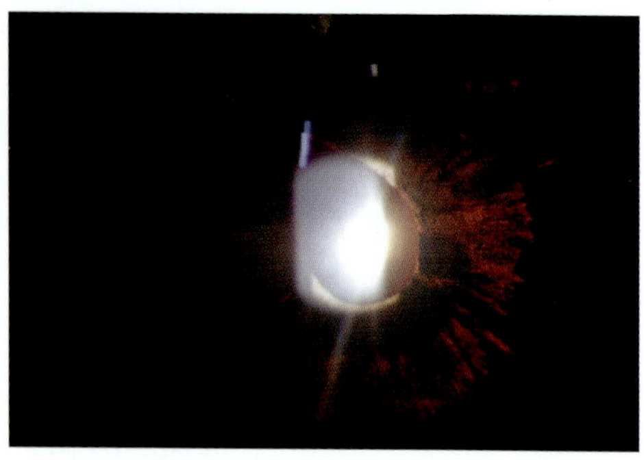

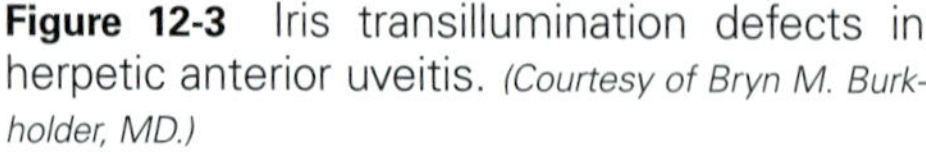

Figure 12-3 Iris transillumination defects in herpetic anterior uveitis. *(Courtesy of Bryn M. Burkholder, MD.)*

Chan NS, Chee SP. Demystifying viral anterior uveitis: A review. *Clin Exp Ophthalmol.* 2019;47(3):320–333.

Cohen EJ, Jeng BH. Herpes zoster: a brief definitive review. *Cornea.* 2021;40(8):943–949.

Terada Y, Kaburaki T, Takase H, et al. Distinguishing features of anterior uveitis caused by herpes simplex virus, varicella-zoster virus, and cytomegalovirus. *Am J Ophthalmol.* 2021;227:191–200.

Tran KD, Falcone MM, Choi DS, et al. Epidemiology of herpes zoster ophthalmicus: recurrence and chronicity. *Ophthalmology.* 2016;123(7):1469–1475.

TREATMENT Treatment for herpetic anterior uveitis includes antiviral therapy as well as topical corticosteroids and cycloplegic agents. Adjunctive IOP-lowering agents are often required throughout the disease course but can sometimes be tapered as the inflammation is better controlled. Recalcitrant cases may require surgical intervention to control IOP elevations.

Initiation of oral antiviral therapy at the onset of HSV-associated and VZV-associated anterior uveitis is typically necessary to control the inflammation. Systemic antiviral drugs such as acyclovir (400–800 mg, 5 times/day), famciclovir (250–500 mg, 3 times/day), and valacyclovir (500 mg to 1 g, 3 times/day) may help treat HSV- or VZV-related intraocular inflammation. The higher doses are usually needed for VZV. Prolonged topical corticosteroid therapy with very gradual tapering may also be required. In addition, systemic corticosteroids are sometimes necessary but should be used only with concurrent systemic antiviral therapy. Long-term, suppressive, low-dose antiviral therapy may be indicated in patients with HSV- and VZV-associated anterior uveitis, but randomized, controlled studies of their efficacy are lacking. The oral prophylactic dosage for patients with herpetic disease is acyclovir, 400 mg 2 times/day (for HSV infection), 800 mg 2 times/day (for VZV infection), or valacyclovir, 1 g/day.

As mentioned previously, HSV- and VZV-associated anterior uveitis should be distinguished from CMV-related disease when antiviral therapy is being considered. CMV-associated anterior uveitis will not respond to the antiviral therapy used for HSV and VZV, as the virus lacks the virally encoded thymidine kinase necessary for drug metabolism. If suspected herpetic anterior uveitis does not improve with empiric acyclovir or valacyclovir, diagnostic polymerase chain reaction (PCR) testing of aqueous fluid for CMV should be considered.

There is no standardized antiviral therapy for CMV-associated anterior uveitis. The infection was previously managed with topical corticosteroids and IOP-lowering agents alone. Additional treatment options include topical ganciclovir 0.15% gel, intravitreal foscarnet or ganciclovir, high-dose oral valganciclovir (see the section "Cytomegalovirus retinitis"), and compounded 2% ganciclovir drops. Long-term systemic antiviral treatment may be limited by drug toxicity or drug resistance, and relapses of CMV-associated anterior uveitis are common after discontinuation of therapy.

La Distia Nora R, Putera I, Mayasari YD, et al. Clinical characteristics and treatment outcomes of cytomegalovirus anterior uveitis and endotheliitis: a systematic review and meta-analysis. *Surv Ophthalmol.* 2022;67(4):1014–1030.

Testi I, Aggarwal K, Jaiswal N, et al. Antiviral therapy for varicella zoster virus (VZV) and herpes simplex virus (HSV)-induced anterior uveitis: a systematic review and meta-analysis. *Front Med (Lausanne).* 2021;8:686427. doi:10.3389/fmed.2021.686427

CLINICAL PEARL

Characteristics of herpesvirus-associated anterior uveitis can include the following:

- unilateral presentation
- ocular hypertension with acute inflammation
- decreased corneal sensation and epithelial/stromal disease (more common with HSV and VZV)
- endotheliitis
- corneal stromal immune ring (more likely with CMV)

Iris atrophy and transillumination defects are a later finding (ie, not seen at initial presentation).

Posterior uveitis and panuveitis The herpetic retinopathies include acute retinal necrosis (ARN), progressive outer retinal necrosis (PORN), and CMV retinitis. Retinal lesions of presumed herpetic etiology that are not consistent with ARN, PORN, or CMV retinitis are grouped under the umbrella designation *nonnecrotizing herpetic retinopathy.* The risk for both types of viral retinitis is increased in immunocompromised patients. HZO can also be associated with vasculitis that can lead to anterior segment ischemia, retinal artery occlusion, and scleritis. Vasculitis in the orbit may cause cranial nerve palsies.

ACUTE RETINAL NECROSIS ARN may occur in healthy adults or children as well as in immunocompromised patients, including those with HIV infection. Acute, fulminant disease may arise without a systemic prodrome, often months or years after primary infection or following cutaneous or systemic herpetic infection such as varicella, herpes zoster, or herpetic encephalitis (HSV-1 or -2). Patients may have a history of recurrent cutaneous herpetic outbreaks. The prevalence of ARN is nearly equal between the sexes, with most cases clustering in patients in the fifth to seventh decades of life.

Patients with ARN usually present with acute unilateral vision loss, photophobia, floaters, and pain. The fellow eye is involved in approximately 36% of cases, usually within 6 weeks of disease onset, but sometimes months or years later. Panuveitis develops, beginning with substantial anterior segment inflammation, KPs, posterior synechiae, and elevated IOP, together with heavy vitreous cellular infiltration and haze. Within 2 weeks, the classic triad of occlusive retinal arteriolitis, vitritis, and a multifocal yellow-white peripheral retinitis evolves. Early on, the peripheral retinal lesions may be discontinuous with

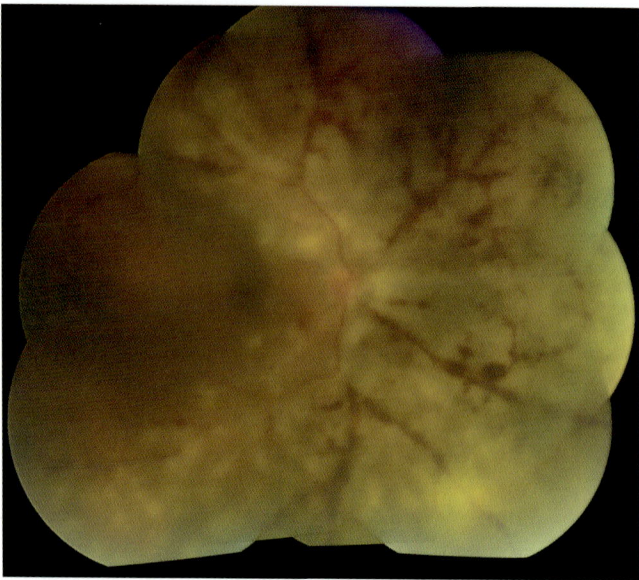

Figure 12-4 Acute retinal necrosis. Fundus photograph montage shows confluent peripheral retinitis with posterior extension. *(Courtesy of H. Nida Sen, MD/National Eye Institute.)*

scalloped edges that appear to arise in the outer retina. Within days, the lesions coalesce to form a confluent 360° cream-colored peripheral retinitis that progresses in a posterior direction, leaving full-thickness retinal necrosis, arteriolitis, phlebitis, and occasional retinal hemorrhage in its wake (Fig 12-4). Widespread necrosis of the peripheral and midzonal retina, multiple posterior retinal breaks, and proliferative vitreoretinopathy may lead to combined tractional–rhegmatogenous retinal detachments in 75% of patients (Fig 12-5). Optic nerve swelling and a relative afferent pupillary defect may also develop.

The differential diagnosis of ARN includes CMV retinitis, atypical toxoplasmic retinochoroiditis, syphilis, lymphoma, leukemia, and autoimmune retinitis with retinal vasculitis (ie, Behçet disease). The American Uveitis Society has established criteria for the diagnosis of ARN solely on the basis of clinical findings and disease progression, independent of viral etiology or host immune status (Table 12-1).

Although the diagnosis of ARN is made clinically, PCR testing of aqueous or vitreous can be used to determine the etiology of ARN and has largely supplanted viral culture, intraocular antibody titers, and serology. For diagnosis of presumed ARN, aqueous (rather than vitreous) sampling is usually sufficient. Quantitative PCR may also add information regarding viral load, disease activity, and response to therapy. In rare cases in which PCR results are negative for necrotizing herpetic retinitis but clinical suspicion is high, endoretinal biopsy may be diagnostic.

Studies using PCR-based assays suggest that the most common cause of ARN is VZV, followed by HSV-1, HSV-2, and in rare cases, CMV. Patients with ARN caused by VZV or HSV-1 infection tend to be older (mean age, 40 years), whereas those with HSV-2 infection tend to be younger (<25 years). The risk of encephalitis and meningitis is higher among patients with ARN caused by HSV-1 than among those with VZV infection.

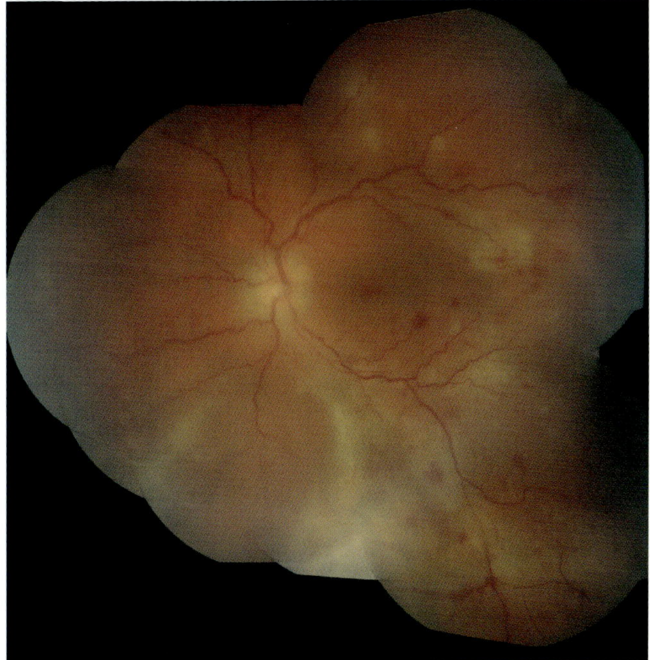

Figure 12-5 Acute retinal necrosis. Fundus photograph montage reveals vitritis, multifocal and confluent areas of retinitis, retinal vasculitis, retinal hemorrhage, optic nerve head edema, and retinal detachment. *(Reproduced from Schoenberger SD, Kim SJ, Thorne JE, et al. Diagnosis and treatment of acute retinal necrosis: a report by the American Academy of Ophthalmology. Ophthalmic Technology Assessment.* Ophthalmology. *2017;124(3):382–392. © 2017 American Academy of Ophthalmology.)*

Table 12-1 American Uveitis Society Criteria for Diagnosis of Acute Retinal Necrosis

One or more foci of retinal necrosis with discrete borders, located in the peripheral retina[a]
Rapid progression in the absence of antiviral therapy
Circumferential spread
Occlusive vasculopathy with arteriolar involvement
Prominent vitritis, anterior chamber inflammation
Supportive, but not required: optic neuropathy/atrophy, scleritis, pain

[a] Macular lesions do not exclude diagnosis in the presence of peripheral retinitis.

Information from Holland GN; the Executive Committee of the American Uveitis Society. Standard diagnostic criteria for the acute retinal necrosis syndrome. *Am J Ophthalmol.* 1994;117(5):663–667.

Initiation of antiviral therapy for ARN should not be delayed while awaiting PCR results. Timely diagnosis and prompt treatment are essential, given the rapidity of disease progression, the frequency of retinal detachment, and the guarded visual prognosis. Intravenous acyclovir, 10 mg/kg every 8 hours for 10–14 days, is effective against HSV and VZV. However, reversible elevations in serum creatinine and liver enzyme levels may occur; in the presence of frank renal insufficiency, the dosage will need to be reduced. As induction therapy for HSV- and VZV-associated retinitis, oral valacyclovir at doses up to 2 g 3 times daily has been a successful alternative to intravenous acyclovir, with similar bioavailability.

After intravenous antiviral induction for VZV infection, treatment with acyclovir at 800 mg orally 5 times daily, valacyclovir (prodrug to acyclovir) at 1–2 g orally 3 times daily, or famciclovir at 500 mg orally 3 times daily should be continued for 3 months. For ARN associated with HSV-1 infection, the oral antiviral dose is one-half that for VZV. Extended antiviral therapy may reduce the incidence of contralateral disease or bilateral ARN by 80% over 1 year.

As first-line therapy for ARN or for disease that fails to respond to systemic treatment, intravitreal ganciclovir (2.0 mg/0.05 or 0.1 mL) and foscarnet (2.4 mg/0.1 mL) may be used with systemic antiviral therapy. An Ophthalmic Technology Assessment report by the American Academy of Ophthalmology suggests that the combination of high-dose oral and intravitreal antiviral therapies may decrease the risk of retinal detachment and severe vision loss, but no randomized clinical trials have investigated this regimen. Given the short intravitreal half-life of these drugs, injections may need to be repeated 2 or 3 times per week until the retinitis is stable, and then weekly if necessary (see Appendix B). Effective treatment should inhibit the development of new lesions and promote lesion regression over 4 days.

After 24–48 hours of antiviral therapy, systemic corticosteroids (prednisone, 1 mg/kg/day, up to 60–80 mg/day) can be introduced to treat intraocular inflammation and then tapered over several weeks. Aspirin and other anticoagulants have been used to treat an associated hypercoagulable state and prevent vascular occlusions, but the results are inconclusive.

Despite treatment, there is a high rate of retinal detachment, which may occur within weeks to months of ARN onset. The use of prophylactic barrier laser photocoagulation in areas of healthy retina at the posterior border of necrotic lesions to prevent retinal detachment is controversial, but it has been employed by some practitioners. When detachment occurs, vitrectomy techniques are preferred over standard scleral buckling. Nevertheless, optic nerve atrophy may be visually limiting even with a favorable retinal anatomical outcome.

Schoenberger SD, Kim SJ, Thorne JE, et al. Diagnosis and treatment of acute retinal necrosis: a report by the American Academy of Ophthalmology. Ophthalmic Technology Assessment. *Ophthalmology.* 2017;124(3):382–392.

PROGRESSIVE OUTER RETINAL NECROSIS PORN is a morphologic variant of ARN that occurs in those who are profoundly immunosuppressed, most commonly owing to advanced AIDS (ie, $CD4^+$ T lymphocytes ≤50 cells/μL). The most common cause of PORN is VZV infection, although HSV has also been isolated. As with ARN, the retinitis begins as patchy areas of outer retinal whitening that coalesce rapidly. In contrast to ARN, the posterior pole may be involved early in the disease course, substantial vitreous cell and haze are typically absent, and the retinal vasculature is minimally involved, at least initially (Fig 12-6). Patients with PORN and HIV/AIDS frequently have a history of cutaneous zoster (67%) and eventually incur bilateral involvement (71%). Similar to ARN, there is a high rate (70%) of retinal detachment. The visual prognosis is poor; in the largest series reported to date, 67% of patients with PORN had a final visual acuity of no light perception. Although PORN is often resistant to treatment with intravenous acyclovir alone, management with combination systemic and intravitreal therapy using foscarnet and ganciclovir has been

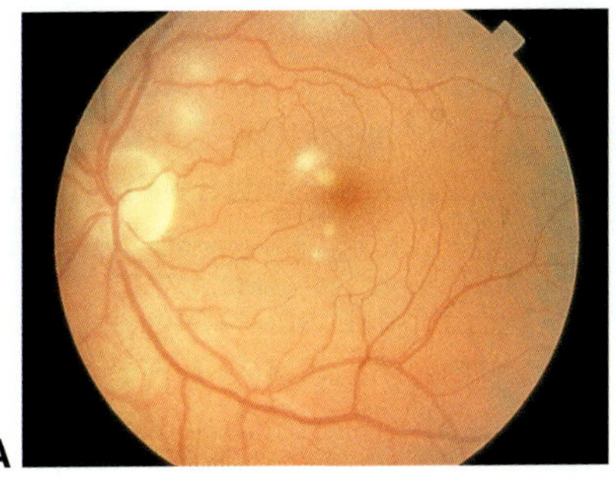

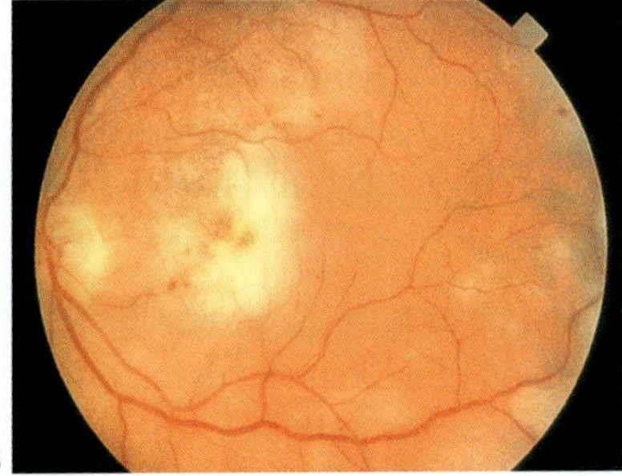

Figure 12-6 Progressive outer retinal necrosis. **A,** Fundus photograph showing multifocal areas of retinitis in the posterior pole. **B,** Fundus photograph taken 5 days later showing rapid disease progression and confluence of the areas of viral retinitis. *(Courtesy of E. Mitchel Opremcak, MD.)*

successful. Long-term suppressive antiviral therapy is required in patients with PORN and HIV/AIDS who are not able to achieve immune reconstitution through antiretroviral treatment. See also BCSC Section 12, *Retina and Vitreous,* for additional discussion of viral retinitis.

Engstrom RE Jr, Holland GN, Margolis TP, et al. The progressive outer retinal necrosis syndrome: a variant of necrotizing herpetic retinopathy in patients with AIDS. *Ophthalmology.* 1994;101(9):1488–1502.

Gore DM, Gore SK, Visser L. Progressive outer retinal necrosis: outcomes in the intravitreal era. *Arch Ophthalmol.* 2012;130(6):700–706.

NONNECROTIZING HERPETIC RETINOPATHY Nonnecrotizing herpetic retinopathy (nonnecrotizing posterior uveitis) may occur in patients with herpetic infections. Examples include acute retinochoroiditis with diffuse hemorrhages after acute VZV infection in children, and chronic choroiditis or retinal vasculitis in adults. In a study using PCR-based assays and local antibody analysis of aqueous fluid samples for herpesviruses in patients with "idiopathic posterior uveitis," 13% of cases had a confirmed viral etiology. Affected patients may be immunocompetent or immunocompromised. Inflammation is typically bilateral, and the disorder may present with uveitic macular edema, as a birdshot-like chorioretinopathy, or as an occlusive bilateral retinitis. The disease is initially resistant to conventional therapy with systemic corticosteroids and/or immunomodulatory therapy (IMT), but the response has been favorable when patients are switched to systemic antiviral medication.

Bodaghi B, Rozenberg F, Cassoux N, Fardeau C, LeHoang P. Nonnecrotizing herpetic retinopathies masquerading as severe posterior uveitis. *Ophthalmology.* 2003;110(9):1737–1743.

Wensing B, de Groot-Mijnes JD, Rothova A. Necrotizing and nonnecrotizing variants of herpetic uveitis with posterior segment involvement. *Arch Ophthalmol.* 2011;129(4):403–408.

Wu XN, Lightman S, Tomkins-Netzer O. Viral retinitis: diagnosis and management in the era of biologic immunosuppression: a review. *Clin Exp Ophthalmol.* 2019;47(3):381–395.

CYTOMEGALOVIRUS RETINITIS CMV causes symptomatic illness in immunocompromised children and adults (eg, those with leukemia, lymphoma, or HIV/AIDS), transplant recipients, and other patients with conditions requiring systemic IMT. In addition, CMV retinitis is the most common ophthalmic manifestation of congenital CMV infection (see BCSC Section 6, *Pediatric Ophthalmology and Strabismus*) as well as of CMV opportunistic coinfection in patients with HIV/AIDS (see Chapter 13). Three distinct clinical variants have been associated with CMV:

- a classic or fulminant retinitis with large areas of retinal hemorrhage against a background of whitened, edematous, or necrotic retina; the retinitis typically appears in the posterior pole, near the vascular arcades, in the distribution of the nerve fiber layer, and associated with blood vessels (Fig 12-7)
- a granular or indolent form found most often in the retinal periphery, characterized by little or no hemorrhage, edema, or vascular sheathing; active retinitis may progress from the borders of the lesion (Fig 12-8)
- a perivascular form often described as a variant of "frosted-branch" angiitis, an undifferentiated retinal perivasculitis initially described in immunocompetent children (Fig 12-9)

CMV reaches the eye hematogenously, with passage of the virus across the blood–ocular barrier, infection of retinal vascular endothelial cells, and cell-to-cell transmission of

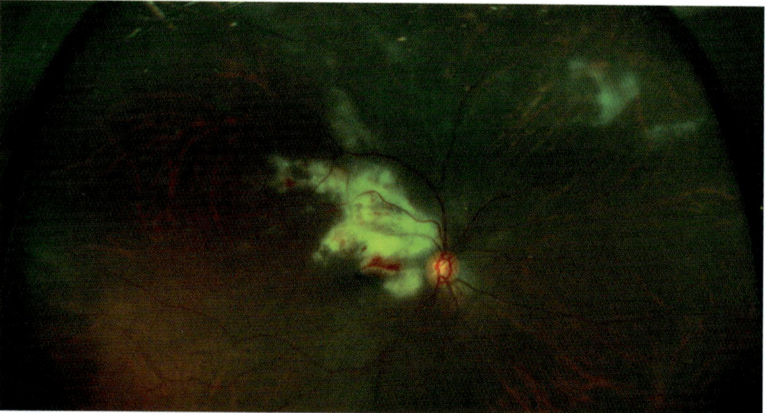

Figure 12-7 Cytomegalovirus retinitis. Wide-field fundus photograph shows fulminant retinitis without vitritis. *(Courtesy of Bryn M. Burkholder, MD.)*

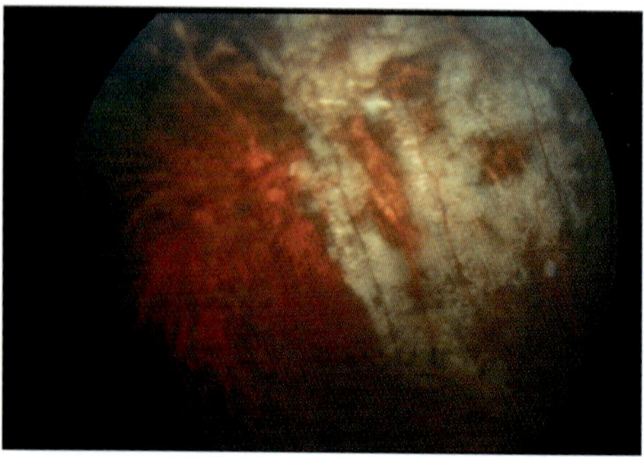

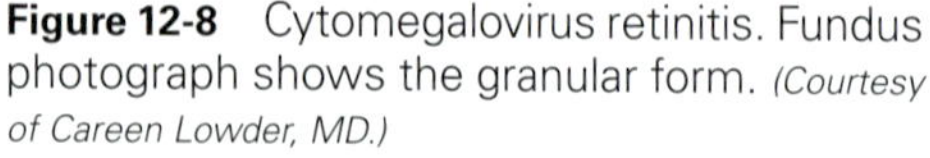

Figure 12-8 Cytomegalovirus retinitis. Fundus photograph shows the granular form. *(Courtesy of Careen Lowder, MD.)*

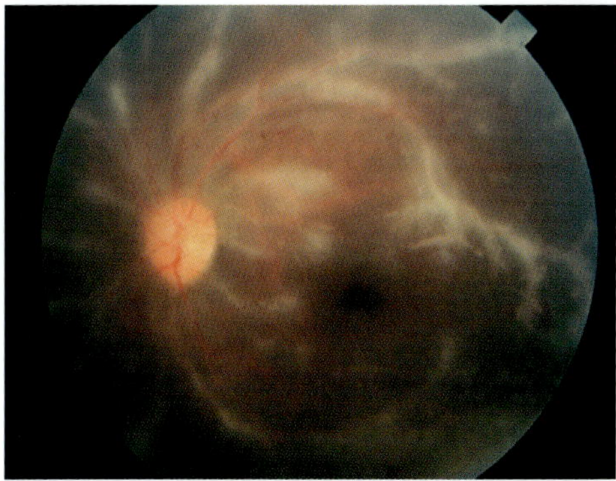

Figure 12-9 Cytomegalovirus retinitis. Fundus photograph shows "frosted-branch" perivasculitis. *(Courtesy of Albert T. Vitale, MD.)*

the virus within the retina. The histologic features of both congenital and acquired disease include a primary, full-thickness, coagulative, necrotizing retinitis and secondary diffuse choroiditis. Infected retinal cells show pathognomonic cytomegalic changes consisting of large eosinophilic intranuclear inclusions and small basophilic cytoplasmic inclusions. Viral inclusions may also be present in the retinal pigment epithelium (RPE) and vascular endothelium. See BCSC Section 4, *Ophthalmic Pathology and Intraocular Tumors,* for examples of CMV histologic findings.

The prevalence of retinitis in children with congenital CMV infection is between 11% and 22%. Systemic manifestations of disseminated infection in this population include fever, thrombocytopenia, anemia, pneumonitis, and hepatosplenomegaly. Diagnosis is suggested by the clinical presentation; positive serum antibodies or PCR testing of urine, saliva, or intraocular fluids; and systemic findings. Serum antibody testing may be useful 5–24 months after the loss of maternal antibodies transferred after pregnancy.

CMV retinitis has also occurred later in life among children who initially had no discernible lesions ophthalmoscopically and with no evidence of systemic disease reactivation. This pattern suggests that even asymptomatic children with congenital CMV infection should be monitored at regular intervals for potential ocular involvement later in childhood. Resolution of the retinitis leaves both pigmented and atrophic lesions, with retinal detachment occurring in up to one-third of these children. Optic atrophy and cataract formation are common sequelae.

In patients who are immunosuppressed or immunocompromised for any reason, CMV retinitis is an opportunistic infection. See Chapter 13 for further discussion.

With the advent of antiretroviral therapy, the incidence of CMV retinitis has decreased by 80% in patients with AIDS who have access to adequate medical resources. CMV retinitis is now more commonly diagnosed in patients immunosuppressed by chemotherapy or those receiving IMT for systemic inflammatory diseases or after solid organ or hematopoietic stem cell transplants. In rare cases, CMV retinitis may develop after a local corticosteroid injection, including intravitreal administration. In patients without AIDS, CMV retinitis is more likely to present as the granular form with substantial anterior chamber and vitreous inflammation and occlusive vasculitis. In patients undergoing systemic immunosuppression or chemotherapy, anti-CMV treatment usually requires close co-management with other medical subspecialists. Although there are no specific screening guidelines for immunosuppressed patients with CMV viremia, indications for an ophthalmic examination can include ocular symptoms and active or recently active multiorgan CMV infection.

Management of CMV retinitis involves antiviral therapy and measures to restore natural immunity, if possible (ie, reducing or discontinuing systemic IMT). Options for treatment include intravenous ganciclovir or foscarnet, oral valganciclovir, and intravitreal ganciclovir or foscarnet. See Chapter 13 for further details about treatment of CMV retinitis.

Months or years after therapy, patients with immune recovery may develop uveitis (eg, immune recovery uveitis) despite the absence of CMV reactivation. Immune recovery uveitis occurs when the reconstituted immune system reacts to residual CMV antigens within the eye. Treatment may include topical, periocular, and oral corticosteroids. See Chapter 13 for further discussion of immune recovery uveitis.

Kempen JH, Min YI, Freeman WR, et al; Studies of Ocular Complications of AIDS Research Group. Risk of immune recovery uveitis in patients with AIDS and cytomegalovirus retinitis. *Ophthalmology.* 2006;113(4);684–694.

Kim DY, Jo J, Joe SG, Kim JG, Yoon YH, Lee JY. Comparison of visual prognosis and clinical features of cytomegalovirus retinitis in HIV and non-HIV patients. *Retina.* 2017;37(2):376–381.

Schneider EW, Elner SG, van Kuijk FJ, et al. Chronic retinal necrosis: cytomegalovirus necrotizing retinitis associated with panretinal vasculopathy in non-HIV patients. *Retina.* 2013;33(9):1791–1799.

Shapira Y, Mimouni M, Vishnevskia-Dai V. Cytomegalovirus retinitis in HIV-negative patients—associated conditions, clinical presentation, diagnostic methods and treatment strategy. *Acta Ophthalmol.* 2018;96(7):e761–e767. doi:10.1111/aos.13553

Su YT, Chen YJ, Lin CP, et al. Clinical characteristics and prognostic factors affecting clinical outcomes in cytomegalovirus retinitis with or without HIV infection. *Retina.* 2023;43(1):57–63. doi:10.1097/IAE.0000000000003631

Epstein-Barr virus

Epstein-Barr virus (EBV) is a ubiquitous double-stranded DNA virus that is commonly associated with infectious mononucleosis (IM) and has been implicated in the pathogenesis of Burkitt lymphoma (especially among African children), nasopharyngeal carcinoma, Hodgkin disease, and Sjögren syndrome. EBV has a tropism for B lymphocytes, the only cells known to have surface receptors for the virus.

Congenital EBV infection may result in congenital cataract. Acquired EBV (eg, IM) is more likely to have ocular manifestations, most commonly a mild, self-limited follicular conjunctivitis. Less frequent anterior segment or external ocular manifestations of IM include epithelial or stromal keratitis; episcleritis; bilateral granulomatous anterior uveitis; dacryoadenitis; and in rare cases, cranial nerve palsies and Parinaud oculoglandular syndrome.

EBV is only rarely associated with posterior segment manifestations such as isolated optic disc edema and optic neuritis, macular edema, retinal hemorrhages, retinitis (including ARN), punctate outer retinitis, choroiditis, multifocal choroiditis with panuveitis (MFCPU), pars planitis and vitritis, progressive subretinal fibrosis, and secondary choroidal neovascularization (CNV). In the absence of systemic EBV-related disease or recently acquired IM, the virus is unlikely to be the cause of these findings. Serum antibody testing against a variety of EBV-specific capsid antigens is rarely useful in proving causality because of the very high seroprevalence of EBV (90%) in the adult population. The presence of EBV DNA or anti-EBV antibodies in ocular fluids has been cited as evidence of the causal role of EBV in ocular inflammation, but an intraocular EBV-associated malignancy, especially when the patient has HIV infection, could masquerade as ocular inflammation.

Most EBV-associated ocular disease is self-limiting. The presence of anterior uveitis may necessitate topical corticosteroids and cycloplegia. Posterior segment inflammation can be treated with systemic corticosteroids. For the management of necrotizing retinitis/ARN in patients with EBV, systemic antiviral therapy with acyclovir or ganciclovir may be considered.

Alba-Linero C, Rocha-de-Lossada C, Rachwani-Anil R, et al. Anterior segment involvement in Epstein-Barr virus: a review. *Acta Ophthalmol.* 2022;100(5):e1052–e1060. doi:10.1111/aos.15061

Cunningham ET, Zierhut M. Epstein-Barr virus and the eye. *Ocul Immunol Inflamm.* 2020;28(4):533–537.

Schaal S, Kagan A, Wang Y, Chan CC, Kaplan HJ. Acute retinal necrosis associated with Epstein-Barr virus: immunohistopathologic confirmation. *JAMA Ophthalmol.* 2014;132(7):881–882.

Smit D, Meyer D, Maritz J, de Groot-Mijnes JDF. Polymerase chain reaction and Goldmann-Witmer coefficient to examine the role of Epstein-Barr virus in uveitis. *Ocul Immunol Inflamm.* 2019;27(1):108–113.

Rubella

The rubella virus is the prototypical teratogenic viral agent that can affect the retina through transplacental transmission (ie, congenital rubella syndrome [CRS]) or acquired infection (ie, German measles). Although rubella infection remains an important cause of blindness in resource-limited regions and nations, the epidemic pattern of the disease was interrupted in the United States in 1969 by introduction of the rubella vaccine. The peak age of incidence has shifted from 5–9 years in the pre-vaccine era to 15–19 years and more recently to 20–24 years. Approximately 5%–25% of women of childbearing age are susceptible to primary infection.

Congenital rubella syndrome

The classic features of CRS are cardiac malformations (eg, patent ductus arteriosus, interventricular septal defects, and pulmonic stenosis), ocular findings (eg, chorioretinitis, pigmentary retinopathy, cataract, corneal clouding, microphthalmia, strabismus, and glaucoma), and deafness (Fig 12-10). Hearing loss is the most common systemic finding. In addition, individuals with CRS are at increased risk for diabetes and diabetic retinopathy later in life. Although the mechanism of rubella embryopathy is not known at the cellular level, the virus is thought to inhibit cellular division and establish a chronic, persistent infection during organogenesis. The persistence of viral replication after birth, with ongoing tissue damage, is central to the pathogenesis of CRS and may explain the appearance of hearing and neurologic and/or ocular deficits long after birth.

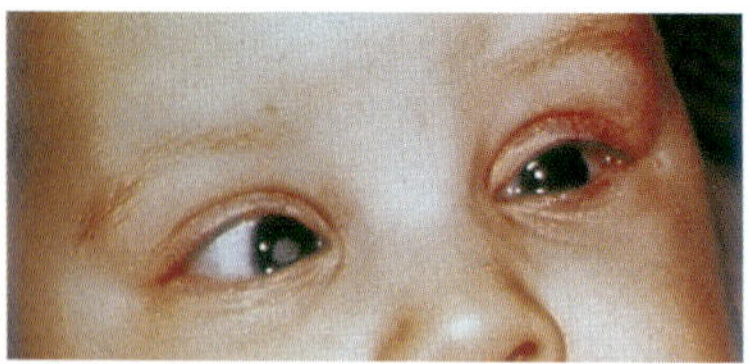

Figure 12-10 Congenital rubella syndrome. External photograph shows a patient who had cataract, esotropia, cognitive impairment, congenital heart disease, and deafness. *(Courtesy of John D. Sheppard Jr, MD.)*

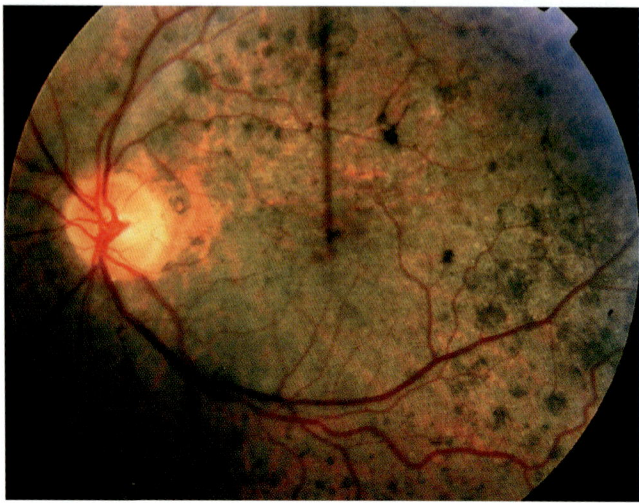

Figure 12-11 Congenital rubella syndrome. Fundus photograph demonstrates a salt and pepper fundus with diffuse retinal pigment epithelial mottling and pigment clumping. *(Courtesy of Albert T. Vitale, MD.)*

The most common ocular manifestation of CRS is a unilateral or bilateral pigmentary retinopathy (25%–50% of cases), followed by cataract (15%) and glaucoma (10%). The pigmentary disturbance, often described as salt and pepper fundus, shows considerable variation, ranging from finely stippled, bone spicule–like, small, black, irregular masses to gross pigmentary irregularities with coarse, blotchy mottling (Fig 12-11). This mottling can be stationary or progressive. Despite loss of the foveal light reflex and prominent pigmentary changes, neither vision nor electroretinogram results are typically affected, and retinal vessels appear normal. The optic nerves are also normal in appearance unless compromised by glaucoma. The most frequent cause of poor visual acuity in CRS is microphthalmia and congenital (nuclear) cataracts. Histologic studies of the lens reveal retained cell nuclei in the embryonic nucleus as well as anterior and posterior cortical degeneration. Although rare, CNV is another cause of vision loss in patients with CRS.

These pigmentary retinal changes and associated systemic findings, together with a history of maternal exposure to rubella, suggest the diagnosis of CRS. Serologic criteria for rubella infection include a fourfold increase in rubella-specific immunoglobulin (Ig) G in paired sera 1–2 weeks apart or the new appearance of rubella-specific IgM. Because the fetus is capable of mounting an immune response to the rubella virus, specific IgM or IgA antibodies to rubella in the cord blood confirm the diagnosis.

The differential diagnosis of congenital rubella retinitis includes the other entities associated with the TORCH syndrome (eg, *t*oxoplasmosis, *o*ther agents, *r*ubella, *c*ytomegalovirus, and *h*erpesviruses). Other viral illnesses, such as mumps, roseola subitum, and postvaccination encephalitis, should also be considered and ruled out by appropriate serologic tests. There is no specific antiviral therapy for congenital rubella, and treatment is supportive.

Arnold JJ, McIntosh ED, Martin FJ, Menser MA. A fifty-year follow-up of ocular defects in congenital rubella: late ocular manifestations. *Aust N Z J Ophthalmol.* 1994;22(1):1–6.

Mets MB, Chhabra MS. Eye manifestations of intrauterine infections and their impact on childhood blindness. *Surv Ophthalmol.* 2008;53(2):95–111.

Acquired rubella

Acquired infection presents with a prodrome of malaise and fever in adolescents and adults before onset of the rubella exanthem. An erythematous, maculopapular rash appears first on the face, spreads toward the hands and feet, involves the entire body within 24 hours, and disappears by the third day. Although the rash is not always prominent and the occurrence of fever is variable, lymphadenopathy is invariably present.

The most frequent ocular complication of postnatally acquired rubella is conjunctivitis (70% of cases), followed by rare occurrences of epithelial keratitis and retinitis. Acquired rubella retinitis has been described in adults presenting with acute-onset decreased vision and multifocal chorioretinitis. Reported findings include large areas of bullous retinal detachment, underlying pigment epithelial detachment involving the entire posterior pole, anterior chamber and preretinal vitreous cells, and dark gray atrophic lesions of the RPE. The retinal vessels and optic nerve typically appear normal, and there are no retinal hemorrhages. The retinal detachments resolve spontaneously, and visual acuity returns to normal. Chronic rubella virus infection has been implicated in the pathogenesis of Fuchs uveitis syndrome (see Chapter 8), as evidenced by the presence of rubella-specific intraocular antibody production and the intraocular persistence of the virus.

Uncomplicated acquired rubella does not require specific therapy; however, rubella retinitis and postvaccination optic neuritis may respond well to systemic corticosteroids.

Matalia J, Vinekar A, Anegondi N, et al. A prospective OCT study of rubella retinopathy. *Ophthalmol Retina.* 2018;2(12):1235–1240.

Lymphocytic Choriomeningitis Virus

Lymphocytic choriomeningitis virus (LCMV) is an under-recognized fetal teratogen that should probably be included among the “other agents” in the TORCH group of congenital infections. The microbe is a single-stranded RNA virus and a member of the family Arenaviridae.

Systemic findings include macrocephaly, hydrocephalus, and intracranial calcifications. Neurologic abnormalities, seizures, and mild cognitive impairment may also occur. Ocular findings include macular and peripheral chorioretinal scars, similar in morphology and distribution to those in congenital toxoplasmosis. Serologic testing of the mother and the infant helps distinguish LCMV from toxoplasmosis. Other findings include optic atrophy, strabismus, and nystagmus.

Mumps

The *Mumps virus* is a member of the family Paramyxoviridae (other members include measles, parainfluenza, and respiratory syncytial virus). A single-stranded RNA virus, mumps is acquired by respiratory droplets and may cause parotitis, aseptic meningitis, and orchitis. In rare cases, mumps may cause inflammation involving the cornea, optic nerve, or retina.

Measles (Rubeola)

Congenital and acquired measles infections are caused by a single-stranded RNA virus of the genus *Morbillivirus* of the family Paramyxoviridae. The virus is highly contagious and is transmitted either directly or via aerosolization of nasopharyngeal secretions to the mucous membranes of the conjunctiva or respiratory tract of susceptible individuals or transplacentally from a pregnant woman to her fetus.

Despite the existence of an effective vaccine, measles remains a leading cause of mortality among children worldwide. Measles is rare in the United States, although there was an outbreak in 2018.

Congenital measles infection may cause cataract, optic disc drusen, and a bilateral diffuse pigmentary retinopathy involving the posterior pole and retinal periphery. The retinopathy may be associated with normal or attenuated retinal vessels, retinal edema, and macular star formation. Electroretinographic results and visual acuity are usually normal.

The most common ocular manifestations of acquired measles are keratitis and a mild, papillary, nonpurulent conjunctivitis. In countries with prevalent malnutrition, corneal scarring may cause post-measles blindness, a significant problem worldwide.

Measles retinopathy is more common in acquired than in congenital disease, presenting with profound loss of vision 6–12 days after the appearance of the characteristic exanthem; it may be accompanied by encephalitis. Acquired measles retinopathy is characterized by attenuated arterioles, diffuse retinal edema, macular star formation, scattered retinal hemorrhages, blurred optic disc margins, and clear media. Optic disc pallor and a secondary pigmentary retinopathy with either a bone spicule or salt-and-pepper appearance may subsequently develop.

The differential diagnosis of congenital measles retinopathy includes the TORCH entities, atypical retinitis pigmentosa, and neuroretinitis. For acquired measles retinopathy, considerations include central serous chorioretinopathy, Vogt-Koyanagi-Harada syndrome (bullous detachments may resolve, leaving extensive RPE disruption), retinitis pigmentosa, syphilis, and other viral retinopathies.

The diagnosis of measles and its ocular sequelae is made clinically and through serologic testing. For patients with acute measles retinopathy, systemic corticosteroids may be considered.

Hübschen JM, Gouandjika-Vasilache I, Dina J. Measles. *Lancet.* 2022;399(10325):678–690.

Lee JH, Agarwal A, Mahendradas P, et al. Viral posterior uveitis. *Surv Ophthalmol.* 2017;62(4): 404–445.

Subacute sclerosing panencephalitis

Subacute sclerosing panencephalitis (SSPE) is a rare, late complication of acquired measles infection. It most often affects unvaccinated children in late childhood or adolescence, 6–8 years after the primary infection. Visual impairment, behavioral disturbances, and memory impairment may insidiously develop, followed by myoclonus and progression to spastic paresis, dementia, and death within 1–3 years.

Ocular findings are reported in up to 50% of patients with SSPE and may precede the neurologic manifestations by several weeks to 2 years. The most consistent finding is a maculopathy consisting of focal retinitis and RPE changes, occurring in 36% of patients with SSPE (Fig 12-12). Retinitis may progress to involve the peripheral retina, but there is usually minimal or no vitritis. Other intraocular findings include optic disc inflammation and papilledema, optic atrophy, macular edema, macular pigment epithelial disturbances, small intraretinal hemorrhages, gliotic scar, white retinal infiltrates, serous macular detachment, drusen, preretinal membranes, and macular hole. Other associations are cortical blindness, hemianopia, horizontal nystagmus, and ptosis.

The diagnosis of SSPE is based on clinical examination, electroencephalographic abnormalities, raised IgG antibody titer against measles in the plasma and cerebrospinal fluid, and/or panencephalitis found on magnetic resonance imaging or brain biopsy.

The differential diagnosis of the ophthalmic findings includes viral retinitis caused by HSV, VZV, and CMV infection. Intermediate uveitis and retinal vasculitis associated with multiple sclerosis may also be considered. Definitive treatment of SSPE remains undetermined.

Yuksel D, Sonmez PA, Yilmaz D, Senbil N, Gurer Y. Ocular findings in subacute sclerosing panencephalitis. *Ocul Immunol Inflamm.* 2011;19(2):135–138.

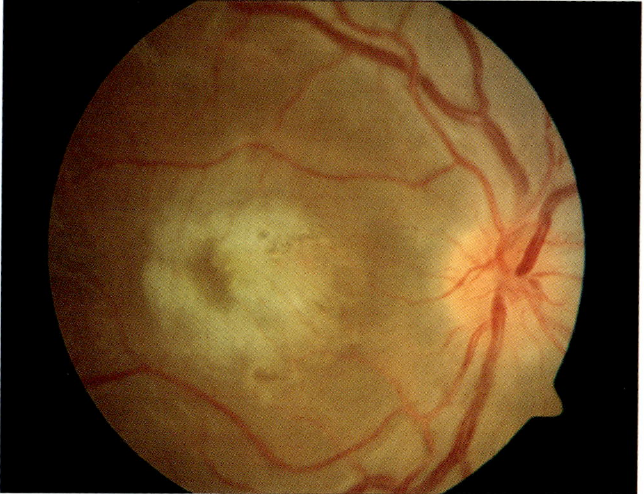

Figure 12-12 Subacute sclerosing panencephalitis in acquired measles infection. Fundus photograph of macular retinitis. *(Courtesy of Emad B. Abboud, MD.)*

West Nile Virus

West Nile virus (WNV) is a single-stranded RNA virus and member of the family Flaviviridae; it belongs to the Japanese encephalitis virus serocomplex and is endemic to Europe, Australia, Asia, and Africa. The virus is transmitted from birds (the natural host) to humans through the bite of an infected mosquito. The peak onset of the disease is late summer, but it can occur anytime between July and December. The incubation period ranges from 3 to 14 days. Eighty percent of WNV infections are subclinical. Twenty percent of infections present as a febrile illness, often accompanied by myalgia, arthralgia, headache, conjunctivitis, lymphadenopathy, and a maculopapular or roseolar rash. Severe neurologic disease (ie, meningitis or encephalitis) may occur, especially in association with diabetes and advanced age.

Presenting ocular symptoms include pain, photophobia, conjunctival hyperemia, and blurred vision. A characteristic multifocal chorioretinitis is present in most affected patients, together with nongranulomatous anterior uveitis and vitreous inflammatory cells. Chorioretinal lesions vary in size (200–1000 μm) and number and may affect the midzone and/or posterior pole, often in linear arrays following the course of retinal nerve fibers (classic appearance). Active lesions appear whitish to yellow, are flat and deep, and evolve with varying degrees of pigmentation and atrophy.

In patients with WNV infection, fluorescein angiography (FA) reveals central hypofluorescence with late staining of active lesions and early hyperfluorescence with late staining of inactive lesions. Inactive or partly active lesions may also have a targetlike appearance with central hypofluorescence caused by blockage from pigment and peripheral hyperfluorescence due to atrophy (Fig 12-13). Indocyanine green angiography reveals hypofluorescent spots, more numerous than those apparent on FA or ophthalmoscopy.

Other findings may include intraretinal hemorrhages, optic disc edema, optic atrophy, and less commonly, focal retinal vascular sheathing and occlusion, cranial nerve VI

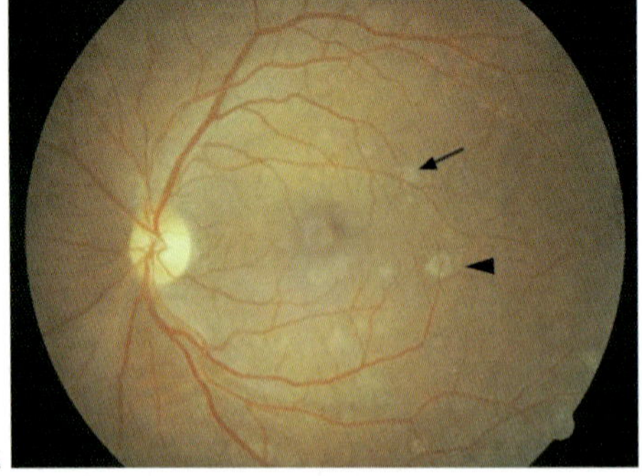

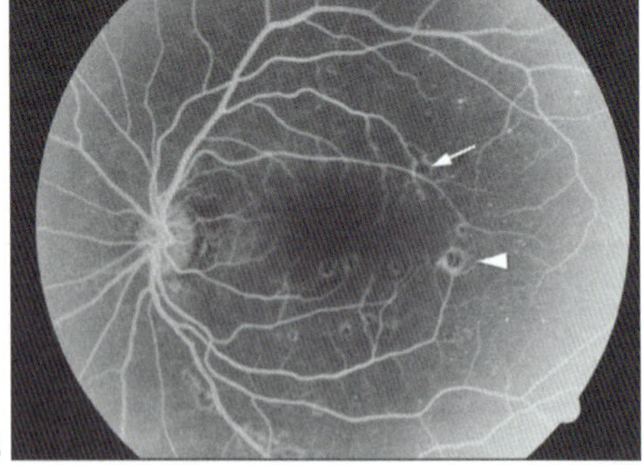

Figure 12-13 West Nile virus chorioretinitis. **A,** Fundus photograph showing multiple active *(arrow)* and partially active *(arrowhead)* discrete cream-colored chorioretinal spots (100–300 μm). **B,** The corresponding fluorescein angiogram shows early hypofluorescence *(arrow)* on the active chorioretinal spots (acute stage) and focal hypofluorescence with a surrounding hyperfluorescent ring *(arrowhead)* on the partially active lesions (subacute stage). On the late-phase angiogram (not shown), there was subsequent staining. *(Reproduced with permission from Chan CK, Limstrom SA, Tarasewicz DG, Ling SG. Ocular features of West Nile virus infection in North America: a study of 14 eyes.* Ophthalmology. *2006;113(9):1539–1546.)*

palsy, and nystagmus. Of note, congenital WNV infection has been reported in an infant who had chorioretinal scarring without intraocular inflammation.

In most patients, intraocular inflammation associated with WNV infection has a self-limiting course, with a return of visual acuity to baseline after several months. In others, loss of vision may occur because of CNV, foveal scar, ischemic maculopathy, vitreous hemorrhage, tractional retinal detachment, optic nerve pathology, and retrogeniculate damage. Diabetes has been implicated as a risk factor for WNV-related death and may increase the risk of WNV-associated ocular involvement.

Ocular findings in patients with systemic symptoms suggestive of WNV infection or with meningoencephalitis may prompt WNV serologic testing. The differential diagnosis includes syphilis, MFCPU, histoplasmosis, sarcoidosis, and tuberculosis.

Currently, there is no vaccine or specific antiviral treatment for WNV infection. Patients receive supportive therapy. Anterior uveitis may be treated with topical corticosteroids. The efficacy of systemic and periocular corticosteroids for chorioretinal manifestations is unknown. Public health strategies directed at prevention are the mainstays of WNV infection control.

Khairallah M, Ben Yahia S, Attia S, Zaouali S, Ladjimi A, Messaoud R. Linear pattern of West Nile virus–associated chorioretinitis is related to retinal nerve fibres organization. *Eye (Lond).* 2007;21(7):952–955.

Khairallah M, Ben Yahia S, Letaief M, et al. A prospective evaluation of factors associated with chorioretinitis in patients with West Nile virus infection. *Ocul Immunol Inflamm.* 2007;15(6):435–439.

Rousseau A, Haigh O, Ksiaa I, Khairallah M, Labetoulle M. Ocular manifestations of West Nile virus. *Vaccines (Basel).* 2020;8(4):641. doi:10.3390/vaccines8040641

Rift Valley Fever

Rift Valley fever is a febrile illness caused by *Rift Valley fever virus,* a member of the family Bunyaviridae. One of 3 clinical syndromes may develop: (1) an uncomplicated, febrile, influenza-like illness; (2) hemorrhagic fever; or (3) encephalitis. Ophthalmic findings may include anterior uveitis, vitritis, a macular or paramacular retinitis (classic finding) (Fig 12-14), retinal hemorrhage, retinal vasculitis, and optic nerve edema. Anterior uveitis

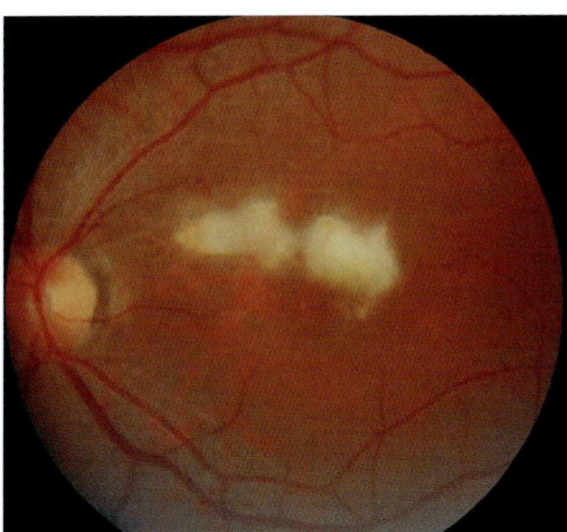

Figure 12-14 Rift Valley fever. Fundus photograph from a 44-year-old male farmer from Saudi Arabia who presented with decreased vision and macular retinitis sparing the fovea. He had a history of fever and contact with animal abortus. *(Courtesy of Albert T. Vitale, MD.)*

occurs in 31% of patients with Rift Valley fever. Patients may also develop macular scarring, vascular attenuation, retinal ischemia, and/or optic atrophy.

The differential diagnosis includes viral entities such as measles, rubella, influenza, dengue fever, and WNV infection as well as bacterial illnesses such as brucellosis, Lyme disease, toxoplasmosis, cat-scratch disease, and rickettsial diseases. The diagnosis of Rift Valley fever is made clinically and serologically.

Al-Hazmi A, Al-Rajhi AA, Abboud EB, et al. Ocular complications of Rift Valley fever outbreak in Saudi Arabia. *Ophthalmology.* 2005;112(2):313–318.

Human T-cell Lymphotropic Virus Type 1

Human T-cell lymphotropic virus type 1 (HTLV-1) is a retrovirus that is endemic in Japan, the Caribbean islands, and parts of Central and South America. It accounts for approximately 1% of uveitis cases in Japan. The diagnosis is made by serologic testing. The major target cell of HTLV-1 is the $CD4^+$ T cell. HTLV-1 infection is the established cause of HTLV-1 uveitis (HU), adult T-cell leukemia/lymphoma (ATL), and HTLV-1–associated myelopathy/tropical spastic paralysis (HAM/TSP).

Most cases of HU (75%) are classified as an intermediate uveitis. Patients present with blurred vision and floaters caused by a mild granulomatous anterior uveitis (20% of HU cases), unilateral vitritis (60%), membranous vitreous opacities, and/or snowballs. Retinal vasculitis (60%), exudative retinal lesions (25%), optic disc abnormalities (20%), and uveitic macular edema (3%) may also be found.

Additional ocular manifestations of HTLV-1 infection include retinal infiltrates caused by secondary ATL (Fig 12-15A). Patients with HAM/TSP may have retinal degeneration, optic neuropathy, and keratoconjunctivitis sicca. HTLV-1–associated keratopathy (previously referred to as *HTLV-1–related chronic interstitial keratitis*) has been described in Brazilian and Caribbean patients but has not been found among Japanese patients. These corneal lesions likely represent lymphoplasmacytic infiltrates and are asymptomatic (Fig 12-15B).

Although HU responds to topical, periocular, or systemic corticosteroids, one-half of patients may experience recurrent disease. For HU cases that progress despite therapy, the clinician should consider mimics of HU such as retinal infiltration caused by ATL (see Fig 12-15A) or retinal degeneration associated with HAM/TSP.

Goto H, Mochizuki M, Yamaki K, Kotake S, Usui M, Ohno S. Epidemiological survey of intraocular inflammation in Japan. *Jpn J Ophthalmol.* 2007;51(1):41–44.

Kamoi K, Watanabe T, Uchimaru K, et al. Updates on HTLV-1 uveitis. *Viruses.* 2022; 14(4):794. doi:10.3390/v14040794

Dengue Fever

Dengue fever, the most common mosquito-borne viral disease in humans, is caused by *Dengue virus,* a member of the family Flaviviridae. The virus is transmitted by the bite of an infected *Aedes aegypti* mosquito and is endemic within more than 100 countries in the tropical and subtropical regions of the globe.

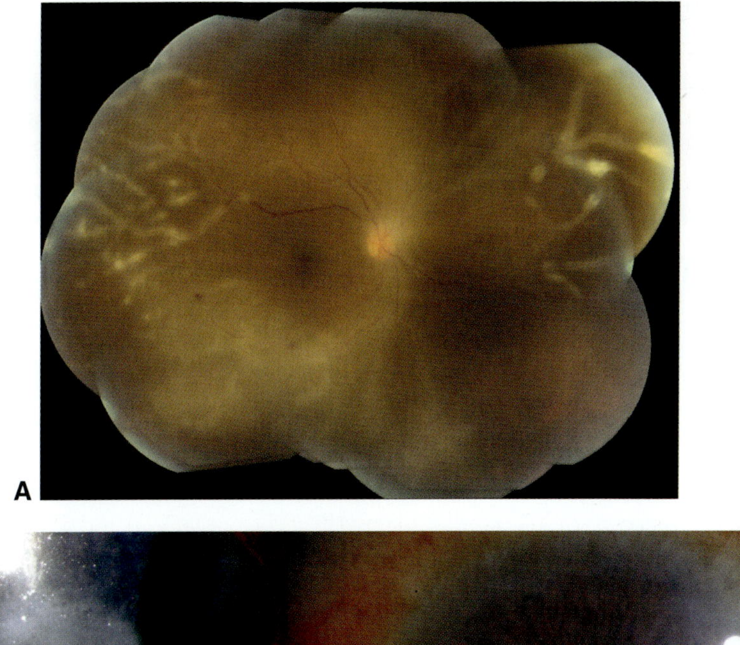

Figure 12-15 Human T-cell lymphotropic virus type 1–associated adult T-cell leukemia/lymphoma. **A,** Fundus photograph montage shows retinal and vascular infiltrates. **B,** Anterior segment photograph of keratopathy. *(Courtesy of H. Nida Sen, MD/National Eye Institute.)*

Systemic signs and symptoms of dengue infection include fever, headache, myalgia, purpuric rash, and other bleeding manifestations secondary to thrombocytopenia. For many patients, this initial infection may be low grade, and they may not mention symptoms unless specifically asked during the history and review of systems. The most common ocular manifestation is petechial subconjunctival hemorrhage. Variable degrees of anterior chamber and vitreous cells may also occur.

One month after the onset of systemic disease, approximately 10% of patients develop maculopathy or "foveolitis" that causes a sudden decrease in vision and central scotoma, often without clinical lesions on examination. FA may show early focal arteriolar knobby hyperfluorescence in the macula with late leakage and/or staining; optical coherence tomography (OCT) angiography may show disruption of the foveal avascular zone (Fig 12-16). OCT may show macular edema, subretinal fluid, or disruption of the inner segment/outer segment junction.

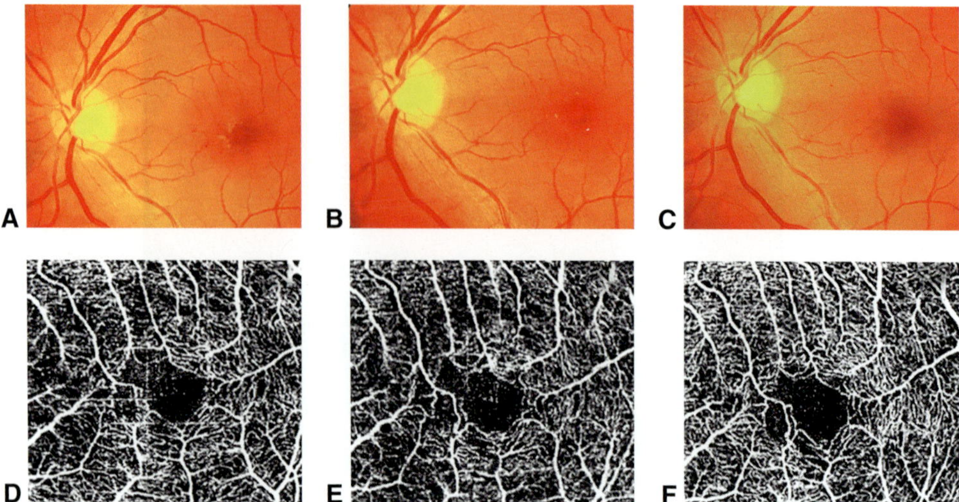

Figure 12-16 Dengue fever. A 46-year-old man presented with decreased vision 1 week after an episode of dengue fever. **A,** Small, white patches of retinal opacification with a few superficial hemorrhages. **B, C,** The lesions gradually resolved after a course of oral corticosteroids. **D–F,** Optical coherence tomography (OCT) angiogram shows enlargement of the foveal avascular zone and loss of retinal superficial capillary plexus, which remained unchanged on follow-up. *(Reproduced with permission from Bajgai P, Singh R, Kapil A. Progression of dengue maculopathy on OCT-angiography and fundus photography.* Ophthalmology. *2017;124(12):1816.)*

The diagnosis of dengue fever is based on clinical findings combined with positive serologic testing. Although the infection is not endemic to the United States, dengue virus–associated maculopathy should be considered in patients presenting with suggestive findings and a history of recent travel to an endemic area. There is no well-defined treatment algorithm for dengue affecting the posterior segment, but local and systemic corticosteroids may be used.

Ng CWK, Tai PY, Oli Mohamed S. Dengue maculopathy associated with choroidopathy and pseudohypopyon: a case series. *Ocul Immunol Inflamm.* 2018;26(5):666–670.

Somkijrungroj T, Kongwattananon W. Ocular manifestations of dengue. *Curr Opin Ophthalmol.* 2019;30(6):500–505.

Vijitha VS, Dave TV, Murthy SI, et al. Severe ocular and adnexal complications in dengue hemorrhagic fever: a report of 29 eyes. *Indian J Ophthalmol.* 2021;69(3):617–622.

Chikungunya Fever

Chikungunya fever is a potentially fatal illness resembling dengue fever that is caused by an arthropod-borne *Alphavirus.* Patients present with fever, headache, fatigue, nausea, vomiting, myalgia, arthralgia, and rash. Chikungunya translates to "that which bends up," a reference to the polyarthropathy, tenosynovitis, and stooped posture of some affected patients. The virus is typically transmitted to humans via mosquito bite. Maternal-fetal

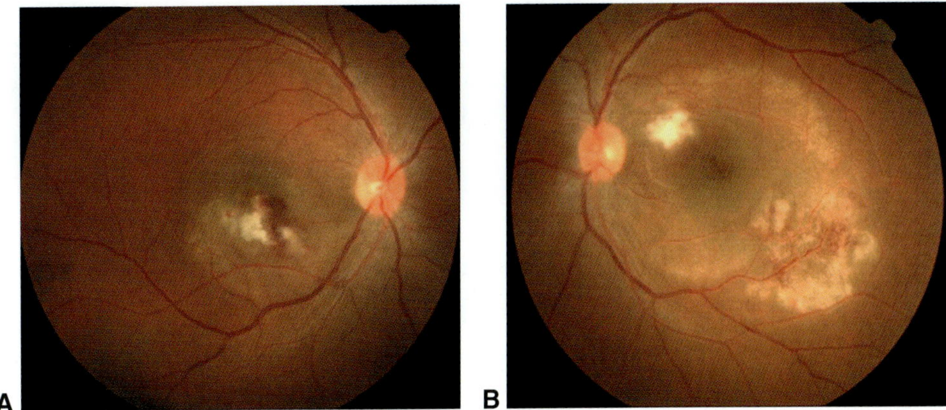

Figure 12-17 Chikungunya fever. Color fundus photographs. **A,** Retinitis with hemorrhages, right eye. **B,** Multifocal retinitis, left eye. *(Reproduced with permission from Mahendradas P, Ranganna SK, Shetty R, et al. Ocular manifestations associated with chikungunya.* Ophthalmology. *2008;115(2):287–291.)*

transmission has also been documented. Recent outbreaks have occurred in Africa, Asia, Europe, and the Americas.

In a 2006 epidemic of chikungunya fever in India, ocular manifestations included both anterior uveitis and retinitis, and less frequently, nodular episcleritis. Each had a typically benign course. Anterior uveitis may be granulomatous or nongranulomatous and is associated with ocular hypertension. Chikungunya retinitis may resemble herpetic retinitis. However, chikungunya retinitis features focal, multifocal, or confluent retinochoroiditis in the posterior pole with retinal hemorrhage and minimal vitritis (Fig 12-17), whereas herpetic retinitis involves the peripheral retina with higher-grade vitritis.

Diagnosis may be confirmed serologically by IgM antibodies, virus isolation, or PCR. Although retinitis has been treated with systemic acyclovir and corticosteroids, no evidence suggests that this therapy improves visual outcome.

Mahendradas P, Avadhani K, Shetty R. Chikungunya and the eye: a review. *J Ophthalmic Inflamm Infect.* 2013;3(1):35. doi:10.1186/1869-5760-3-35

Zika Virus

Zika virus (ZIKV), an arbovirus and member of the family Flaviviridae, is named after a forest in Uganda. Similar to dengue and chikungunya viruses, ZIKV is transmitted to humans by mosquito (often *Aedes aegypti*) bite. Coinfection with any of these 3 distinct viral diseases may occur in endemic areas. A large proportion of patients infected with ZIKV have no symptoms or minimal symptoms (ie, fever, headache, rash, arthralgia, myalgia, conjunctivitis) that typically resolve within a week.

Acute ZIKV infection in adults has caused individual cases of conjunctivitis, anterior uveitis, posterior uveitis with numerous chorioretinal lesions, and unilateral acute maculopathy. There is no defined treatment, but topical, systemic, or local corticosteroids may be considered.

Brazil experienced an epidemic of ZIKV that began in April 2015. A 20-fold spike in newborns with microcephaly was noted in the ensuing months, suggesting congenital ZIKV infection. The US Centers for Disease Control and Prevention (CDC) has defined *congenital Zika syndrome* as having 5 features:

- microcephaly
- structural brain abnormalities
- ocular findings
- congenital contractures such as clubfoot
- hypertonia restricting body movement soon after birth

No reports of uveitis have been associated with congenital ZIKV infection. Instead, observed ocular abnormalities have included microphthalmia, cataract, glaucoma, iris coloboma, retinal pigment mottling, chorioretinal atrophy, and optic nerve hypoplasia or atrophy (Fig 12-18). No vaccine exists to prevent Zika infection at this time. In the United States, where mosquito-borne transmission of ZIKV has been reported, current prevention efforts focus on education and mosquito control. See also BCSC Section 1, *Update on General Medicine.*

De Paula Freitas B, de Oliveira Dias JR, Prazeres J, et al. Ocular findings in infants with microcephaly associated with presumed Zika virus congenital infection in Salvador, Brazil. *JAMA Ophthalmol.* 2016;134(5):529–535.

De Paula Freitas B, Ventura CV, Maia M, Belfort R Jr. Zika virus and the eye. *Curr Opin Ophthalmol.* 2017;28(6):595–599.

Furtado JM, Espósito DL, Klein TM, Teixeira-Pinto T, da Fonseca BA. Uveitis associated with Zika virus infection. *N Engl J Med.* 2016;375(4):394–396.

Kodati S, Palmore TN, Spellman FA, Cunningham D, Weistrop B, Sen HN. Bilateral posterior uveitis associated with Zika virus infection. *Lancet.* 2017;389(10064):125–126.

Parke DW III, Almeida DR, Albini TA, Ventura CV, Berrocal AM, Mittra RA. Serologically confirmed Zika-related unilateral acute maculopathy in an adult. *Ophthalmology.* 2016; 123(11):2432–2433.

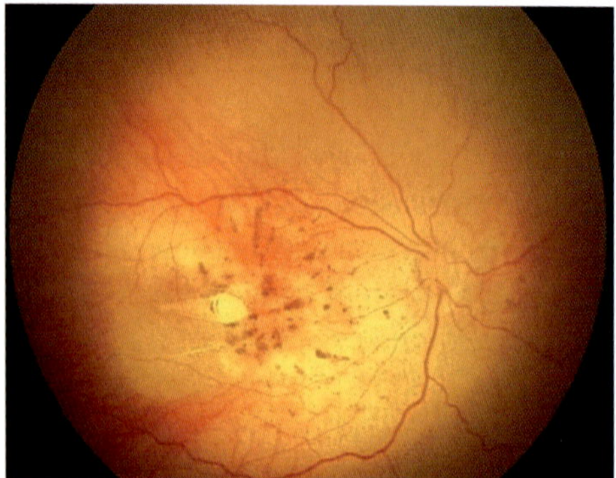

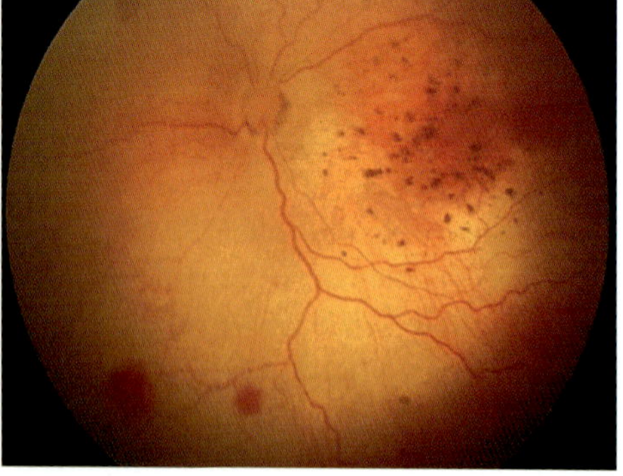

Figure 12-18 Congenital Zika syndrome. Fundus photographs show bilateral pigmentary clumping within the macula. *(Reproduced with permission from Miranda HA II, Costa MC, Frazão MAM, Simão N, Franchischini S, Moshfeghi DM. Expanded spectrum of congenital ocular findings in microcephaly with presumed Zika infection.* Ophthalmology. *2016;123(8):1788–1794.)*

Ebola Virus

Ebola virus disease (EVD) was first discovered in 1976 near the Ebola River in the Democratic Republic of the Congo. The virus is transmitted through direct contact with infected blood and/or body fluids. Sexual transmission has also occurred in survivor populations. EVD is characterized as a hemorrhagic fever; other acute symptoms are easy bruising, headache, weakness and fatigue, nausea and vomiting, and diarrhea. Patients with acute EVD may also experience conjunctivitis, subconjunctival hemorrhage, and acute vision loss of unclear etiology. Symptoms may appear 2–21 days after initial exposure.

Survivors of EVD may experience "post–Ebola virus disease syndrome," which can include arthralgias, myalgias, fatigue, weight loss, headache, neurocognitive deficits, psychosocial issues, and eye disease. One of the most common ophthalmic manifestations affecting Ebola survivors is uveitis. Patients may also have episcleritis, interstitial keratitis, anterior uveitis, chorioretinal lesions, or optic neuropathy. In one patient, a unilateral acute hypertensive anterior uveitis appeared 9 weeks after systemic viremia had resolved, and Ebola virus was isolated from the aqueous humor. This patient also developed iris heterochromia and uveal edema that eventually resolved (Fig 12-19). RPE cells also may be a potential reservoir for the virus. In a prospective longitudinal cohort, recurrent uveitis occurred more frequently in Ebola survivors when compared with a control population.

PREVAIL III Study Group, Sneller MC, Reilly C, Badio M, et al. A longitudinal study of Ebola sequelae in Liberia. *N Engl J Med.* 2019;380(10):924–934.

Varkey JB, Shantha JG, Crozier I, et al. Persistence of Ebola Virus in ocular fluid during convalescence. *N Engl J Med.* 2015;372(25):2423–2427. Published correction appears in *N Engl J Med.* 2015;372(25):2469.

SARS-CoV-2 and COVID-19

To date, millions of cases of COVID-19 and subsequent deaths have been reported worldwide. Systemic infection ranges from asymptomatic to severe respiratory distress and failure of multiple organ systems. In various studies, SARS-CoV-2 has been found in tears from 0%–57% of patients with the disease. The implications of viral transmission via the ocular surface have yet to be elucidated. Ophthalmic manifestations of COVID-19 are relatively rare and range from mild conjunctivitis and subconjunctival hemorrhage to retinopathy and vascular occlusions. The pathogenesis of the retinal vascular disease may be related to widespread systemic inflammation and derangements in coagulation parameters as well as direct viral infection.

COVID-19 dashboard by the Center for Systems Science and Engineering (CSSE) at Johns Hopkins University (JHU). Accessed December 7, 2022. https://coronavirus.jhu.edu/map.html

D'Alessandro E, Kawasaki A, Eandi CM. Pathogenesis of vascular retinal manifestations in COVID-19 patients: a review. *Biomedicines.* 2022;10(11):2710. doi:10.3390/biomedicines10112710

Guan WJ, Ni ZY, Hu Y, et al. Clinical characteristics of coronavirus disease 2019 in China. *N Engl J Med.* 2020;382(180):1708–1720.

Xia J, Tong J, Liu M, et al. Evaluation of coronavirus in tears and conjunctival secretions of patients with SARS-CoV-2 infection. *J Med Virol.* 2020;92(6):589–594.

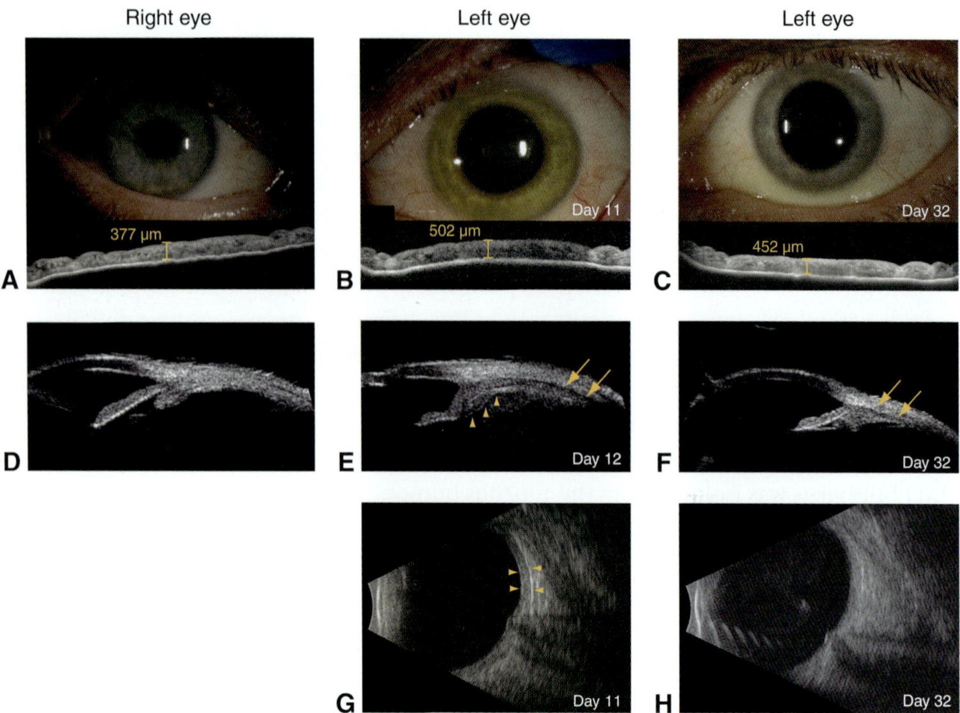

Figure 12-19 Late-onset panuveitis and iris heterochromia in an Ebola survivor. **A,** Slit-lamp photograph of right eye with corresponding anterior segment OCT at baseline. **B,** At day 11, the iris of the left eye had turned green and showed edema. **C,** By day 32, the iris had reverted to its original blue color, and the iris edema had improved. **D,** Ultrasound biomicroscopy (UBM) image shows normal ciliary body anatomy of the right eye. **E,** At day 12, UBM of the left eye shows ciliary body swelling *(arrowheads)* and supraciliary/choroidal effusion *(arrows)* consistent with progressive panuveitis, choroiditis, and evolving hypotony. **F,** Subsequent UBM shows decreased ciliary body swelling and resolution of supraciliary/choroidal effusion *(arrows)* by day 32. **G,** B-scan ultrasonography shows choroidal thickening at day 11 *(arrowheads)*. **H,** At day 32, the choroidal thickening had resolved. *(Reproduced with permission from Shantha JG, Crozier I, Varkey JB, et al. Long-term management of panuveitis and iris heterochromia in an Ebola survivor.* Ophthalmology. *2016;123(12):2626–2628.e2.)*

Other Viral Diseases

Acute anterior uveitis may also occur with other viral infections. The uveitis observed with influenza, adenovirus infection, and infectious mononucleosis is mild and transient. Synechiae and ocular damage seldom occur. Uveitis associated with adenovirus infection is usually secondary to corneal disease (see BCSC Section 8, *External Disease and Cornea).*

Fungal Uveitis

Candidiasis and aspergillosis are covered in Chapter 14. For a discussion of cryptococcosis, see Chapter 13.

Ocular Histoplasmosis Syndrome

Ocular histoplasmosis syndrome (OHS) is a multifocal chorioretinitis presumed to be caused by *Histoplasma capsulatum*. Primary infection occurs after inhalation of the fungal spores, and ocular disease likely arises from hematogenous dissemination to the choroid. OHS is usually found in *Histoplasma* endemic areas such as the Ohio and Mississippi River valleys, but it may occur in nonendemic areas as well. Most affected patients are of northern European descent, and men and women are equally at risk.

Initial choroidal infection is usually asymptomatic and subsides, leaving multiple small atrophic scars and depigmentation of the RPE *(histo spots)*. The choroiditis may disrupt Bruch membrane, choriocapillaris, and RPE, allowing proliferation of subretinal vessels and development of CNV years later. The diagnosis of OHS is suggested by the clinical triad of histo spots without vitreous cells, peripapillary pigment changes, and macular CNV. Histo spots may appear in the macula or periphery, are discrete and punched out, and are usually asymptomatic (Fig 12-20). Approximately 1.5% of patients from endemic areas exhibit typical peripheral histo spots, often first appearing during adolescence. Linear equatorial streaks are present in 5% of patients (Fig 12-21).

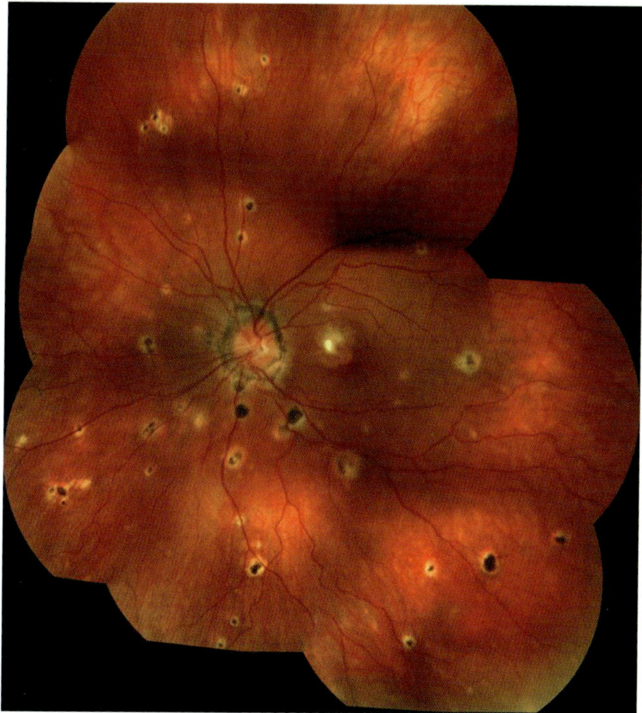

Figure 12-20 Ocular histoplasmosis syndrome. Fundus photograph montage shows peripapillary pigmentary scarring; midperipheral chorioretinal scars, or histo spots (some pigmented and fibrotic); and spontaneously regressed, nasal, juxtafoveal choroidal neovascular membrane in the absence of vitreous cells. Visual acuity was 20/25. *(Courtesy of Ramana S. Moorthy, MD.)*

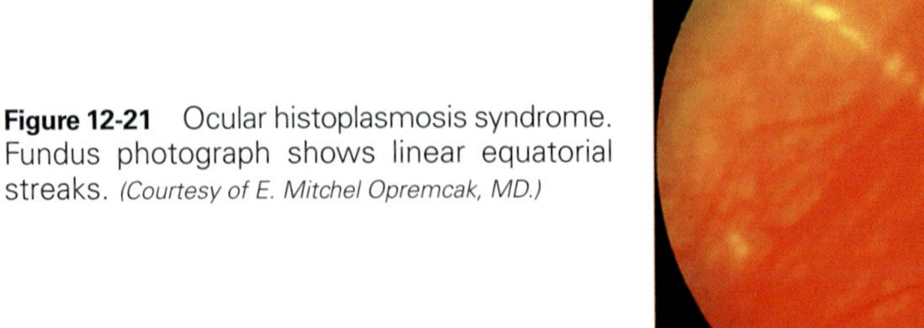

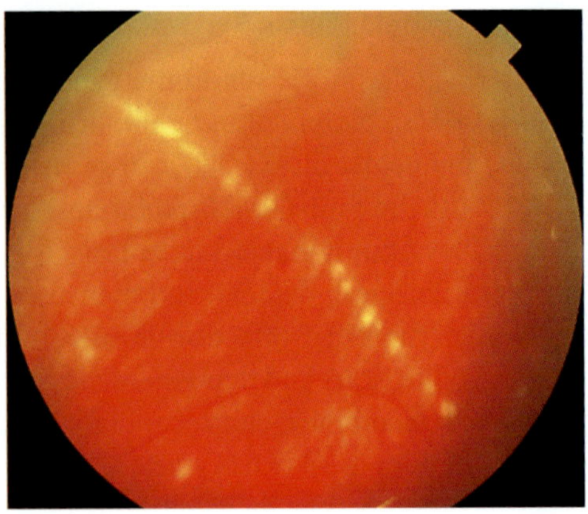

Figure 12-21 Ocular histoplasmosis syndrome. Fundus photograph shows linear equatorial streaks. *(Courtesy of E. Mitchel Opremcak, MD.)*

The early, acute granulomatous lesions of OHS are rarely seen but may be treated with oral or regional (periocular) corticosteroids. The foci of active choroiditis hypofluoresce on early FA and then hyperfluoresce in a staining pattern late in the imaging study. In contrast, areas of active CNV hyperfluoresce early and then exhibit hyperfluorescent leakage pattern in later FA.

Over time, new choroidal scars develop in more than 20% of patients; however, only 3.8% of these cases progress to CNV. When histo spots appear in the macular area, the patient has a 15% chance of developing CNV within 5 years; if no spots are observed, the probability falls to 5%.

Macular CNV is heralded by metamorphopsia and a profound reduction in central vision, which typically brings the patient to the attention of the ophthalmologist. The mean age of patients presenting with maculopathy is 41 years. Ophthalmoscopy of active neovascular lesions reveals a yellow-green subretinal membrane typically surrounded by a pigment ring. There may be associated intraretinal or subretinal fluid and subretinal hemorrhage. Massive subretinal exudation, hemorrhage, and retinal detachment can lead to subretinal fibrosis. Intravitreal vascular endothelial growth factor (VEGF) inhibitors are the primary treatment for OHS-associated macular CNV. See BCSC Section 12, *Retina and Vitreous*, for further details about VEGF inhibitors and alternative treatments for CNV, including thermal laser photocoagulation, photodynamic therapy, intravitreal corticosteroids, and submacular surgery.

The differential diagnosis for OHS includes disorders associated with CNV, such as age-related macular degeneration, myopic degeneration, angioid streaks, choroidal rupture, undifferentiated CNV, MFCPU, and punctate inner choroidopathy. Granulomatous fundus lesions (eg, toxoplasmosis, tuberculosis, coccidioidomycosis, syphilis, sarcoidosis, and toxocariasis) may mimic the scarring of OHS.

Cionni DA, Lewis SA, Petersen MR, et al. Analysis of outcomes for intravitreal bevacizumab in the treatment of choroidal neovascularization secondary to ocular histoplasmosis. *Ophthalmology*. 2012;119(2):327–332.

Diaz RI, Sigler EJ, Rafieetary MR, Calzada JI. Ocular histoplasmosis syndrome. *Surv Ophthalmol*. 2015;60(4):279–295.

Spencer WH, Chan CC, Shen DF, Rao NA. Detection of *Histoplasma capsulatum* DNA in lesions of chronic ocular histoplasmosis syndrome. *Arch Ophthalmol.* 2003;121(11): 1551–1555.

Toussaint BW, Kitchens JW, Marcus DM, et al. Intravitreal aflibercept injection for choroidal neovascularization due to presumed ocular histoplasmosis syndrome: The HANDLE Study. *Retina.* 2018;38(4):755–763.

Xu TT, Reynolds MM, Hodge DO, Smith WM. Epidemiology and clinical characteristics of presumed ocular histoplasmosis in Olmsted County, Minnesota. *Ocul Immunol Inflamm.* 2022;30(5):1039–1043.

Coccidioidomycosis

Coccidioidomycosis is a disease produced by the dimorphic soil fungus *Coccidioides immitis,* which is endemic to the San Joaquin Valley of central California, parts of the southwestern United States, and portions of Central and South America. Infection follows inhalation of dust-borne arthrospores, most commonly resulting in pulmonary infection and secondary dissemination to the central nervous system, skin, skeleton, and eyes. Approximately 40% of infected patients become symptomatic, with most presenting with a mild upper respiratory tract infection or pneumonitis approximately 3 weeks after exposure to the organism. Erythema nodosum or multiforme may appear days to weeks after the onset of symptoms. Disseminated infection is rare, occurring in fewer than 1% of patients with pulmonary coccidioidomycosis.

Ocular coccidioidomycosis is likewise uncommon, even with disseminated disease. Ocular manifestations include blepharitis, keratoconjunctivitis, phlyctenular and granulomatous conjunctivitis, episcleritis and scleritis, and cranial nerve palsies and orbital infection. Uveal involvement is rarer still. Intraocular manifestations include unilateral or bilateral granulomatous anterior uveitis, iris granulomas, and a multifocal chorioretinitis characterized by multiple discrete, yellow-white lesions usually less than 1 disc diameter located in the postequatorial fundus. These choroidal granulomas may resolve, leaving punched-out chorioretinal scars. Vitreous cellular infiltration, vascular sheathing, retinal hemorrhage, serous retinal detachment, and involvement of the optic nerve have also been reported (Fig 12-22).

In the correct clinical context, the diagnosis of coccidioidomycosis is established by seropositive results for anti-coccidioidal antibodies in the serum, cerebrospinal fluid, vitreous, and aqueous, as well as by skin testing for exposure to coccidioidin.

The Infectious Diseases Society of America recommends initiating treatment for coccidioidomycosis with an oral azole antifungal drug such as fluconazole or itraconazole. Surgical debulking of anterior chamber granulomas, pars plana vitrectomy, and intraocular injections of amphotericin and voriconazole may be required. With systemic disease, much higher doses and a longer duration of intravenous amphotericin therapy or oral voriconazole therapy may be needed. Despite aggressive treatment, visual outcomes are often poor, and enucleation may be necessary for pain and blindness.

Shields RA, Tang PH, Bodnar ZM, Smith SJ, Silva AR. Optical coherence tomography angiography highlights chorioretinal lesions in ocular coccidioidomycosis. *Ophthalmic Surg Lasers Imaging Retina.* 2019;50(3):e71–e73. doi:10.3928/23258160-20190301-14

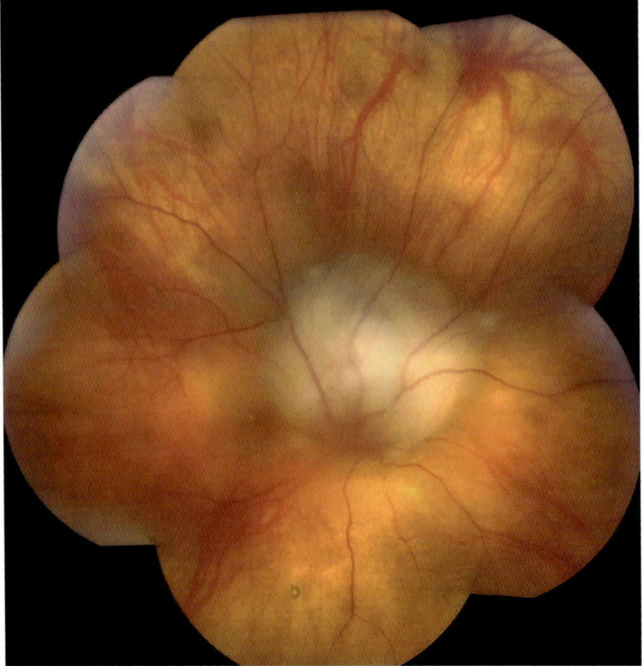

Figure 12-22 Ocular coccidioidomycosis. Fundus photograph montage shows a subretinal lesion involving the optic nerve and peripapillary retina. Associated subretinal fluid extended into the subfoveal region. *(Courtesy of Henry Wiley, MD, and Jared E. Knickelbein, MD, PhD.)*

Toomey CB, Gross A, Lee J, Spencer DB. A case of unilateral coccidioidal chorioretinitis in a patient with HIV-associated meningoencephalitis. *Case Rep Ophthalmol Med.* 2019 Oct 7;2019:1475628. doi:10.1155/2019/1475628

Vasconcelos-Santos DV, Lim JI, Rao NA. Chronic coccidioidomycosis endophthalmitis without concomitant systemic involvement: A clinicopathological case report. *Ophthalmology*. 2010;117(9):1839–1842.

Protozoal Uveitis

Toxoplasmosis

Ocular toxoplasmosis is the most common form of infectious posterior uveitis in adults and children. It is caused by the parasite *Toxoplasma gondii,* a single-cell, obligate, intracellular, apicomplexan parasite with a worldwide distribution. Felines are the definitive hosts of *T gondii;* humans and a variety of other animals serve as intermediate hosts. *T gondii* has a complex life cycle and exists in 3 major forms:

- the oocyst, or soil form (10–12 μm), which contains sporozoites
- the tachyzoite, or infectious form (4–8 μm)
- the tissue cyst, or latent form (10–200 μm), which contains as many as 3000 bradyzoites (Fig 12-23)

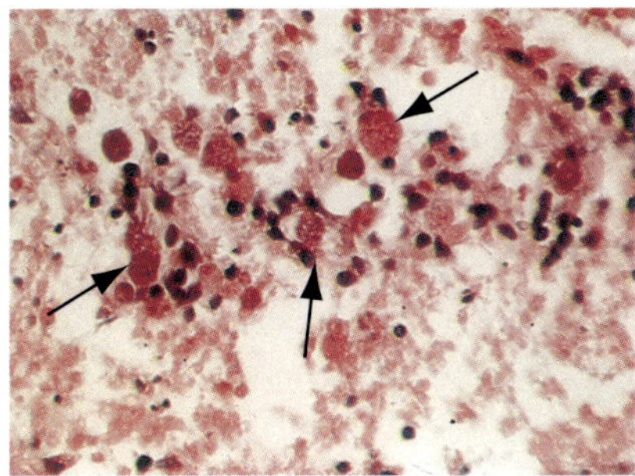

Figure 12-23 Ocular toxoplasmosis. Histologic examination of *Toxoplasma gondii* infection of the retina. Note the cysts *(arrows)* in the necrotic retina.

Transmission of *T gondii* to humans and other animals may occur with all 3 forms of the parasite through a variety of vectors. Tachyzoites, the proliferative form of the parasite, are found in the circulatory system and may invade nearly all host tissues. In an immunocompetent host, tachyzoite proliferation eventually stops. However, some microorganisms may persist as dormant bradyzoites within intercellular tissue cysts (see Fig 12-23).

The reported seropositivity rates of toxoplasmosis among healthy adults vary considerably worldwide. As of this writing, the CDC estimates that 11% of the US population aged 6 years and older is infected with *T gondii.* Of that group, 2% may develop ocular toxoplasmosis. In contrast, an estimated 80% of the population in southern Brazil is infected with *T gondii,* and up to 18% of these individuals may develop eye disease. Some studies show a greater genotypic heterogeneity of parasites in Brazil than in North America. Such differences may contribute to variance in disease severity and ocular involvement in different regions of the world.

Human infection by *T gondii* may be either congenital or acquired. The principal modes of transmission include

- ingestion of undercooked infected meat containing tissue cysts
- ingestion of contaminated water, fruit, or vegetables with oocysts
- contact with cat feces, cat litter, or soil containing oocysts
- primary infection during pregnancy resulting in transplacental transmission
- blood transfusion or organ transplantation

Data collected from the 2009–2010 National Health and Nutrition Examination Survey (NHANES) showed an age-adjusted seroprevalence of *T gondii* of 9.1% among women of childbearing age (15–44 years) in the United States. Thus, most women of childbearing age in the United States are at risk for primary *T gondii* infection. The American Academy of Pediatrics estimates that the incidence of primary infection during pregnancy in the United States is approximately 0.2–1.1 per 1000 pregnant women, translating to 800–4400 women with acute *T gondi* infection among the 4 million annual pregnancies in the country.

Overall, 40% of primary maternal infections result in congenital infection, with transplacental transmission highest during the third trimester. The risk of severe disease developing in the fetus is inversely proportional to gestational age. Disease acquired early in pregnancy may result in spontaneous abortion, stillbirth, or severe congenital disease, whereas disease acquired later in gestation may produce latent infection in an asymptomatic, healthy-appearing infant. Chronic or recurrent maternal infection during pregnancy probably does not confer a major risk of congenital toxoplasmosis because maternal immunity protects against fetal transmission; however, congenital toxoplasmosis may occur in an immune pregnant mother reinfected with a new, more virulent strain.

Centers for Disease Control and Prevention, Division of Parasitic Diseases and Malaria. Toxoplasmosis. Accessed September 8, 2022. https://www.cdc.gov/dpdx/toxoplasmosis/

Furtado JM, Winthrop KL, Butler NJ, Smith JR. Ocular toxoplasmosis I: parasitology, epidemiology and public health. *Clin Exp Ophthalmol.* 2013;41(1):82–94.

Presentation

The classic presentation of congenital toxoplasmosis, which includes retinochoroiditis, hydrocephalus or microcephaly, intracranial calcifications, and cognitive impairment (Sabin's tetrad), occurs in fewer than 10% of infected children. The most common abnormality in patients with congenital toxoplasmosis is retinochoroidal lesions, found in up to 80% of cases. Lesions are bilateral in approximately 85% of affected individuals and tend to occur in the posterior pole and macula (Fig 12-24). Posterior segment involvement may be subclinical and chronic. As many as 85% of infected children develop retinochoroiditis after a mean of 3.7 years, and 25% of these become blind in one or both eyes. For newborns with congenital toxoplasmosis during the first year of life, most experts recommend antiparasitic therapy to reduce disease burden, regardless of the presence of ocular and/or systemic signs.

Although toxoplasmosis after infancy was previously considered reactivation of congenital disease, it is now recognized that ocular toxoplasmosis in children and adults may represent newly acquired infection in a substantial proportion of cases. In one study, acquired postnatal infection accounted for up to two-thirds of cases of ocular toxoplasmosis.

Depending on the location of the retinochoroidal lesion, presenting symptoms of acquired toxoplasmosis frequently include unilateral blurred or hazy vision and floaters. A mild to moderate granulomatous anterior uveitis is often observed, and up to 20% of patients have acutely elevated IOP at presentation. Classically, ocular toxoplasmosis

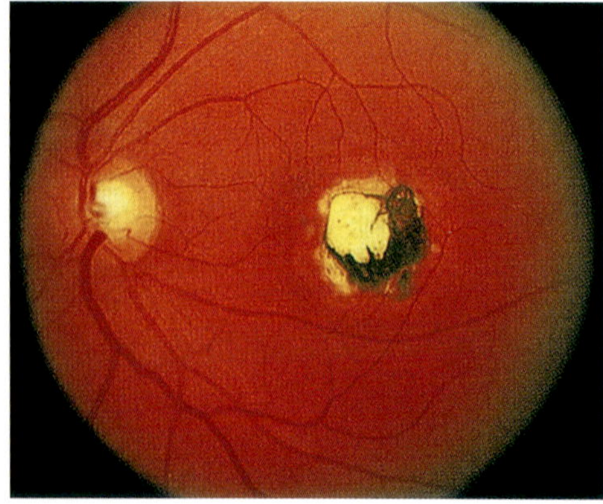

Figure 12-24 Congenital toxoplasmosis. Fundus photograph of quiescent, partially pigmented congenital toxoplasmic macular scar. This patient has 20/400 visual acuity. *(Courtesy of John D. Sheppard Jr, MD.)*

appears as a focal, white retinochoroiditis often adjacent to a pigmented retinochoroidal scar (Fig 12-25), with moderate overlying vitreous inflammation ("headlight in the fog") (Fig 12-26). In the absence of a retinochoroidal scar, recently acquired disease often presents as a focal retinochoroiditis (Fig 12-27). Retinochoroiditis lesions occur more commonly in the posterior pole, but they are occasionally found immediately adjacent to or directly involving the optic nerve, where they may be mistaken for optic neuritis. Retinal vessels in the vicinity of an active lesion may show perivasculitis with diffuse venous sheathing and segmental arterial plaques (previously known as Kyrieleis arteriolitis). Vascular occlusions may also be present. Additional ocular complications include cataract, persistent vitreous opacities, macular edema, retinal detachment, epiretinal membranes, optic atrophy, and CNV.

In immunocompromised and older patients, retinochoroiditis may present with atypical findings, including large, multiple, and/or bilateral lesions with or without associated retinochoroidal scars. This more severe clinical picture can also occur in patients who receive corticosteroids without concomitant antiparasitic therapy (Fig 12-28). Ocular

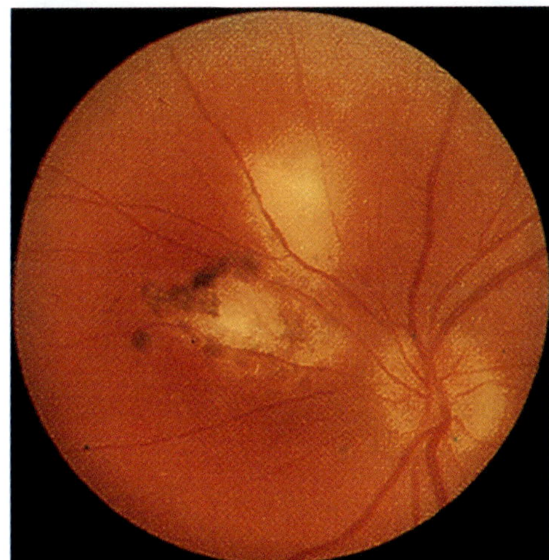

Figure 12-25 Ocular toxoplasmosis. Fundus photograph shows active retinochoroiditis adjacent to a partially pigmented retinochoroidal scar.

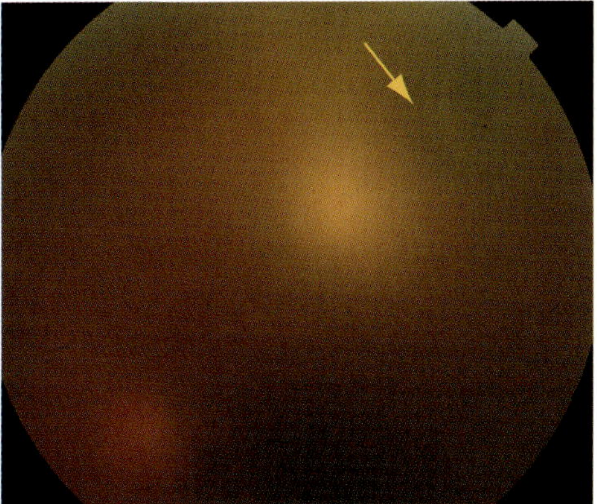

Figure 12-26 Ocular toxoplasmosis. Fundus photograph shows focal retinitis adjacent to a pigmented scar *(arrow)* with dense overlying vitritis, producing a "headlight in the fog" appearance. *(Courtesy of Emillio M. Dodds, MD.)*

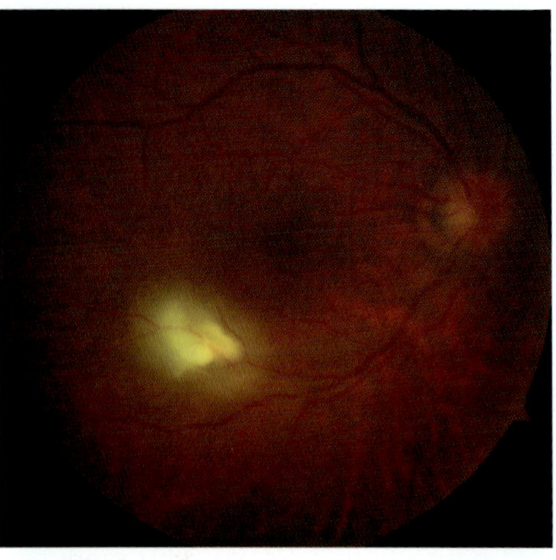

Figure 12-27 Ocular toxoplasmosis. Fundus photograph shows toxoplasmic retinochoroiditis in the absence of a previous retinochoroidal scar. *(Originally published in the Retina Image Bank website. Gregg T. Kokame, MD, and James C. Lai, MD, Retina Consultants of Hawaii. Photograph by Jaclyn Pisano, Retina Consultants of Hawaii. Retina Image Bank; 2012. Image number 1346. © American Society of Retina Specialists.)*

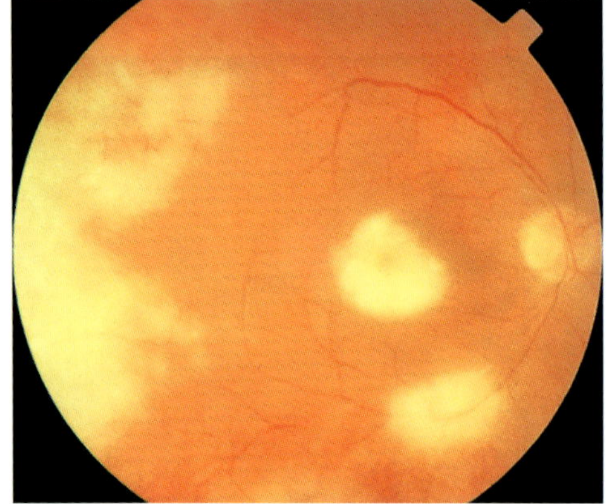

Figure 12-28 Ocular toxoplasmosis. Fundus photograph shows widespread retinal necrosis and multiple patches of retinochoroiditis after periocular corticosteroid injection. *(Courtesy of E. Mitchel Opremcak, MD.)*

toxoplasmosis may simulate herpetic ARN. Other atypical presentations include neuroretinitis, unilateral pigmentary retinopathy simulating retinitis pigmentosa, and other forms of intraocular inflammation in the absence of retinochoroiditis, as well as punctate outer retinal toxoplasmosis (PORT). Characteristics of PORT include small, multifocal lesions at the level of the outer retina, with exudation to the subretinal space and scant overlying vitreal inflammation (Fig 12-29).

Butler NJ, Furtado JM, Winthrop KL, Smith JR. Ocular toxoplasmosis II: clinical features, pathology and management. *Clin Exp Ophthalmol.* 2013;41(1):95–108.

Goh EJH, Putera I, La Distia Nora R, et al. Ocular toxoplasmosis. *Ocul Immunol Inflamm.* 2022 Sep 12:1–20. Epub ahead of print. doi:10.1080/09273948.2022.2117705

Jones JL, Bonetti V, Holland GN, et al. Ocular toxoplasmosis in the United States: recent and remote infections. *Clin Infect Dis.* 2015;60(2):271–273.

Diagnosis

In most cases, toxoplasmic retinochoroiditis is clinically diagnosed on the basis of the characteristic fundus lesion. Positive serologic testing for anti–*T gondii* IgG or IgM confirms

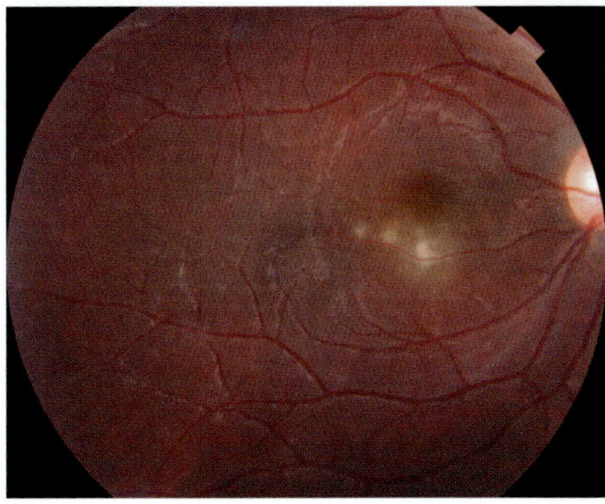

Figure 12-29 Punctate outer retinal toxoplasmosis. Fundus photograph shows deep retinal lesions. *(Courtesy of Emilio M. Dodds, MD.)*

exposure to the parasite. IgG antibodies appear after the first 2 weeks of infection, typically remain detectable for life at variable levels, and cross the placenta. In contrast, IgM antibodies increase in number early during the acute phase of the infection, typically remain detectable for less than 1 year, and do not cross the placenta. In the appropriate clinical context, the presence of anti–*T gondii* IgG antibodies supports the diagnosis of toxoplasmic retinochoroiditis. The presence of IgM confirms congenital infection in newborns but indicates newly acquired disease in adults. In cases of diagnostic uncertainty, PCR testing of aqueous humor and vitreous fluid may be performed.

Greigert V, Di Foggia E, Filisetti D, et al. When biology supports clinical diagnosis: review of techniques to diagnose ocular toxoplasmosis. *Br J Ophthalmol.* 2019;103(7):1008–1012.

Maldonado YA, Read JS; AAP Committee on Infectious Diseases. Diagnosis, treatment, and prevention of congenital toxoplasmosis in the United States. *Pediatrics.* 2017;139(2): e20163860. doi:10.1542/peds.2016-3860

Treatment

Ocular toxoplasmosis is a progressive and recurrent disease. New lesions may occur at the margins of old scars as well as elsewhere in the fundus, and toxoplasmic cysts may be present in a normal-appearing retina. In the immunocompetent patient, the disease may have a self-limiting course. Without treatment, the borders of the lesions become sharper and less edematous over a 6- to 8-week period, and RPE hyperplasia occurs gradually over a period of months. In the immunocompromised patient, the disease is often more severe and progressive.

Although numerous medications may be used to treat toxoplasmosis, there is no consensus regarding the most efficacious regimen. Most antibiotics have efficacy against the active tachyzoite only, not the tissue-encysted bradyzoite. In immunocompetent patients, firm evidence showing that antimicrobial therapy alters the natural history of toxoplasmic retinochoroiditis is limited. Thus, in this population, some clinicians may elect to observe small lesions in the retinal periphery that are not associated with a notable decrease in vision or vitritis.

Other clinicians treat virtually all patients in an effort to reduce the number of subsequent recurrences and minimize structural complications associated with intraocular inflammation. Treatment may also shorten the duration of parasitic replication, accelerating cicatrization and ultimately reducing retinochoroidal scars.

In addition, treatment is indicated for the following populations: immunocompromised patients (ie, those with HIV/AIDS, with neoplastic disease, or receiving IMT), patients with congenital toxoplasmosis, and pregnant women with recently acquired disease.

Other relative treatment indications include

- lesions threatening the optic nerve, fovea, or major vasculature
- decreased vision
- lesions associated with moderate to severe vitreous inflammation
- lesions greater than 1 disc diameter
- persistence of disease for more than 1 month
- presence of multiple active lesions

Table 12-2 summarizes treatment options for toxoplasmosis. Many ophthalmologists use trimethoprim-sulfamethoxazole (160 mg/800 mg, 2 times/day) because of its accessibility, simplicity of administration, and cost. Intravitreal clindamycin (1 mg/0.1 mL) with or without periocular dexamethasone 400 mg/0.1 mL may also be injected as an off-label use, either in combination with systemic therapy or as monotherapy in patients who do not tolerate systemic therapy (see Appendix B).

In immunocompetent patients, systemic corticosteroids (approximately 0.25–0.75 mg/kg, typically not more than 60 mg/day) may be considered after 48 hours of antimicrobial therapy. The use of systemic corticosteroids without appropriate antimicrobial coverage or the use of long-acting periocular and intravitreal corticosteroid formulations such as triamcinolone acetonide is contraindicated because of the potential for severe panophthalmitis, blindness, and loss of the eye (see Fig 12-28). However, topical corticosteroids can be used liberally in the presence of prominent anterior segment inflammation. Systemic corticosteroid treatment may be used for 3–5 weeks or until inflammation begins to subside and the retinal lesion shows signs of early cicatrization. Antimicrobial coverage should be continued for the entire period of systemic corticosteroid use.

In cases of newly acquired toxoplasmosis during pregnancy, treatment is given to prevent infection of the fetus or limit fetal damage if infection has already occurred, as well as to limit the destructive sequelae of intraocular disease in the mother. Spiramycin (treatment dose, 400 mg 3 times/day) reduces the rate of tachyzoite transmission to the fetus and may be used safely without major risk of teratogenicity. This drug has limited availability in the United States, but it can be directly obtained from the US Food and Drug Administration. Substitutions for spiramycin include azithromycin, clindamycin, and atovaquone. Sulfonamides may be used safely in the first 2 trimesters of pregnancy. Alternatively, intravitreal clindamycin and short-acting periocular corticosteroids (eg, dexamethasone) may be used in women who are pregnant to reduce adverse effects of systemic treatment (see preceding paragraphs and Appendix B).

Patients with HIV/AIDS and toxoplasmosis require extended systemic treatment given the frequent association of ocular disease with cerebral involvement (56% of cases)

Table 12-2 Systemic Treatment of Toxoplasmosis

Medication	Dosing	Indication	Adverse Effects
Pyrimethamine, sulfadiazine, and folinic acid	Pyrimethamine: loading dose, 50–100 mg; treatment dose, 25–50 mg/day for 4–8 weeks; sulfadiazine: treatment dose, 1 g, 4 times/day; and folinic acid: 5–10 mg/day	Classic triple therapy	Pyrimethamine: myelosuppression, leukopenia, thrombocytopenia Sulfa compounds: rash, gastrointestinal intolerance, crystalluria, kidney stones, and Stevens-Johnson syndrome Monitor with complete blood count every 2 weeks
Clindamycin	300 mg, 4 times/day	Used alone or as a substitution for sulfa medication in triple therapy	Pseudomembranous colitis
Azithromycin	500 mg daily or 500 mg ×1 day, then 250 mg daily	Used alone or in place of other medications	
Atovaquone	750 mg, 2–4 times/day	Used alone or in place of other medications	
Trimethoprim-sulfamethoxazole	160 mg/800 mg, 2 times/day	Used alone	Stevens-Johnson syndrome
Pyrimethamine, sulfadiazine, and folinic acid	Pyrimethamine: 2 mg/kg for 1 day, then 1 mg/kg daily; sulfadiazine: 50 mg/kg 2 times/day; and folinic acid, 7.5 mg/day	Congenital toxoplasmosis	See classic triple therapy
Spiramycin	400 mg 3 times/day	Used in pregnancy	

and the frequency of recurrent ocular disease when anti-*Toxoplasma* medication is discontinued. The best regimen for secondary prophylaxis is undetermined; however, atovaquone acts synergistically with pyrimethamine and sulfadiazine and thus may be useful for reducing the dose and toxicity of these drugs in the treatment of patients with AIDS and toxoplasmosis. The management of ocular toxoplasmosis in association with HIV/AIDS is also covered in Chapter 13.

Among patients with recurrent toxoplasmic retinochoroiditis, long-term intermittent trimethoprim-sulfamethoxazole treatment (160 mg/800 mg 3 times per week) was shown to decrease the risk of reactivation over a 20-month period. Similarly, the utility of prophylactic antimicrobial treatment shortly before and after intraocular surgery in patients with inactive *Toxoplasma* scars—particularly scars close to the optic disc or fovea—was raised by a report describing an association between cataract surgery and increased risk of reactivation of otherwise inactive toxoplasmic retinochoroiditis. However, there is no consensus regarding this treatment approach or the optimal antibiotic regimen in this clinical situation.

Feliciano-Alfonso JE, Muñoz-Ortiz J, Marín-Noriega MA, et al. Safety and efficacy of different antibiotic regimens in patients with ocular toxoplasmosis: systematic review and meta-analysis. *Syst Rev.* 2021;10(1):206. doi:10.1186/s13643-021-01758-7

Fernandes Felix JP, Cavalcanti Lira RP, Grupenmacher AT, et al. Long-term results of trimethoprim-sulfamethoxazole versus placebo to reduce the risk of recurrent *Toxoplasma gondii* retinochoroiditis. *Am J Ophthalmol.* 2020;213:195–202.

Kim SJ, Scott IU, Brown GC, et al. Interventions for toxoplasma retinochoroiditis: a report by the American Academy of Ophthalmology. *Ophthalmology.* 2013;120(2):371–378.

Soheilian M, Ramezani A, Azimzadeh A, et al. Randomized trial of intravitreal clindamycin and dexamethasone versus pyrimethamine, sulfadiazine, and prednisolone in treatment of ocular toxoplasmosis. *Ophthalmology.* 2011;118(1):134–141.

Helminthic Uveitis

Helminths (derived from the Greek word for *worms*) are multicellular organisms that can be free living or parasitic. Approximately 280 species are recognized.

Toxocariasis

Ocular toxocariasis (OT) is a zoonotic infection caused by *Toxocara canis* and *Toxocara cati.* Dogs and cats, the definitive hosts of the roundworms, pass eggs via their feces into the environment (often into the soil). According to the CDC, 30% of dogs younger than 6 months are infected with *T canis,* and 25% of cats are infected with *T cati.* Transmission to humans occurs through ingestion of viable *T canis* eggs in soil or food or via the fecal–oral route. Risk factors include exposure to playgrounds, sandboxes, kittens, and puppies, as well as the pica eating disorder. In rare cases, humans may acquire the infection from undercooked meat.

NHANES data from 2011–2014 suggested an overall *Toxocara* seroprevalence of 5.1% in the United States. In children, the rate of antibody positivity has been associated with lack of health insurance. In a large population treated for uveitis at tertiary care centers in northern California, the prevalence of OT was recently estimated to be 1%.

In humans, *Toxocara* organisms grow in the small intestine, enter the portal circulation, and disseminate hematogenously to various parts of the body, including the liver, heart, lungs, brains, or muscles (known as *visceral toxocariasis,* or *VT*) as well as the eyes. The larvae do not undergo further development in the human but rather cause a local inflammatory reaction. Ova are not shed in the gastrointestinal tract, so stool analysis for larvae is not helpful for diagnosis.

VT usually affects children younger than 3 years. Symptoms may include fever, coughing, enlarged liver, pneumonia, and meningoencephalitis. Peripheral eosinophilia may also be present. OT is found in older children, typically without substantial eosinophilia. OT and VT rarely present simultaneously.

Ophthalmic presentations include a chronic endophthalmitis (25% of OT cases), a posterior pole granuloma (25%; Fig 12-30), or a peripheral granuloma (50%), sometimes with fibrous bands in the vitreous that may extend posteriorly (Fig 12-31). Any of these presentations may produce leukocoria. Uncommon variants include unilateral pars planitis with diffuse peripheral inflammatory exudates, granulomas involving the optic nerve, and diffuse unilateral subacute neuroretinitis. Table 12-3 summarizes the patterns of manifestation of ocular toxocariasis.

OT is principally a clinical diagnosis. Serologic testing may suggest prior exposure, although patients with OT may also have negative serology results. Antibody testing of ocular fluids may be positive despite negative serology results. PCR testing is not readily available for OT; however, vitrectomy specimens have yielded larvae (Fig 12-32). In cases with media opacity, B-scan ultrasonography and/or computed tomography (CT) may show vitreous membranes and/or tractional detachment and may confirm the absence of calcium, a potential finding in retinoblastoma.

The differential diagnosis of OT includes retinoblastoma, infectious endophthalmitis, Coats disease, familial exudative vitreoretinopathy, persistent fetal vasculature, toxoplasmosis, undifferentiated intermediate uveitis/pars planitis, retinopathy of prematurity, combined hamartoma of the retina and RPE, and diffuse unilateral subacute neuroretinitis.

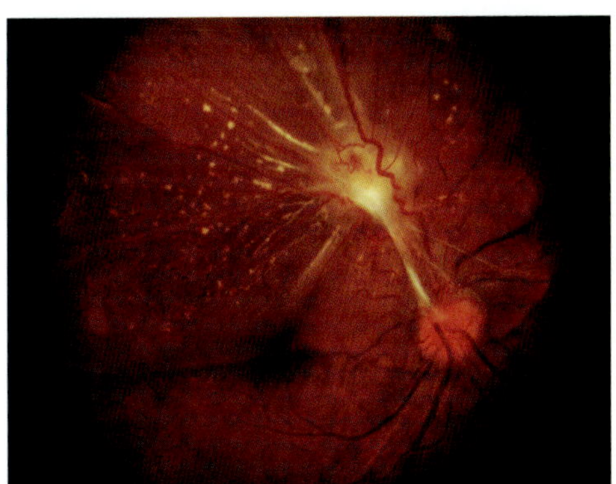

Figure 12-30 Ocular toxocariasis. Fundus photograph shows *Toxocara* posterior pole granuloma causing macular pucker. *(Originally published in the Retina Image Bank website. Photograph by H. Michael Lambert, MD. Retina Image Bank; 2015. Image number 23430. © American Society of Retina Specialists.)*

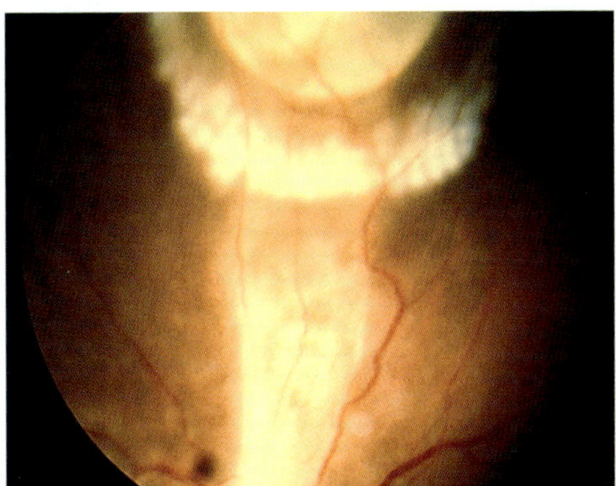

Figure 12-31 Ocular toxocariasis. Fundus photograph shows *Toxocara* peripheral granuloma. *(Originally published in the Retina Image Bank website. Thomas M. Aaberg, MD, and Thomas M. Aaberg Jr; image number 3508. © American Society of Retina Specialists.)*

Table 12-3 Patterns of Manifestation of Ocular Toxocariasis

Syndrome	Age at Onset, y	Characteristic Lesion
Chronic endophthalmitis	2–9	Chronic unilateral uveitis, cloudy vitreous, cyclitic membrane
Localized granuloma	6–14	Occurs in the macula and peripapillary region Solitary, white, retinal elevation; minimal reaction; 1–2 disc diameter
Peripheral granuloma	6–40	Peripheral hemispheric masses with dense connective tissue strands in the vitreous cavity that may connect to the disc Rarely bilateral

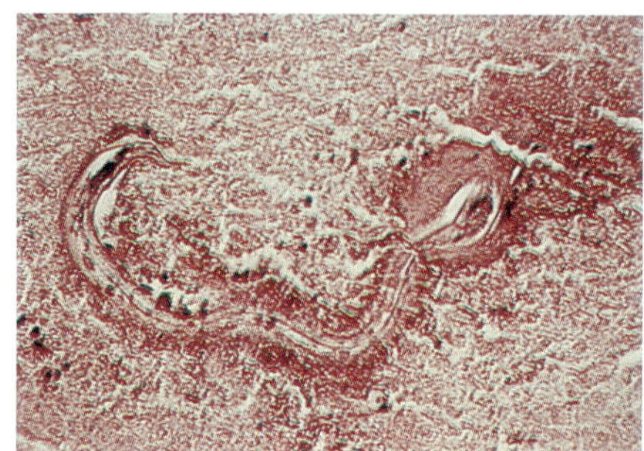

Figure 12-32 Ocular toxocariasis. Histologic examination of an eosinophilic vitreous abscess. The organism is in the center of the abscess.

The migrating larvae of other helminths such as *Baylisascaris procyonis* may also simulate OT. In contrast to children with OT, children with retinoblastoma are typically younger, lack substantial inflammation, and show lesion growth.

Patients with VT are usually treated with oral albendazole. For OT, the use of anthelminthic therapy is not established but may be considered if the larvae appear active. Typically, local and systemic corticosteroids are used to reduce inflammation and minimize structural complications, which may later be amenable to vitreoretinal surgical techniques.

Ahn SJ, Woo SJ, Jin Y, et al. Clinical features and course of ocular toxocariasis in adults. *PLoS Negl Trop Dis.* 2014;8(6):e2938. doi:10.1371/journal.pntd.0002938

Arevalo JF, Espinoza JV, Arevalo FA. Ocular toxocariasis. *J Pediatr Ophthalmol Strabismus.* 2013;50(2):76–86.

Centers for Disease Control and Prevention. Ocular toxocariasis—United States, 2009–2010. *MMWR.* 2011;60(22):734–736.

Farmer A, Beltran T, Choi YS. Prevalence of *Toxocara* species infection in the U.S.: results from the National Health and Nutrition Examination Survey, 2011–2014. *PLoS Negl Trop Dis.* 2017;11(7):e0005818. doi:10.1371/journal.pntd.0005818

Li S, Sun L, Liu C, et al. Clinical features of ocular toxocariasis: a comparison between ultra-wide-field and conventional camera imaging. *Eye (Lond).* 2021;35(10):2855–2863.

Ma G, Holland CV, Wang T, et al. Human toxocariasis. *Lancet Infect Dis.* 2018;18(1):e14–e24. doi:10.1016/S1473-3099(17)30331-6

Woodhall D, Starr MC, Montgomery SP, et al. Ocular toxocariasis: epidemiologic, anatomic, and therapeutic variations based on a survey of ophthalmic subspecialists. *Ophthalmology.* 2012;119(6):1211–1217.

Cysticercosis

Cysticercosis is the most common ocular tapeworm infection. Human infection is caused by *Cysticercus cellulosae,* the larval stage of the cestode *Taenia solium,* which is endemic to Mexico, Africa, Southeast Asia, eastern Europe, Central and South America, and India. Humans acquire the disease via fecal–oral transmission or by consuming undercooked infected pork. The eggs mature into larvae, penetrate the intestinal mucosa, and spread hematogenously to the eye via the posterior ciliary arteries.

Ocular cysticercosis usually affects individuals between the ages of 10 and 30 years, without sex predilection. Cysticercosis may affect any structure of the eye, orbit, or adnexa, but it most frequently involves the subretinal space (Fig 12-33). Larvae may perforate the retina, gaining access to the vitreous cavity (Fig 12-34). Other presentations include a subconjunctival or eyelid nodule.

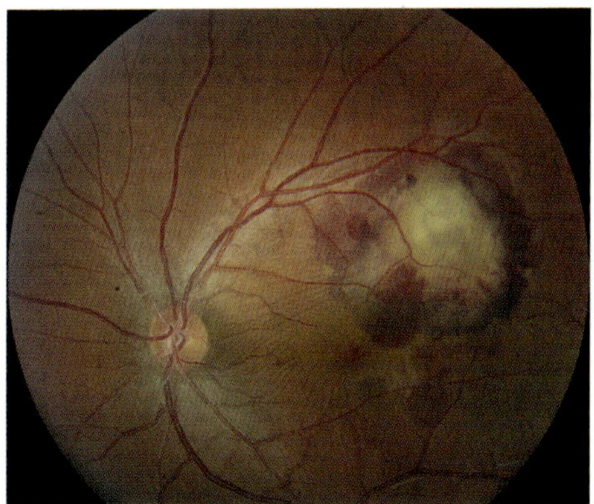

Figure 12-33 Ocular cysticercosis. Fundus photograph shows a subretinal lesion. *(Courtesy of Preema Abraham, MD, and the Retina Image Bank. © American Society of Retina Specialists.)*

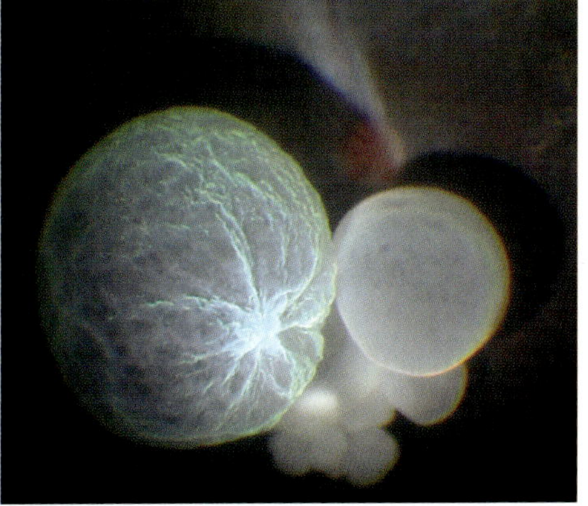

Figure 12-34 Ocular cysticercosis. Fundus photograph of multiple intravitreal cysts. *(Courtesy of Vishal Agrawal, MD, and the Retina Image Bank. © American Society of Retina Specialists.)*

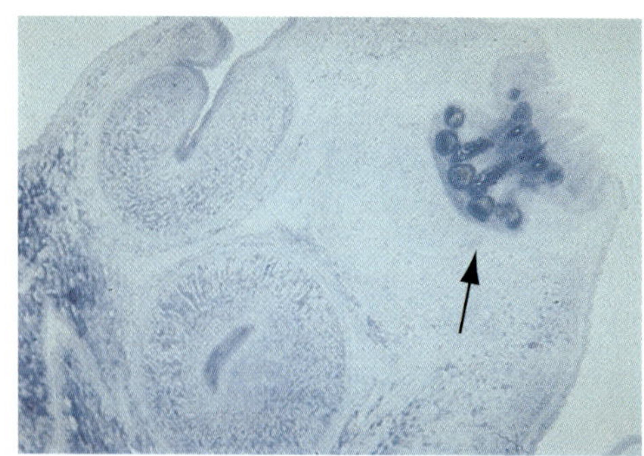

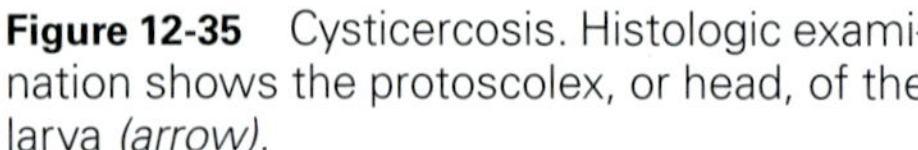

Figure 12-35 Cysticercosis. Histologic examination shows the protoscolex, or head, of the larva *(arrow).*

Patients may be asymptomatic with relatively good vision or may report floaters, mobile foreign body sensations, ocular pain, photophobia, redness, and decreased vision. Larvae are observed in the vitreous or subretinal space in up to 46% of infected patients. A globular translucent cyst is seen, with an invaginated or evaginated head, or scolex, that undulates in response to the examining light (Fig 12-35; see also Fig 12-34). Exudative, rhegmatogenous, or tractional retinal detachment may occur. In patients with neural cysticercosis, CT may reveal intracerebral calcification or hydrocephalus.

The differential diagnosis for cysticercosis includes conditions associated with leukocoria (retinoblastoma, Coats disease, retinopathy of prematurity, persistent fetal vasculature, toxocariasis, and retinal detachment) and diffuse unilateral subacute neuroretinitis.

Larvae death provokes panuveitis. Laser photocoagulation alone may also provoke severe inflammation. Hence, early removal of intraocular larvae, often via vitreoretinal surgical techniques with perioperative systemic corticosteroids, is advocated. Anthelminthic drugs plus systemic corticosteroids may be used for extraocular disease.

Pujari A, Bhaskaran K, Modaboyina S, et al. Cysticercosis in ophthalmology. *Surv Ophthalmol.* 2022;67(2):544–569.

Sheemar A, Gaur N, Thakur PS, et al. Optical coherence tomography features of ocular cysticercosis: a review of literature with observer variation. *Ophthalmic Surg Lasers Imaging Retina.* 2022;53(8):446–454.

Diffuse Unilateral Subacute Neuroretinitis

Diffuse unilateral subacute neuroretinitis (DUSN) is an uncommon but important disease likely caused by infection with a nematode that migrates through the subretinal space. The mean age of affected patients is 14 years (range, 11–65 years). Evidence to date suggests that DUSN can be caused by 2 types of nematodes that differ in size and geographic region. The smaller worm, measuring 400–1000 µm in length, has been proposed to be either *Ancylostoma caninum* (the dog hookworm) or *T canis,* although there are no reports of the latter being isolated from an eye with DUSN. The larger worm is believed to be *Baylisascaris procyonis* (the raccoon roundworm), which measures 1500–2000 µm in length and has been found in the northern midwestern United States and Canada. The disease has also been reported outside North America.

The clinical course of DUSN is characterized by the insidious unilateral loss of vision from recurrent episodes of focal, multifocal, or diffuse inflammation of the retina, RPE, and optic nerve. The early stages of the disease are marked by moderate to severe vitritis; optic disc edema; and multiple, focal, gray-white lesions in the postequatorial fundus that range from 1200 µm to 1500 µm in size (Fig 12-36A). These lesions are transient and may be associated with overlying exudative retinal detachment. The worm may be visualized in the subretinal space, especially in the early stages (Fig 12-36B). Diffuse outer retinal disruption may be observed on OCT (Fig 12-36C). Differential diagnosis at this phase of the disease includes sarcoidosis-associated uveitis, MFCPU, acute posterior multifocal placoid pigment epitheliopathy, multiple evanescent white dot syndrome, serpiginous choroiditis, Behçet disease, toxocariasis, OHS, nonspecific optic neuritis, and papillitis. Later disease stages are typified by retinal arteriolar narrowing, optic atrophy, diffuse pigment epithelial degeneration, and abnormal electroretinographic results (Fig 12-37). These findings may be confused with those of posttraumatic chorioretinopathy, occlusive vascular disease, toxic retinopathy, and retinitis pigmentosa. Rare bilateral cases have been reported, and cases of DUSN have also been associated with neurologic disease (neural larva migrans).

The diagnosis is based on clinical findings and is most strongly supported by the observation of a worm in the subretinal space (Video 12-1). Results of systemic and laboratory evaluations are typically negative for patients with DUSN.

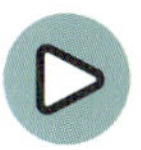

VIDEO 12-1 How to find a live worm in diffuse unilateral subacute neuroretinitis.
Courtesy of Carlos A. A. Garcia, MD.

In patients with DUSN, medical therapy with corticosteroids alone may only transiently control inflammation. Direct laser photocoagulation of the worm in the early phases of the disease does not appear to be inflammatory and may be highly effective in halting progression of the disease (Fig 12-38). Successful treatment and immobilization of the subretinal worm have been reported with oral thiabendazole (22 mg/kg twice daily for 2–4 days with a maximum dose of 3 g) or albendazole (200 mg twice daily for 30 days), which may be a better-tolerated alternative. If the worm cannot be visualized, patients may undergo a course of anthelminthic therapy to increase the chance of identifying and treating the nematode. If inflammation does not improve after laser therapy alone, anthelminthic therapy may be used to treat a presumed second undetected nematode.

de Amorim Garcia Filho CA, Bezerra Gomes AH, de A Garcia Soares AC, de Amorim Garcia CA. Clinical features of 121 patients with diffuse unilateral subacute neuroretinitis. *Am J Ophthalmol.* 2012;153(4):743–749.

Mazzeo TJMM, Dos Santos Motta MM, Curi ALL. Diffuse unilateral subacute neuroretinitis: review article. *J Ophthalmic Inflamm Infect.* 2019;9(1):23. doi:10.1186/s12348-019-0191-x

Souza EC, Casella AM, Nakashima Y, Monteiro ML. Clinical features and outcomes of patients with diffuse unilateral subacute neuroretinitis treated with oral albendazole. *Am J Ophthalmol.* 2005;140(3):437–445. Published correction appears in *Am J Ophthalmol.* 2006;141(4):795–796.

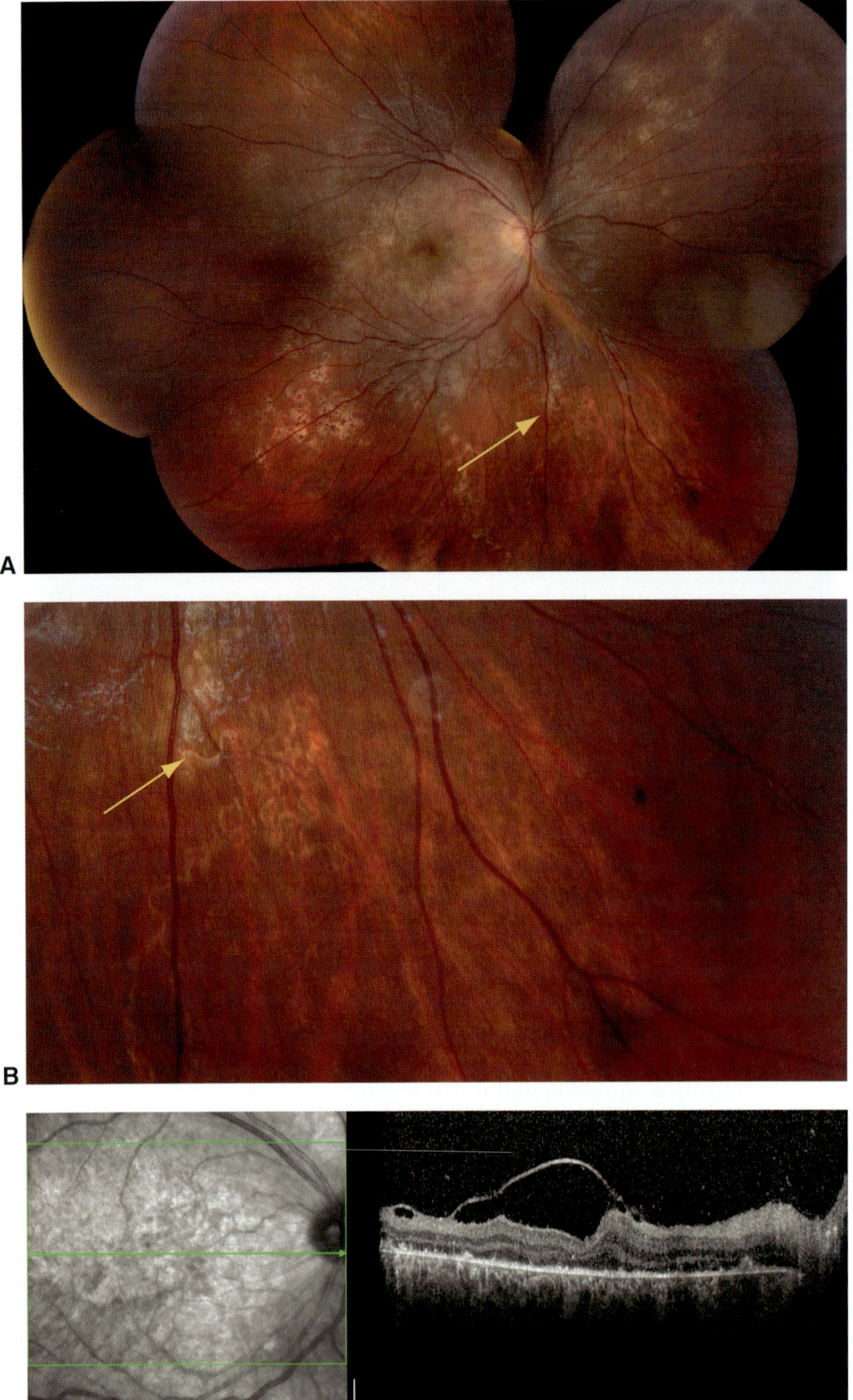

Figure 12-36 Diffuse unilateral subacute neuroretinitis. **A,** Fundus photograph montage shows diffuse whitening in the macula with discrete whiplike deep tracks in the periphery *(arrow)*. **B,** The nematode is moving in the subretinal space *(arrow)*. **C,** OCT through the fovea shows traction from preretinal membranes and irregular disruption of outer retinal structures. *(Courtesy of Wendy M. Smith, MD.)*

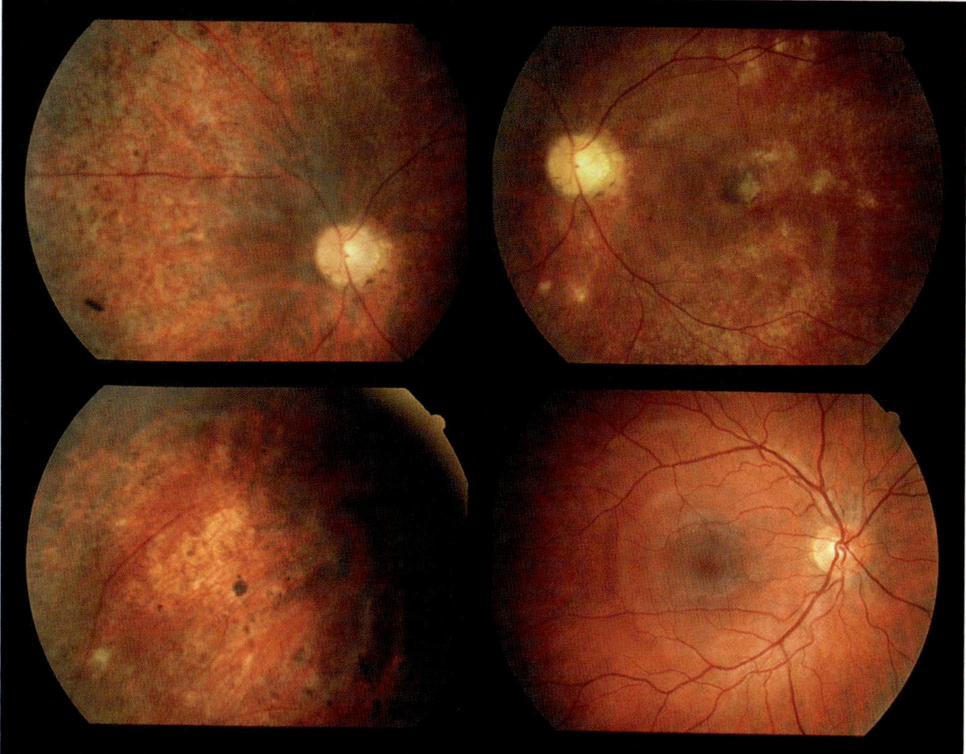

Figure 12-37 Diffuse unilateral subacute neuroretinitis. Fundus photographs from a 23-year-old man. *(Originally published in the Retina Image Bank website. Howard Schatz, MD. Retina Image Bank; 2013. Image number 6039. © American Society of Retina Specialists.)*

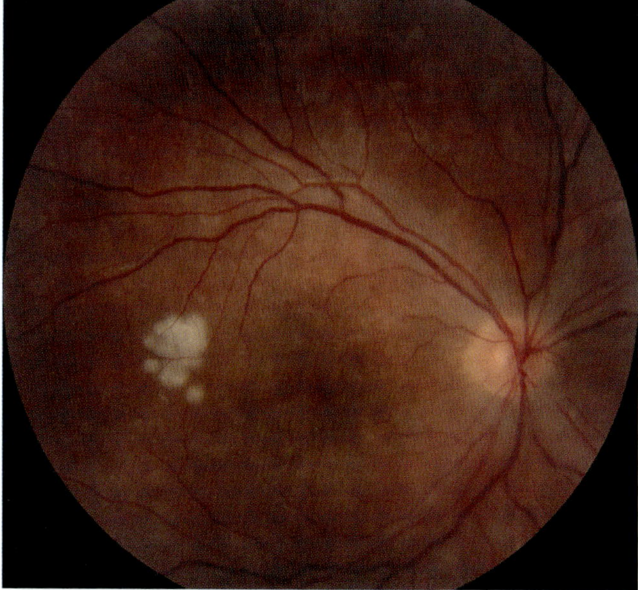

Figure 12-38 Diffuse unilateral subacute neuroretinitis. Fundus photograph from the same patient shown in Figure 12-36 after the nematode was visualized and treated with laser photocoagulation. *(Courtesy of Wendy M. Smith, MD.)*

Onchocerciasis

Onchocerciasis, commonly known as *River Blindness,* is endemic in many areas of sub-Saharan Africa and in isolated foci in Central and South America. Worldwide, at least 25 million people are infected, including almost 300,000 who are blind and 800,000 who are visually impaired. Humans are the only host for the *Onchocerca volvulus* parasite. As the vector, female black flies that breed near rivers bite an infected human and ingest microfilariae. The infective larvae are then transmitted to another human with a subsequent black fly bite. Microfilariae probably reach the eye by various routes:

- direct invasion of the cornea from the conjunctiva
- penetration of the sclera, both directly and through the vascular bundles
- hematogenous spread (possibly)

Microfilariae can be observed swimming freely in the anterior chamber. They may also be seen in the cornea, where dead microfilariae can cause stromal punctate keratitis. Anterior uveitis may lead to synechiae, secondary glaucoma, and cataract. In the posterior segment, RPE disruption and focal atrophy may occur. Advanced disease often manifests as severe chorioretinal and optic atrophy (Fig 12-39).

A diagnosis of onchocerciasis is suspected on the basis of the clinical appearance and a history of pathogen exposure in an endemic area. It is confirmed by detecting microfilariae in small skin biopsies or in the eye. Ivermectin, the treatment of choice, is given every 3–6 months as long as there is evidence of skin or eye infection. Topical corticosteroids can be used to control associated anterior uveitis.

Ivermectin effectively kills the microfilariae, but it does not have a permanent effect on the adult worms. Concomitant doxycycline therapy helps kill the adult worms by eradicating the symbiotic partner—*Wolbachia* bacteria. Lastly, patients coinfected with *O volvulus* and *Loa loa* are at risk of a fatal encephalitic reaction to ivermectin,

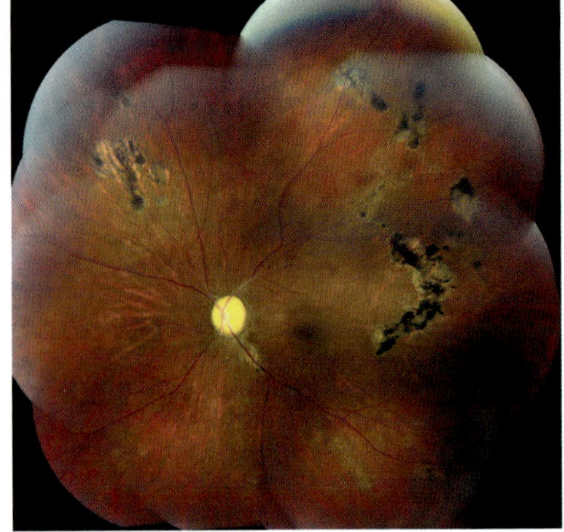

Figure 12-39 Onchocerciasis. Fundus photograph montage shows optic nerve pallor and extensive chorioretinal scars involving both the periphery and the posterior pole. *(Courtesy of H. Nida Sen, MD/National Eye Institute.)*

so consultation with a specialist in infectious diseases should be obtained for these individuals.

Brattig NW, Cheke RA, Garms R. Onchocerciasis (river blindness) - more than a century of research and control. *Acta Trop.* 2021 Jun;218:105677. doi:10.1016/j.actatropica.2020.105677

Ejere HO, Schwartz E, Wormald R, Evans JR. Ivermectin for onchocercal eye disease (river blindness). *Cochrane Database Syst Rev.* 2012;8:CD002219.

CHAPTER 13

Ocular Involvement in HIV Infection and AIDS

Highlights

- AIDS causes a microangiopathy known as *HIV retinopathy* that is associated with higher viral loads and lower $CD4^+$ T lymphocyte counts.
- Uveitis due to opportunistic infections—such as cytomegalovirus (CMV) retinitis, *Pneumocystis jirovecii* choroiditis, and *Cryptococcus neoformans* choroiditis—has become less common since the introduction of antiretroviral therapy.
- Immune recovery uveitis is sterile intraocular inflammation that develops after CMV retinitis when antiretroviral therapy improves the T-lymphocyte count.
- Malignant neoplasms such as vitreoretinal lymphoma and Kaposi sarcoma are associated with AIDS.

Acquired Immunodeficiency Syndrome

AIDS is caused by HIV, which infects and depletes $CD4^+$ helper T lymphocytes. The loss of $CD4^+$ T lymphocytes causes profound immune deficiency with subsequent opportunistic infections. See BCSC Section 1, *Update on General Medicine,* for a full discussion of HIV infection and AIDS.

Ophthalmic Manifestations

Ophthalmic manifestations may be the first sign of disseminated systemic HIV infection/AIDS and have been reported in up to 70% of infected people. These manifestations include

- HIV-related microangiopathy of the retina
- opportunistic viral, bacterial, parasitic, and fungal infections
- Kaposi sarcoma of the eyelid and conjunctiva
- lymphomas involving primarily the retina and/or vitreous (vitreoretinal lymphoma), adnexal structures, and orbit
- squamous cell carcinoma of the conjunctiva

Reports also suggest that HIV infection itself may cause anterior or intermediate uveitis that is unresponsive to corticosteroids but improves with antiretroviral therapy (ART).

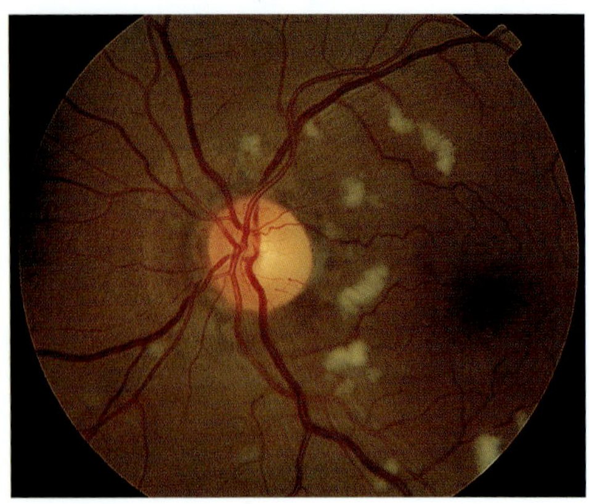

Figure 13-1 HIV retinopathy. Fundus photograph shows numerous cotton-wool spots. *(Reproduced with permission from Cunningham ET Jr, Belfort R Jr.* HIV/AIDS and the Eye: A Global Perspective. *Ophthalmology Monograph 15. American Academy of Ophthalmology; 2002:55.)*

The most common ocular finding in patients with AIDS is HIV retinopathy, a microangiopathy characterized mainly by cotton-wool spots (Fig 13-1) but also by microaneurysms and retinal hemorrhages. HIV has been isolated from the human retina, and its antigen has been detected in retinal endothelial cells. The HIV endothelial infection may play a role in the development of cotton-wool spots and other vascular alterations. In addition, accelerated aging may be a part of AIDS-associated eye disease, with earlier onset of macular degeneration and cataracts.

Other infectious agents that can affect the eye in patients with AIDS include cytomegalovirus (CMV), herpes simplex viruses types 1 and 2 (HSV-1, HSV-2), varicella-zoster virus (VZV), *Toxoplasma gondii, Treponema pallidum, Mycobacterium tuberculosis, Mycobacterium avium-intracellulare, Cryptococcus neoformans, Pneumocystis jirovecii, Histoplasma capsulatum, Candida* species, molluscum contagiosum virus, and microsporidia. These pathogens can infect the ocular adnexa, anterior segment, or posterior segment. However, visual morbidity occurs primarily with posterior segment involvement, particularly retinitis caused by infection with CMV, HSV, VZV, *T gondii,* or *T pallidum.*

Agarwal A, Invernizzi A, Acquistapace A, et al; OCTA Study Group. Analysis of retinochoroidal vasculature in human immunodeficiency virus infection using spectral-domain OCT angiography. *Ophthalmol Retina.* 2017;1(6):545–554.

Kalyani PS, Fawzi AA, Gangaputra S, et al; Studies of the Ocular Complications of AIDS Research Group. Retinal vessel caliber among people with acquired immunodeficiency syndrome: relationships with visual function. *Am J Ophthalmol.* 2012;153(3):428–433.

Peters RPH, Kestelyn PG, Zierhut M, Kempen JH. The changing global epidemic of HIV and ocular disease. *Ocul Immunol Inflamm.* 2020;28(7):1007–1014.

Cytomegalovirus Retinitis

Before the availability of potent antiretroviral treatment regimens, disseminated CMV infection was the most common opportunistic infection in people with AIDS, and retinal infection was its most clinically important manifestation, occurring in up to 40% of patients with AIDS, usually those with $CD4^+$ T-lymphocyte counts less than 50 cells/μL. CMV infection is now uncommon in areas of the world where potent combination ART is available. However, CMV retinitis remains the most common opportunistic ocular infection in patients with

AIDS, and it is occasionally the first AIDS-defining infection diagnosed. CMV infection remains an increasing problem in resource-limited regions, particularly in Southeast Asia.

Early CMV retinitis may manifest as a small, white retinal infiltrate that resembles the cotton-wool spots seen in HIV-associated retinopathy. However, unlike HIV-associated retinopathy, CMV retinitis progresses without treatment. Patients with $CD4^+$ cell counts less than 50 cells/μL should be monitored every 3 months for development of CMV retinitis because it can be asymptomatic. In patients whose disease is not responding to therapy, polymerase chain reaction (PCR) testing of aqueous or vitreous fluids may help differentiate CMV from necrotizing retinitis secondary to HSV-1, HSV-2, or VZV infection. Of note, toxoplasmosis and syphilis may masquerade as a viral retinitis.

Management of CMV retinitis requires anti-CMV therapy and measures to restore immune function. Anti-CMV therapy is particularly important, as CMV retinitis signifies a twofold-increased mortality risk in patients with a $CD4^+$ T-cell count less than 100 cells/μL (an effect not observed with counts ≥100 cells/μL). Resistant CMV infection is further associated with increased mortality in patients with HIV infection/AIDS and CMV retinitis. Options for systemic coverage include high-dose induction therapy with either intravenous ganciclovir (5 mg/kg twice daily) or foscarnet (90 mg/kg twice daily) for 2 weeks, followed by maintenance therapy with daily dosing of either antiviral; or oral valganciclovir (900 mg twice daily) for 3 weeks, followed by maintenance therapy (900 mg/day).

Intraocular disease is treated effectively with intravitreal injection of ganciclovir or foscarnet (see Appendix B). In patients with vision-threatening retinitis, intravitreal injection may be used as an adjunct to systemic antiviral treatment (Fig 13-2). Intravitreal treatment may be the only treatment option in patients who cannot tolerate systemic therapy because of myelotoxicity from valganciclovir or ganciclovir or because of nephrotoxicity associated with foscarnet.

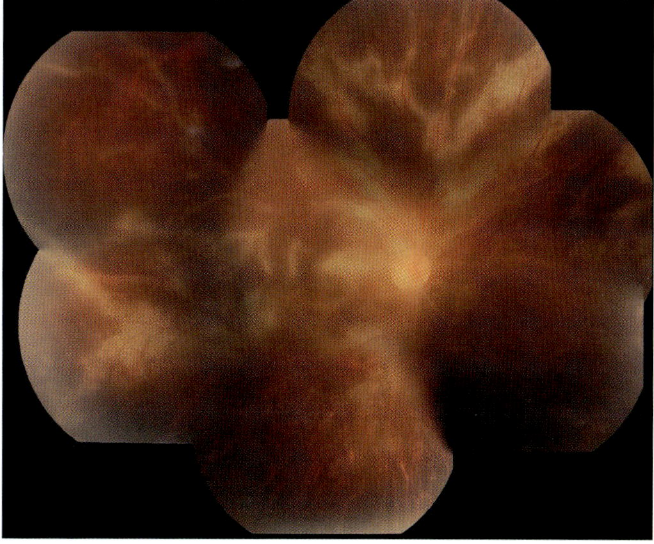

Figure 13-2 Cytomegalovirus retinitis. Montage of color fundus photographs shows diffuse retinitis with "frosted-branch" angiitis in a patient with AIDS. *(Courtesy of Emilio M. Dodds, MD.)*

HIV-infected patients with CMV retinitis who have sustained immune recovery (ie, CD4+ T-lymphocyte count ≥100 cells/μL for 3–6 months) can safely discontinue systemic anti-CMV maintenance therapy. ART-naive patients may require only 6 months of anti-CMV therapy if they have good immune reconstitution, whereas ART-experienced patients may require long-term maintenance therapy. Despite immune recovery, patients with a history of CMV retinitis who discontinue anti-CMV maintenance therapy remain at risk for recurrence and should be monitored at 3-month intervals.

Ford N, Shubber Z, Saranchuk P, et al. Burden of HIV-related cytomegalovirus retinitis in resource-limited settings: a systematic review. *Clin Infect Dis.* 2013;57(9):1351–1361.

Holland GN, Vaudaux JD, Shiramizu KM, et al; Southern California HIV/Eye Consortium. Characteristics of untreated AIDS-related cytomegalovirus retinitis. II. Findings in the era of highly active antiretroviral therapy (1997 to 2000). *Am J Ophthalmol.* 2008;145(1):12–22.

Jabs DA, Martin BK, Forman MS; Cytomegalovirus Retinitis and Viral Resistance Research Group. Mortality associated with resistant cytomegalovirus among patients with cytomegalovirus retinitis and AIDS. *Ophthalmology.* 2010;117(1):128–132.

Jabs DA, Van Natta ML, Holland GN, Danis R; Studies of the Ocular Complications of AIDS Research Group. Cytomegalovirus retinitis in patients with acquired immunodeficiency syndrome after initiating antiretroviral therapy. *Am J Ophthalmol.* 2017;174:23–32.

Immune recovery uveitis

Immune recovery uveitis (IRU) is an inflammatory process that affects patients with a history of CMV retinitis and AIDS whose immune status improves with ART. The risk factors for developing inflammation depend on the extent of CMV retinitis (CMV retinitis surface area of 25% or more), amount of intraocular CMV antigen, degree of immune reconstitution, and previous treatment (higher risk in patients treated with cidofovir). Manifestations of IRU include anterior uveitis, vitritis, uveitic macular edema, epiretinal membrane formation, papillitis, and neovascularization of the optic disc or retina.

Inflammation in the anterior chamber is treated with topical corticosteroids. When IRU is an isolated mild vitritis, treatment is observation, as the vitreous inflammation can be transient. IRU with more severe vitreous inflammation and/or uveitic macular edema can be treated with periocular corticosteroids or short courses of oral corticosteroids. Intravitreal corticosteroids can also be used for treatment of severe IRU or uveitis macular edema; however, reactivation of CMV retinitis may occur.

El-Bradey MH, Cheng L, Song MK, Torriani FJ, Freeman WR. Long-term results of treatment of macular complications in eyes with immune recovery uveitis using a graded treatment approach. *Retina.* 2004;24(3):376–382.

Kempen JH, Min YI, Freeman WR, et al; Studies of Ocular Complications of AIDS Research Group. Risk of immune recovery uveitis in patients with AIDS and cytomegalovirus retinitis. *Ophthalmology.* 2006;113(4):684–694.

Urban B, Bakunowicz-Łazarczyk A, Michalczuk M. Immune recovery uveitis: pathogenesis, clinical symptoms, and treatment. *Mediators Inflamm.* 2014;2014:971417. doi:10.1155/2014/971417

Retinal detachment

Retinal detachment occurs in up to 50% of patients with AIDS and CMV retinitis and may develop during active disease or after successful treatment of the retinitis. With potent antiretroviral regimens available, the rate of retinal detachment has been reduced to 0.06 per patient-year. Risk factors for developing retinal detachment include involvement of all 3 retinal zones, lower CD4$^+$ T-lymphocyte count, and more extensive retinitis. Because eyes with CMV retinitis have extensive retinal necrosis and multiple posterior holes, most of these detachments require pars plana vitrectomy with long-term silicone oil tamponade. Anatomical reattachment can be achieved in 90% of patients.

Jabs DA, Van Natta ML, Thorne JE, et al; Studies of Ocular Complications of AIDS Research Group. Course of cytomegalovirus retinitis in the era of highly active antiretroviral therapy: 2. Second eye involvement and retinal detachment. *Ophthalmology*. 2004;111(12):2232–2239.

Necrotizing Herpetic Retinitis

Patients with HIV infection may develop necrotizing herpetic retinitis, which appears to manifest as a spectrum of disease; the severity is directly proportional to the degree of immunologic compromise. These patients may develop typical acute retinal necrosis or progressive outer retinal necrosis (PORN; see Chapter 12). In its early stages, PORN may be difficult to distinguish from peripheral CMV retinitis (Fig 13-3).

Wons J, Kempen J, Garweg JG. HIV-induced retinitis. *Ocul Immunol Inflamm*. 2020;28(8): 1259–1268.

Toxoplasma Retinochoroiditis

In immunocompetent patients, ocular toxoplasmosis classically appears as a focal retinochoroiditis often adjacent to a retinochoroidal scar. In patients with AIDS, it may be more difficult to diagnose ocular toxoplasmosis because of manifestations that differ from the classic presentation. For example, the ocular toxoplasmosis lesions are larger, and bilateral

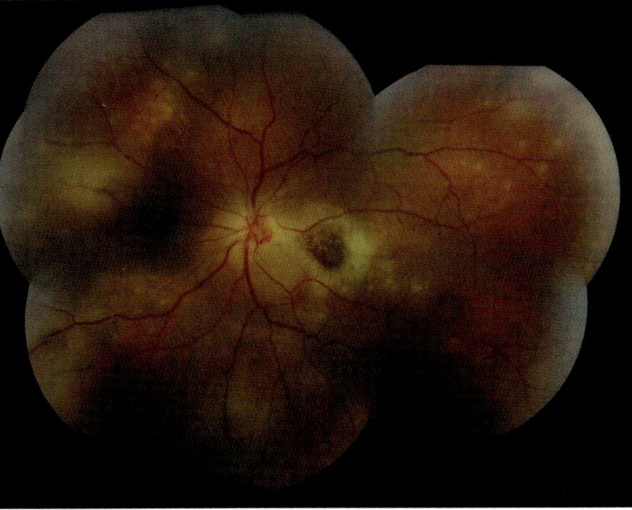

Figure 13-3 Progressive outer retinal necrosis. Montage of color fundus photographs shows extensive retinitis with relative preservation of vessels and early involvement of the posterior pole in a patient with AIDS. *(Courtesy of H. Nida Sen, MD/National Eye Institute.)*

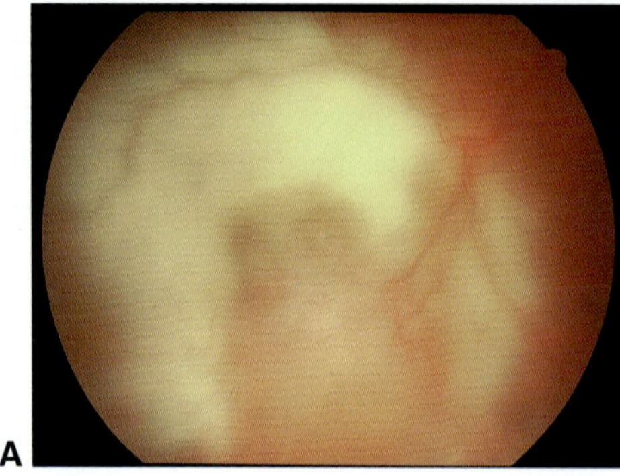

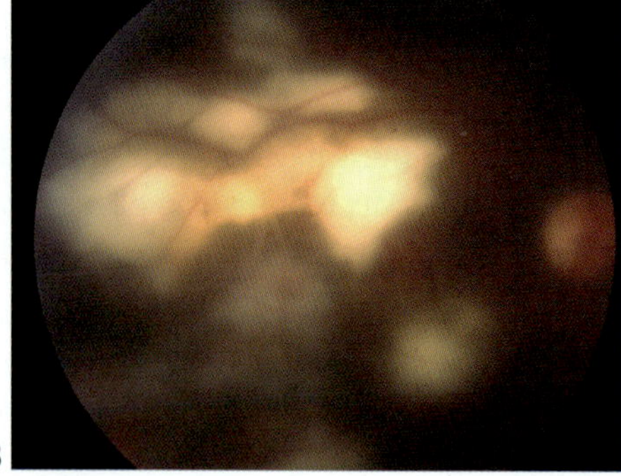

Figure 13-4 *Toxoplasma* retinochoroiditis. **A,** Fundus photograph shows a large area of macular *Toxoplasma* retinochoroiditis in a patient with AIDS. **B,** Fundus photograph from a different patient with AIDS demonstrates multifocal *Toxoplasma* retinochoroiditis. *(Courtesy of Emilio M. Dodds, MD.)*

disease occurs in up to 40% of cases. Solitary or multifocal patterns of retinitis have also been observed in these patients (Fig 13-4). In general, the inflammation in the choroid, retina, and vitreous is less prominent in patients with AIDS than in immunocompetent patients (see also Chapter 12). Also, trophozoites and cysts can be found in greater numbers within areas of retinitis, and *T gondii* organisms are occasionally seen invading the choroid, a finding not observed in immunocompetent patients.

Ocular toxoplasmosis may result from newly acquired *T gondii* infection or from reactivation of chronic infection within the retina or nonocular sites. In patients with AIDS, newly acquired *T gondii* infections and dissemination from nonocular sites are the most likely causes, although reactivation of quiescent toxoplasmosis also occurs. Thus, the retinochoroidal scars that are commonly associated with the active lesions of *Toxoplasma* retinochoroiditis may be absent. Further, ocular toxoplasmosis in patients with AIDS may be difficult to distinguish from acute retinal necrosis, necrotizing herpetic retinitis, or syphilitic retinitis. Definitive diagnosis may require aqueous and vitreous samples for culture and PCR analysis.

The prompt diagnosis of ocular toxoplasmosis is especially important in patients who are immunocompromised because the condition inevitably progresses if left untreated. In addition, ocular toxoplasmosis in these patients may be associated with cerebral or disseminated toxoplasmosis, both of which are important causes of morbidity and mortality in patients with AIDS. For patients with AIDS who have active ocular toxoplasmosis, computed tomography and/or magnetic resonance imaging of the head, as well as consultation with specialists in infectious diseases should be pursued to rule out central nervous system (CNS) involvement (Fig 13-5).

Anti-*Toxoplasma* therapy with a synergistic combination of pyrimethamine, sulfadiazine, sulfamethoxazole and trimethoprim, azithromycin, atovaquone, and/or clindamycin is required. Because of the risk of further immunosuppression in this population, corticosteroids should be used with caution and only when there is appropriate antimicrobial coverage. In selecting the therapeutic regimen, the physician should consider the possibility of coexisting cerebral or disseminated toxoplasmosis as well as the toxic effects of pyrimethamine and sulfadiazine on bone marrow. Continued maintenance therapy may be necessary for patients with poor immune status that is not improving. See Chapter 12 for more detailed discussion of treatment.

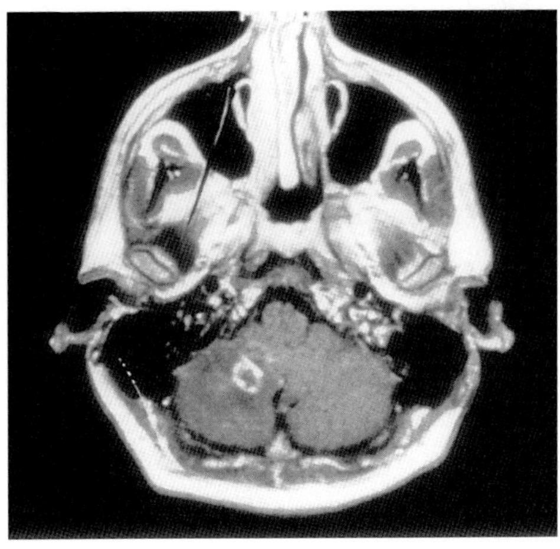

Figure 13-5 Central nervous system toxoplasmosis. Enhanced computed tomography scan reveals a cerebellar *Toxoplasma* lesion in a patient with AIDS who presented with ataxia. *(Courtesy of John D. Sheppard Jr, MD.)*

de-la-Torre A, Gómez-Marín J. Disease of the year 2019: ocular toxoplasmosis in HIV-infected patients. *Ocul Immunol Inflamm.* 2020;28(7):1031–1039.

Ocular Syphilis

Syphilis, which is due to *T pallidum* infection, is reemerging globally, particularly in association with HIV coinfection. The clinical presentation of ocular syphilis includes scleritis; anterior, intermediate, posterior, or panuveitis; and optic neuritis. Patients may also have mucocutaneous and CNS symptoms. In patients with AIDS, vitritis without chorioretinitis can be the first manifestation of syphilis. In contrast to patients without HIV infection, these patients are also more likely to present with optic neuritis or neuroretinitis. A classic manifestation of syphilis in patients with AIDS is unilateral or bilateral pale-yellow, placoid retinal lesions that preferentially involve the macula (syphilitic posterior placoid chorioretinitis). The presence of discrete creamy-yellow superficial retinal precipitates overlying areas of retinitis is very suggestive of syphilis; however, these precipitates can occur regardless of HIV status. For discussion of other manifestations of syphilis, see Chapter 11.

The course of syphilis may be more aggressive in HIV-infected patients. These patients require treatment with 18–24 million units of intravenous penicillin G administered daily for 10–14 days, followed by 2.4 million units of intramuscular benzathine penicillin G administered weekly for 3 weeks. Monitoring of results from the quantitative rapid plasma reagin test is recommended, as symptomatic disease can recur.

Queiroz RP, Smit DP, Peters RPH, Vasconcelos-Santos DV. Double trouble: challenges in the diagnosis and management of ocular syphilis in HIV-infected individuals. *Ocul Immunol Inflamm.* 2020;28(7):1040–1048.

Multifocal Choroiditis and Systemic Dissemination

The choroid is often a site of opportunistic disseminated infections. Multifocal choroidal lesions resulting from ocular infection are found in up to 10% of patients with AIDS; discovery of these lesions should prompt an exhaustive workup because they can be a sign of disseminated infection. Common etiologic agents are *C neoformans, P jirovecii, M tuberculosis,* and atypical mycobacteria. Because of the profound immunosuppression in patients with AIDS, multiple infectious agents may cause simultaneous infectious multifocal choroiditis.

Pneumocystis jirovecii *choroiditis*

Patients with AIDS are at increased risk for *P jirovecii* pneumonia. In rare cases, this infection can result in a choroiditis with infiltrates that contain the microorganisms. The choroidal lesions are slightly elevated, plaquelike, and yellow white with minimal vitritis (Fig 13-6). On fluorescein angiography, these lesions tend to be hypofluorescent in the early phase and hyperfluorescent in the later phases. If disseminated *P jirovecii* infection is suspected, an extensive evaluation should be conducted by a specialist in infectious diseases.

Treatment of *P jirovecii* choroiditis involves a 3-week regimen of intravenous trimethoprim (20 mg/kg/day) and sulfamethoxazole (100 mg/kg/day) or pentamidine (4 mg/kg/day). Within 3–12 weeks after treatment, most of the yellow-white lesions disappear, leaving mild overlying pigmentary changes. Vision is usually not affected.

Cryptococcosis

Cryptococcus neoformans is a yeast found worldwide in high concentrations in soil and pigeon feces. Infection is acquired through inhalation of the aerosolized fungus. It has a predilection for the CNS and may produce severe disseminated disease in immunocompromised or debilitated patients. Although overall it remains an uncommon disease, cryptococcosis is the most common cause of fungal meningitis as well as the most frequent fungal eye infection in patients with AIDS. The fungus probably reaches the eye hematogenously; however, the frequent association of ocular cryptococcosis with meningitis suggests that direct extension of infection from the optic nerve may result in ocular infection. Ocular infections may occur months after the onset of meningitis or, in rare instances, before the onset of clinically apparent CNS disease.

Ocular findings associated with cryptococcal meningitis include optic nerve edema followed by optic atrophy. Other manifestations include nystagmus and cranial nerve palsies associated with diplopia, ptosis, and ophthalmoplegia.

The most frequent presentation of ocular cryptococcosis that is not directly related to meningitis is multifocal choroiditis (Fig 13-7). Associated findings include granulomatous anterior chamber inflammation, variable degrees of vitritis, vascular sheathing, exudative

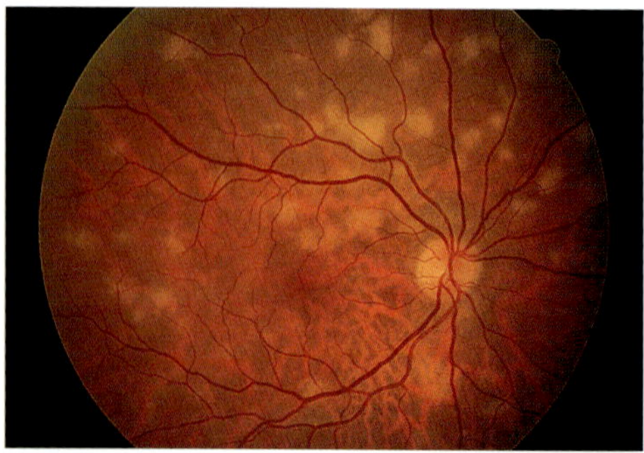

Figure 13-6 *Pneumocystis jirovecii* choroiditis. Fundus photograph shows multiple choroidal lesions. Findings were similar for the fellow eye. *(Reproduced with permission from Cunningham ET Jr, Belfort R Jr.* HIV/AIDS and the Eye: A Global Perspective. *Ophthalmology Monograph 15. American Academy of Ophthalmology; 2002:67.)*

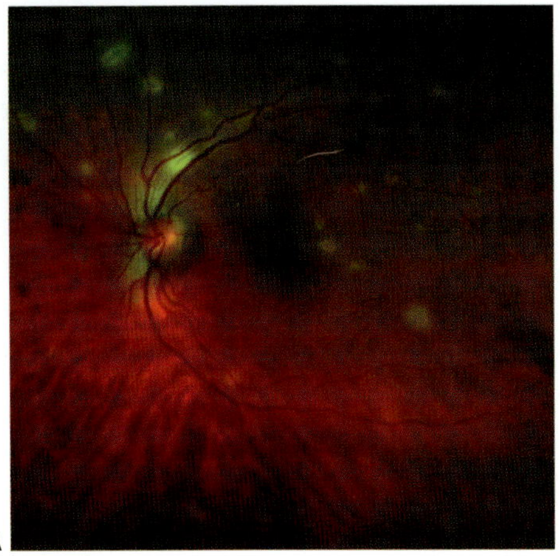

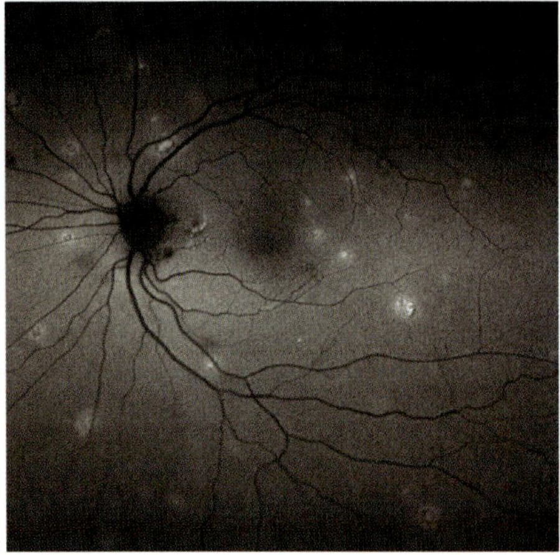

Figure 13-7 Cryptococcal choroiditis. Fundus photograph **(A)** and fundus autofluorescence image **(B)** show multifocal chorioretinal lesions. *(Originally published in the Retina Image Bank. Akshay S. Thomas, MD, MS. Retina Image Bank; 2018. Image number 28299. © American Society of Retina Specialists.)*

retinal detachment, and papilledema. It has been hypothesized that the infection begins as a focus in the choroid, with subsequent extension and secondary involvement of overlying tissues. Severe intraocular infection that progresses to endophthalmitis may occur in the absence of meningitis or clinically apparent systemic disease.

Diagnosis requires a high degree of clinical suspicion and is supported by demonstration of the organism with India ink stains or by positive *C neoformans* cultures of vitreous, chorioretinal biopsy specimens, or cerebrospinal fluid. Intravenous amphotericin B and oral flucytosine are required in order to halt disease progression. Systemic and intravitreal voriconazole may also be considered. With optic nerve or macular involvement, the prognosis for visual recovery is poor.

Aderman CM, Gorovoy IR, Chao DL, Bloomer MM, Obeid A, Stewart JM. Cryptococcal choroiditis in advanced AIDS with clinicopathologic correlation. *Am J Ophthalmol Case Rep.* 2018 Jan 31;10:51–54.

Kestelyn P, Taelman H, Bogaerts J, et al. Ophthalmic manifestations of infections with *Cryptococcus neoformans* in patients with the acquired immunodeficiency syndrome. *Am J Ophthalmol.* 1993;116(6):721–727.

Wykoff CC, Albini TA, Couvillion SS, Dubovy SR, Davis JL. Intraocular cryptococcoma. *Arch Ophthalmol.* 2009;127(5):700–702.

External Eye Manifestations

Other ophthalmic conditions associated with infection that occur in persons with AIDS include Kaposi sarcoma; molluscum contagiosum; herpes zoster ophthalmicus; and keratitis, which can be due to various viral or protozoal infections, conjunctival infections, and microvascular abnormalities. All of these conditions affect mainly the anterior segment of the globe and the ocular adnexa. These conditions are also discussed in BCSC Section 8, *External Disease and Cornea.*

Kaposi sarcoma

Human herpesvirus 8 is associated with Kaposi sarcoma. Two aggressive variants of this tumor have been described: an endemic variety especially prevalent in Kenya and Nigeria and a second variant, epidemic Kaposi sarcoma, which was first noted in renal transplant recipients and in patients with AIDS.

AIDS-associated Kaposi sarcoma may be found in visceral organs (the gastrointestinal tract, lung, and liver) in up to 50% of patients. Before the availability of potent ART, involvement of the ocular adnexa (orbit, eyelid, lacrimal gland, or conjunctiva) occurred in approximately 20% of patients with AIDS-associated systemic Kaposi sarcoma (Fig 13-8). Histologic investigation shows spindle cells mixed with vascular structures. Treatment of Kaposi sarcoma consists of excision, cryotherapy, radiotherapy, or a combination of these methods and is based on the clinical stage of the tumor as well as its location and the presence or absence of disseminated lesions.

Ong Beng Seng M, Meyer D, Gichuhi S, et al. Ocular surface disorders in patients with human immunodeficiency virus (HIV) infection. *Ocul Immunol Inflamm.* 2020;28(7): 1015–1021.

Molluscum contagiosum

Molluscum contagiosum is caused by infection with a poxvirus (family Poxviridae), which is a double-stranded DNA virus. The characteristic skin lesions are raised with central umbilication. In immunocompetent individuals, the eyelid lesions are few and unilateral. In contrast, in patients with AIDS, molluscum contagiosum eyelid lesions may be numerous and bilateral; if they are symptomatic or cause conjunctivitis, surgical excision may be necessary. These lesions may also resolve after ART.

Herpes zoster ophthalmicus

Herpes zoster ophthalmicus is caused by reactivation of latent VZV in the ophthalmic division of the trigeminal nerve. Testing for HIV should be considered for patients younger than 50 years who present with herpes zoster lesions of the face or eyelids. Corneal involvement can cause a persistent, chronic epithelial keratitis. Treatment consists of systemic and topical acyclovir. These patients should receive periodic monitoring with retinal examinations to ensure that posterior segment involvement does not occur.

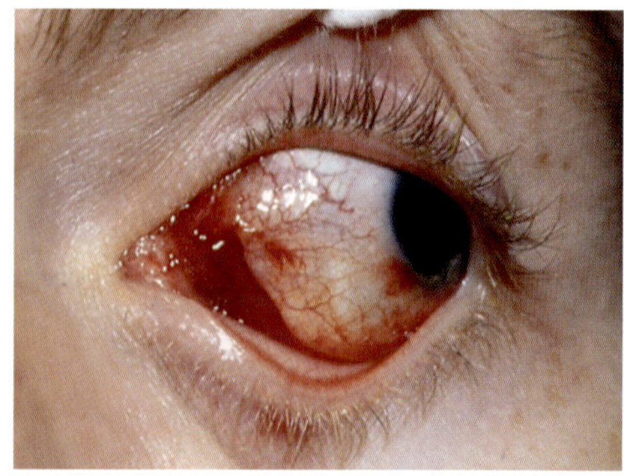

Figure 13-8 Kaposi sarcoma. External photograph shows a hemorrhagic conjunctival tumor. *(Courtesy of Elaine Chuang, MD.)*

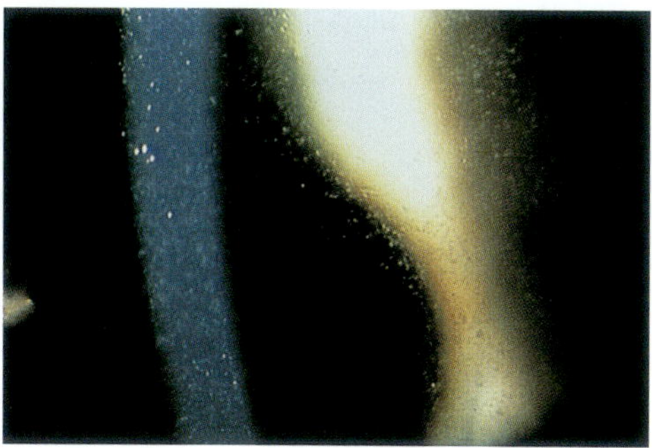

Figure 13-9 Microsporidia. Slit-lamp photograph of cornea shows punctate epithelial keratitis caused by microsporidia.

Other infections

Infection with HIV does not appear to predispose patients to bacterial keratitis, although bacterial and fungal keratitis can occur in patients with AIDS who have no obvious predisposing factors such as trauma or topical corticosteroid use. Infections can be more severe and are more likely to cause corneal perforation in patients with AIDS than in immunocompetent patients. Similarly, while patients with AIDS do not have a higher incidence of herpes simplex keratitis, they may have a protracted disease course or multiple recurrences, and the keratitis may involve the limbus. Microsporidial infection has been shown to cause a coarse punctate epithelial keratitis with minimal conjunctival reaction in patients with AIDS (Fig 13-9). Electron microscopy of epithelial scrapings has revealed the organism, which is an obligate intracellular protozoal parasite.

Solitary granulomatous conjunctivitis caused by cryptococcal or mycotic infection or by tuberculosis can occur in HIV-infected persons. Aggressive investigation for and treatment of dissemination, if present, is critical.

CHAPTER 14

Endophthalmitis

Highlights

- Chronic postoperative endophthalmitis may be difficult to diagnose and may require invasive diagnostic testing; treatment may include antibiotic or antifungal injection and, in many cases, explantation of an intraocular lens.
- Endogenous endophthalmitis should be suspected in immunosuppressed patients and in patients with a recent history of infection, surgery, diabetes, or intravenous drug use who are found to have anterior and posterior segment inflammation. The diagnosis can be definitively established by cultures, stains, or molecular studies (eg, polymerase chain reaction analysis) of vitreous aspirate.
- Endogenous endophthalmitis requires evaluation for a systemic source of infection and treatment with intravitreal antibiotic or antifungal injection and often systemic antimicrobials.

Definitions

Endophthalmitis is a clinical diagnosis made when intraocular inflammation involving both the anterior and posterior segments is attributable to bacterial or fungal infection within the eye. The retina or the choroid may be involved. Occasionally, concomitant infectious scleritis or keratitis is present. Endophthalmitis may be either exogenous, as in postoperative or posttraumatic cases, or endogenous, as in hematogenous spread from a systemic infection. Acute postoperative endophthalmitis and posttraumatic endophthalmitis are typically manifested by aggressive intraocular inflammation within days of ocular surgery or trauma. Their incidence varies between 0.04% and 0.2%. In contrast, chronic postoperative endophthalmitis occurs weeks or months after surgery and can be caused by a myriad of bacteria and fungi. Because this condition often goes undiagnosed for long periods, its incidence has not been established. Endogenous endophthalmitis occurs when bacteria or fungi are hematogenously disseminated into the ocular circulation from a systemic infection.

Acute postoperative and posttraumatic endophthalmitis are covered in BCSC Section 12, *Retina and Vitreous,* and are not discussed further here. For a detailed discussion of post–cataract surgery endophthalmitis, including proper surgical techniques and perioperative antibiotic prophylaxis, see BCSC Section 11, *Lens and Cataract.*

Chronic Postoperative Endophthalmitis

Clinical Findings

Chronic postoperative endophthalmitis has a distinctive clinical course, with multiple recurrences of chronic indolent inflammation in an eye that has previously undergone surgery, typically cataract extraction. Unlike the explosive onset of acute postoperative endophthalmitis, in chronic disease the initial inflammation may occur at any point during the postoperative course; however, it is often delayed by many months. Chronic anterior segment inflammation, hypopyon, keratic precipitates, intracapsular plaques, and/or vitritis may be present (Fig 14-1). Inflammation may respond to corticosteroid therapy but often recurs after corticosteroids are tapered. In the most severe cases, inflammation may cause corneal decompensation or even iris neovascularization.

Chronic postoperative endophthalmitis can be divided into bacterial and fungal varieties. Chronic postoperative bacterial endophthalmitis is most commonly caused by *Cutibacterium acnes* (formerly *Propionibacterium acnes*). Gram-positive bacteria with limited virulence (eg, *Staphylococcus epidermidis* and *Corynebacterium* species), gram-negative bacteria, or *Mycobacterium* species may also be causative agents. *C acnes,* a commensal, anaerobic, pleomorphic, gram-positive rod, is commonly found on the eyelid skin or conjunctiva. The organism may also sequester itself between an intraocular lens (IOL) implant and the posterior capsule. In this relatively anaerobic environment, *C acnes* grows and forms colonies, which manifest as whitish plaques between the posterior capsule and the IOL implant. Nd:YAG capsulotomy may trigger chronic endophthalmitis in these eyes by liberating the organism into the vitreous cavity, resulting in more severe vitreous inflammation and exacerbation of the underlying infection.

Chronic postoperative fungal endophthalmitis may have a presentation similar to that of *C acnes–related disease.* Numerous fungal organisms have been implicated in this chronic inflammatory process, including *Candida parapsilosis, Aspergillus flavus, Torulopsis candida,* and *Paecilomyces lilacinus,* as well as *Verticillium* species. Certain clinical signs may be helpful in differentiating a fungal from a bacterial etiology, including the presence of corneal infiltrate or edema, a mass in the iris or ciliary body, or development of necrotizing scleritis. The

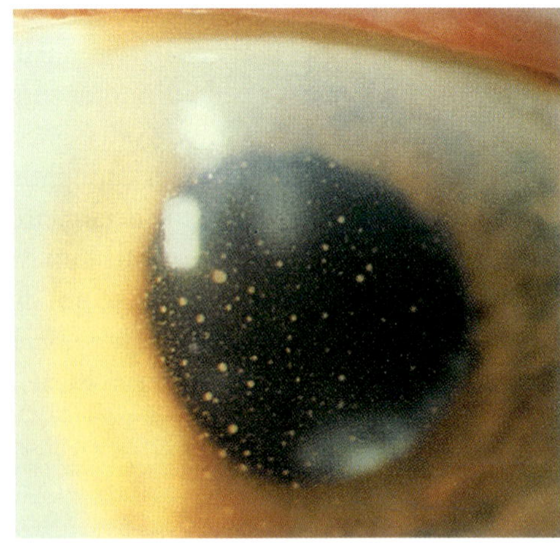

Figure 14-1 Chronic postoperative endophthalmitis caused by *Cutibacterium acnes* infection. Anterior segment photograph shows keratic precipitates and white plaque in the capsular bag. *(Courtesy of David Meisler, MD.)*

presence of vitreous snowballs with a "string-of-pearls" appearance in the vitreous may also be indicative of a fungal infection. The intraocular inflammation may worsen after topical, periocular, or intraocular corticosteroid therapy, which should automatically raise suspicion for a fungal infection.

Maalouf F, Abdulaal M, Hamam RN. Chronic postoperative endophthalmitis: a review of clinical characteristics, microbiology, treatment strategies, and outcomes. *Int J Inflam.* 2012:313248. doi:10.1155/2012/313248

Shirodkar AR, Pathengay A, Flynn HW Jr, et al. Delayed- versus acute-onset endophthalmitis after cataract surgery. *Am J Ophthalmol.* 2012;153(3):391–398.e2.

Diagnosis

The diagnosis of chronic postoperative endophthalmitis is based on clinical suspicion and confirmed by obtaining aerobic, anaerobic, and fungal cultures of intraocular fluids. The aqueous, capsular plaques (if present), and vitreous should be sampled using needle aspiration or pars plana vitrectomy. Gram and fungal stains should also be obtained. The value of such stains should not be underestimated, especially in cases of fungal endophthalmitis. In addition, polymerase chain reaction (PCR) testing with primers for *C acnes* and pan-fungal and pan-bacterial targets may be helpful. The bacterial and fungal stains or PCR may yield information rapidly, enabling the clinician to tailor therapy and improve clinical prognosis long before the results of the cultures become positive. Because of the slow-growing and fastidious nature of the organisms that cause chronic endophthalmitis, cultures must be retained by the microbiology laboratory for 2 or more weeks. If initial cultures are negative for infection but clinical suspicion remains high, cultures may need to be repeated.

The differential diagnosis of chronic postoperative endophthalmitis includes noninfectious causes such as lens-induced uveitis (from retained cortical material or retained intravitreal lens fragments), uveitis-glaucoma-hyphema syndrome (IOL malposition leading to iris chafing and intraocular inflammation), sympathetic ophthalmia (if the fellow eye has had prior surgery or trauma), and masquerade syndromes such as vitreoretinal lymphoma. See the Clinical Pearl for the differential diagnosis of chronic postsurgical intraocular inflammation.

Lai J-Y, Chen K-H, Lin Y-C, Hsu W-M, Lee S-M. *Propionibacterium acnes* DNA from an explanted intraocular lens detected by polymerase chain reaction in a case of chronic pseudophakic endophthalmitis. *J Cataract Refract Surg.* 2006;32(3):522–525.

Meisler DM, Mandelbaum S. *Propionibacterium*-associated endophthalmitis after extracapsular cataract extraction: review of reported cases. *Ophthalmology.* 1989;96(1):54–61.

CLINICAL PEARL

The differential diagnosis for chronic postoperative intraocular inflammation includes the following conditions:

- persistent postoperative noninfectious inflammation
- chafing by an intraocular lens, including uveitis-glaucoma-hyphema syndrome
- viral anterior uveitis
- chronic infectious endophthalmitis

Treatment

Treatment of chronic postoperative bacterial endophthalmitis ranges from intravitreal antibiotic alone (see Appendix B) to pars plana vitrectomy and intravitreal antibiotic with or without partial capsulectomy. These measures may not completely eradicate the infection, especially if the microorganism is sequestered in the equatorial lens capsule. In such cases, IOL explantation, complete capsulectomy, and intravitreal vancomycin injection may be curative. The decision to explant an IOL is made on a case-by-case basis depending on the clinical course, the severity of the intraocular inflammation, and the level of vision loss. Although there is no preferred method for treating this chronic infection, existing literature suggests that more than one surgical procedure may be necessary to eradicate it.

The treatment of chronic fungal endophthalmitis is more difficult and requires the use of weekly intravitreal antifungal injections (amphotericin or voriconazole) and possibly systemic antifungal drugs in the most severe cases. In vitrectomized eyes, antifungals are often injected twice a week. Multiple vitrectomies may be necessary.

Clark WL, Kaiser PK, Flynn HW Jr, Belfort A, Miller D, Meisler DM. Treatment strategies and visual acuity outcomes in chronic postoperative *Propionibacterium acnes* endophthalmitis. *Ophthalmology.* 1999;106(9):1665–1670.

Endogenous Endophthalmitis

Endogenous Bacterial Endophthalmitis

Endogenous bacterial endophthalmitis is caused by hematogenous dissemination of the organisms, resulting in intraocular infection. This disease is uncommon and accounts for less than 10% of all endophthalmitis cases. Patients who have compromised immune systems are most at risk for endogenous endophthalmitis. Predisposing conditions include type 1 and type 2 diabetes, systemic malignancy, sickle cell anemia, and systemic lupus erythematosus. Endogenous endophthalmitis may also develop in patients with immunosuppression from HIV infection; however, it is unclear whether HIV infection is an independent risk factor. In addition, extensive gastrointestinal surgery, endoscopy, dental procedures, and intravenous drug use may increase the risk of endogenous endophthalmitis. Systemic immunomodulatory therapy and chemotherapy may also put patients at risk. Although the eye may be the only location where the infection is found, an extraocular focus exists in as many as 90% of cases. Possible sources of infection include cellulitis, tooth abscess, pneumonia, endocarditis, urinary tract infection, bacterial meningitis, and liver abscess. Previous use of an indwelling line or port may also be related.

A wide variety of bacteria can cause endogenous endophthalmitis. The most common gram-positive organisms are *Streptococcus* species (endocarditis), *Staphylococcus aureus* (cutaneous infections), *Bacillus* species (from intravenous drug use), and *Nocardia* species (in immunocompromised patients, discussed in further detail in Chapter 11). The most common gram-negative organisms are *Neisseria meningitidis, Haemophilus influenzae,* and enteric organisms such as *Escherichia coli* and *Klebsiella* species. In Asia, the most common cause of endogenous endophthalmitis is infection from *Klebsiella* species in liver abscesses.

Jackson TL, Paraskevopoulos T, Georgalas I. Systematic review of 342 cases of endogenous bacterial endophthalmitis. *Surv Ophthalmol.* 2014;59(6):627–635.

Clinical findings

Although some patients with endogenous bacterial endophthalmitis are ambulatory and afebrile, others may show signs of an ongoing systemic infection, such as fever greater than 101.5°F, elevated peripheral leukocyte count, and positive bacterial cultures from extraocular sites (blood, urine, sputum). Patients who present with endogenous endophthalmitis may also be ill and undergoing treatment for a primary underlying disease, such as cancer treated with prolonged intravenous chemotherapy or other chronic infections that may subsequently sequester in the eye. A nonocular infection serving as a nidus for bacterial dissemination to the eye may be very difficult to diagnose, especially in cases of osteomyelitis, sinusitis, or pneumonia misdiagnosed as a simple upper respiratory tract infection. In these situations, laboratory tests cannot substitute for a detailed history and review of systems.

Ocular symptoms of endogenous bacterial endophthalmitis include acute onset of eye pain, photophobia, and blurred vision. Examination usually reveals severely reduced visual acuity. Substantial inflammation may be seen in the anterior chamber, including fibrin and hypopyon, as well as in the vitreous cavity (Fig 14-2). Both eyes may be affected simultaneously. Chorioretinal abscess and retinal hemorrhages, including white-centered Roth spots, may also be present (Fig 14-3). Very rarely, there is periorbital and eyelid edema.

Morbidity due to endogenous bacterial endophthalmitis can be significant. If the associated systemic infection is missed, sepsis may develop and the patient may die. Recurrent or persistent intraocular infection may require numerous surgical procedures and repeated injections of intravitreal antibiotics. In the most severe cases, complications such as cataract development, retinal detachment, suprachoroidal hemorrhage, vitreous hemorrhage, macular scar, hypotony, and phthisis bulbi can also occur. The prognosis is directly related to the offending organism and the systemic status of the patient.

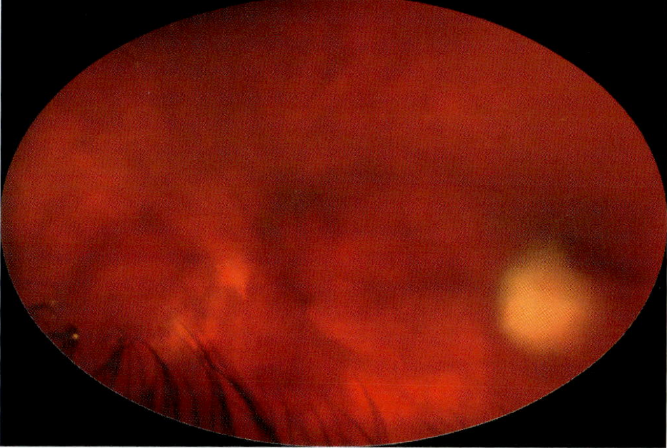

Figure 14-2 Endogenous bacterial endophthalmitis. Fundus photograph of the left eye shows substantial vitreous haze with a large chorioretinal abscess and associated hemorrhage in the temporal periphery. *(Courtesy of Jared E. Knickelbein, MD, PhD.)*

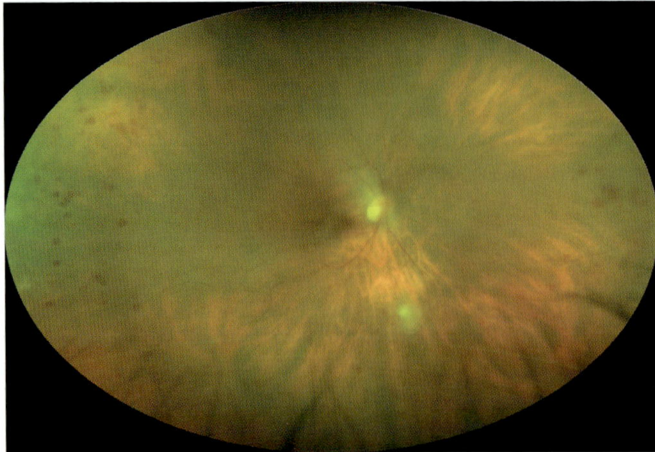

Figure 14-3 Endogenous bacterial endophthalmitis. Fundus photograph shows vitreous haze, a small chorioretinal abscess in the inferior midperiphery, and peripheral intraretinal hemorrhages. *(Courtesy of Jared E. Knickelbein, MD, PhD.)*

Diagnosis

Endogenous bacterial endophthalmitis is diagnosed on the basis of vitreous and aqueous cultures and appropriate stains. PCR evaluation of ocular fluids with pan-bacterial primers can also be useful. Vitrectomy may be required. Cultures of blood and other body fluids can help confirm the diagnosis and establish therapy.

Treatment

Intravitreal antibiotics, typically vancomycin and ceftazidime, are given at the time of vitreous sampling (see Appendix B). When fungal organisms may be involved, empiric treatment of both fungal and bacterial causes is indicated. Patients with endogenous bacterial endophthalmitis should be evaluated by a specialist in infectious diseases to identify and treat the systemic source of infection. Intravenous antibiotic treatment may be needed for several weeks, depending on the organism isolated. Initial antimicrobial choices may be empiric and subsequently tailored to the culture results.

Endogenous Fungal Endophthalmitis

Endogenous fungal endophthalmitis develops acutely to subacutely and is associated with poor visual outcomes. Affected patients often have a history of type 1 or type 2 diabetes, immunosuppression, or intravenous drug use. Ocular infection stems from hematogenous spread from a systemic source and usually begins in the choroid, appearing as yellow-white chorioretinal lesions with indistinct borders that can range in size from <1 mm to several disc diameters. Organisms can subsequently break through into the vitreous, producing localized cellular and fungal aggregates overlying the original site(s). Chorioretinal lesions may be difficult to detect on initial presentation, with vitreous inflammation being the main sign of infection. Anterior segment inflammation, including keratic precipitates and hypopyon, as well as iris nodules and rubeosis, may also be observed.

Endogenous fungal endophthalmitis may be mistaken for noninfectious uveitis and treated with corticosteroids alone. This treatment usually worsens the clinical course of the disease, necessitating further investigation to establish the correct diagnosis. The condition requires aggressive systemic and local antifungal therapy and often surgical intervention. Co-management with a specialist in infectious diseases is essential.

Endogenous fungal endophthalmitis is most commonly caused by *Candida* species, followed by *Aspergillus* species (see the following sections for further discussion). *Cryptococcus neoformans, Coccidioides immitis, Histoplasma capsulatum, Sporothrix schenckii,* and *Blastomyces dermatitidis* are less common causes.

Sridhar J, Flynn HW Jr, Kuriyan AE, Miller D, Albini T. Endogenous fungal endophthalmitis: risk factors, clinical features, and treatment outcomes in mold and yeast infections. *J Ophthalmic Inflamm Infect.* 2013;3(1):60.

Candida *endophthalmitis*

Candida species are an important cause of nosocomial infections and are the most common cause of endogenous fungal endophthalmitis. *Candida albicans,* a yeast naturally found on the skin and mucous membranes as well as in the gut, is the most common pathogenic species, but non-*albicans* species (eg, *Candida glabrata*) have also been identified in patients with fungal endophthalmitis. Fungal organisms reach the eye hematogenously through metastasis to the choroid. Fungi may then break through Bruch membrane, form subretinal abscesses, and secondarily involve the retina and vitreous. Histologically, *Candida* species are recognized as budding yeast with a characteristic pseudohyphate appearance (Fig 14-4; see also BCSC Section 4, *Ophthalmic Pathology and Intraocular Tumors*).

In patients with candidemia, the reported prevalence rates of *Candida* endophthalmitis vary widely. In a systematic review that included a rigorous definition of endophthalmitis and involved more than 1,000 prospectively identified patients with candidemia, the endophthalmitis rate was <1%. Of note, patients with candidemia often have major comorbidities, such as anemia, thrombocytopenia, and hypertension. These comorbidities

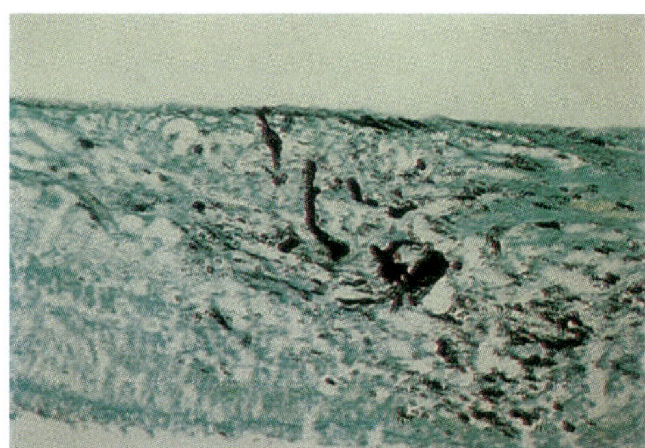

Figure 14-4 *Candida* retinitis in fungal endophthalmitis. Histologic examination with a Gomori methenamine silver stain reveals fungi *(black)* in the retina.

may cause ocular findings, including intraretinal hemorrhages (and Roth spots) and cotton-wool spots, which do not necessarily represent intraocular infection.

Predisposing conditions associated with candidemia and the development of intraocular infection include the following:

- intravenous drug use
- immunosuppressive therapy
- prolonged neutropenia
- organ transplant
- poorly controlled chronic diseases (eg, diabetes)
- use of indwelling catheters
- history of recent major gastrointestinal surgery
- hospitalized neonates
- hyperalimentation
- bacterial sepsis
- systemic antibiotic use

Breazzano MP, Day HR Jr, Bloch KC, et al. Utility of ophthalmologic screening for *Candida* bloodstream infections: a systematic review. *JAMA Ophthalmol.* 2019;137(6):698–710.

Shah CP, McKey J, Spirn MJ, Maguire J. Ocular candidiasis: a review. *Br J Ophthalmol.* 2008;92(4):466–468.

Clinical findings Patients with *Candida* endophthalmitis may present with floaters or blurred vision resulting from vitreous opacities or macular chorioretinal involvement. Patients may also have eye pain arising from associated anterior uveitis, which may be severe. Typically, *Candida* chorioretinitis is characterized by multiple, bilateral, white, well-circumscribed lesions less than 1 mm in diameter. Lesions are typically distributed throughout the postequatorial fundus and are associated with overlying vitreous inflammation (Fig 14-5). The chorioretinal lesions may be associated with vascular sheathing and intraretinal hemorrhages. The vitreous opacities may assume a string-of-pearls appearance.

Rao NA, Hidayat AA. Endogenous mycotic endophthalmitis: variations in clinical and histopathologic changes in candidiasis compared with aspergillosis. *Am J Ophthalmol.* 2001;132(2):244–251.

Diagnosis The diagnosis of ocular candidiasis is suggested by the presence of chorioretinitis or endophthalmitis in the appropriate clinical context and is confirmed by positive results from blood or vitreous culture. It has been suggested that all patients with candidemia undergo baseline dilated ophthalmoscopic examinations and monitoring for the development of metastatic ocular candidiasis for at least 2 weeks after an initial eye examination. However, the American Academy of Ophthalmology currently recommends ophthalmic consultation only for patients with a clinical rationale, such as signs or symptoms concerning for endophthalmitis, or those who are intubated or otherwise unable to communicate ocular symptoms; routine screening for all patients with candidemia is not necessary.

The presence of vitreous snowballs and endophthalmitis may require diagnostic and therapeutic vitrectomy, especially with severe disease or when systemic infection has yet to be confirmed. Fungal stains and cultures on Sabouraud agar plates, as well as pan-fungal

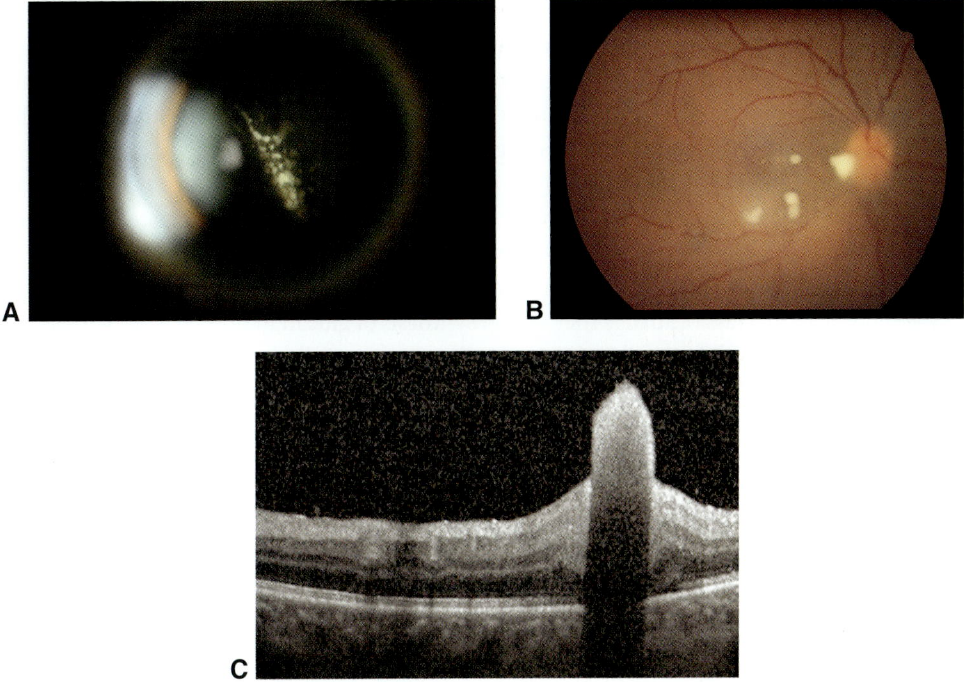

Figure 14-5 Endogenous *Candida* endophthalmitis. **A,** Slit-lamp photograph shows a "string of pearls" in the vitreous. **B,** Fundus photograph shows vitreous opacities and underlying white chorioretinal lesions. **C,** Optical coherence tomography line scan shows a fungal lesion breaking through the retina into the vitreous cavity. *(Part A courtesy of H. Nida Sen, MD, and Henry Wiley, MD/National Eye Institute; part B courtesy of Debra A. Goldstein, MD; part C courtesy of Jared E. Knickelbein, MD, PhD.)*

PCR and PCR for *Candida* species if available, should be obtained on undiluted vitreous fluid samples. Blood cultures should also be obtained if systemic infection has yet to be confirmed.

The differential diagnosis of *Candida* endophthalmitis includes infection with other fungi or bacteria as well as *Toxoplasma* retinochoroiditis, which can exhibit similar posterior pole lesions. *Candida* snowball lesions may also resemble pars planitis.

Breazzano MP, Bond JB III, Bearelly S, et al; for the American Academy of Ophthalmology. American Academy of Ophthalmology recommendations on screening for endogenous *Candida* endophthalmitis. *Ophthalmology*. 2022;129(1):73–76.

Hidalgo JA, Alangaden GJ, Eliott D, et al. Fungal endophthalmitis diagnosis by detection of *Candida albicans* DNA in intraocular fluid by use of a species-specific polymerase chain reaction assay. *J Infect Dis*. 2000;181(3):1198–1201.

Treatment The treatment of intraocular candidiasis includes systemic and often intravitreal administration of antifungal drugs. Consultation with a specialist in infectious diseases is essential. Chorioretinal lesions not yet involving the vitreous body may be treated effectively with the oral triazole antifungal drugs fluconazole or voriconazole (200 mg, twice daily, for 2–4 weeks), with vigilant monitoring for evidence of progression. Voriconazole is often preferred as it has good oral bioavailability, achieving therapeutic intravitreal levels with a broad spectrum of antifungal activity. When the vitreous body is involved, intravitreal injection of antifungal drugs (amphotericin B, 5–10 μg/0.1 mL, or voriconazole, 100 μg/0.1 mL; see Appendix B) should be considered, usually in conjunction with pars plana vitrectomy. Long-acting corticosteroid injections should be avoided. Vitrectomy may be useful diagnostically by providing intraocular fluid for microbiologic and molecular analyses and therapeutically by debulking the pathogen load and clearing the vitreous inflammation.

More severe infections may require intravenous amphotericin B with or without flucytosine. Major dose-limiting toxicities (renal, cardiac, and neurologic) associated with conventional amphotericin B therapy have been greatly reduced by the use of liposomal lipid complex formulations. Finally, intravenously administered caspofungin, an antifungal drug in the echinocandin class (ie, drugs that inhibit synthesis of glucan in the cell wall) with activity against *Candida* and *Aspergillus* species, has been successfully employed in a small number of patients with *Candida* endophthalmitis; however, some treatment failures have also been reported with this drug. Another echinocandin agent, intravenous micafungin, is also available in the United States and Europe for treatment of candidiasis. Oral voriconazole, flucytosine, fluconazole, or rifampin may be administered in addition to intravenous amphotericin B or caspofungin. Systemic antifungal treatment may be necessary for 6 weeks or longer.

Hariprasad SM, Mieler WF, Holz ER, et al. Determination of vitreous, aqueous, and plasma concentration of orally administered voriconazole in humans. *Arch Ophthalmol.* 2004;122(1):42–47.

Paulus YM, Cheng S, Karth PA, Leng T. Prospective trial of endogenous fungal endophthalmitis and chorioretinitis rates, clinical course, and outcomes in patients with fungemia. *Retina.* 2016;36(7):1357–1363.

Riddell J IV, Comer GM, Kauffman CA. Treatment of endogenous fungal endophthalmitis: focus on new antifungal agents. *Clin Infect Dis.* 2011;52(5):648–653.

Aspergillus *endophthalmitis*

Aspergillus species are molds found in soils and decaying vegetation. The spores of these ubiquitous saprophytic molds become airborne and seed the lungs and paranasal sinuses of humans. Human exposure is very common, but infection is rare and depends on the virulence of the fungal pathogen and immunocompetence of the host. Ocular disease occurs via hematogenous spread of *Aspergillus* organisms to the choroid.

Endogenous *Aspergillus* endophthalmitis is a rare disorder associated with disseminated aspergillosis among patients with severe chronic pulmonary diseases, cancer, organ transplant, endocarditis, severe immunocompromise, or intravenous drug use. In isolated instances, *Aspergillus* endophthalmitis occurs in immunocompetent patients with no apparent predisposing factors. Disseminated infection most commonly involves the lungs; the eye is the second most common site of infection. *Aspergillus fumigatus* and *A flavus* are the species most frequently isolated from patients with intraocular infection.

Clinical findings Endogenous *Aspergillus* endophthalmitis results in rapid onset of pain and loss of vision. A confluent yellowish infiltrate is often present in the posterior pole, beginning in the choroid and subretinal space (Fig 14-6A). A hypopyon can develop in the subretinal or subhyaloidal space. Retinal hemorrhages, retinal vascular occlusions, and full-thickness retinal necrosis may occur. The infection can spread, producing a dense vitritis and variable degrees of cells, flare, and hypopyon in the anterior chamber. When healed, the macular lesions form a central atrophic scar.

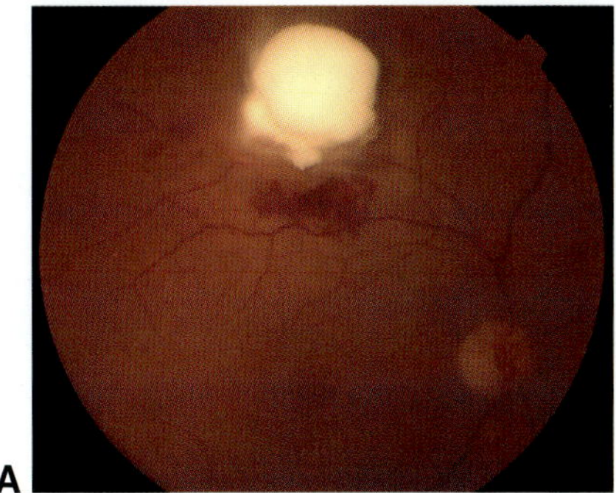

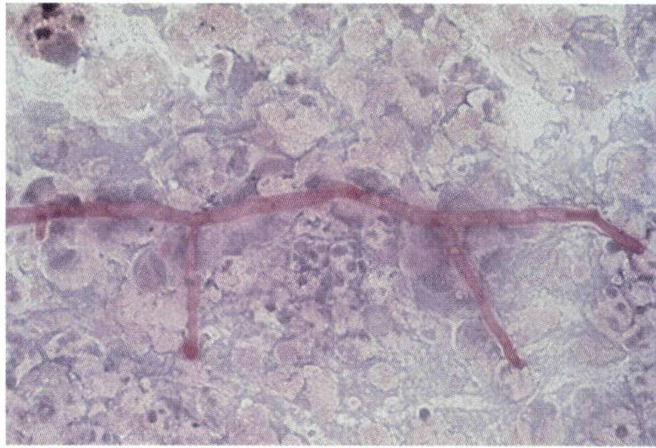

Figure 14-6 *Aspergillus* endophthalmitis. **A,** Fundus photograph shows a large granuloma in the posterior pole. **B,** Histologic specimen shows septate hyphae. *(Courtesy of Ramana S. Moorthy, MD.)*

Diagnosis The diagnosis of endogenous *Aspergillus* endophthalmitis is based on clinical findings combined with positive results from vitreous biopsy and cultures as well as results from Gram and fungal stains. Coexisting systemic aspergillosis can be a strong clue of dissemination to the eye, especially among high-risk patients. The diagnosis requires a high degree of suspicion within the correct clinical context and is confirmed by the demonstration of dichotomously branching septate hyphae on analysis of vitreous fluid specimens (Fig 14-6B). *Aspergillus* organisms may be difficult to culture from the blood.

The differential diagnosis of endogenous *Aspergillus* endophthalmitis includes *Candida* endophthalmitis, cytomegalovirus retinitis, *Toxoplasma* retinochoroiditis, coccidioidomycotic choroiditis or endophthalmitis, and bacterial endophthalmitis. In contrast to the lesions associated with *Candida* chorioretinitis and endophthalmitis, lesions produced by *Aspergillus* species are larger and more likely to be hemorrhagic, and they commonly invade the retinal and choroidal vessels, which may result in broad areas of ischemic infarction.

Rao NA, Hidayat A. A comparative clinicopathologic study of endogenous mycotic endophthalmitis: variations in clinical and histopathologic changes in candidiasis compared to aspergillosis. *Trans Am Ophthalmol Soc.* 2000;98:183–193; discussion 193–194.

Treatment Endogenous *Aspergillus* endophthalmitis usually requires aggressive treatment with diagnostic and therapeutic pars plana vitrectomy combined with intravitreal injection of amphotericin B or voriconazole. Intravitreal corticosteroids may be used in conjunction with these drugs. Because most patients with this condition have disseminated aspergillosis, systemic treatment with oral voriconazole, intravenous amphotericin B, or caspofungin is often required. Other systemic antifungal drugs, such as itraconazole, miconazole, fluconazole, and ketoconazole, may also be used. Systemic aspergillosis should be managed by a specialist in infectious diseases. Despite aggressive treatment, the visual prognosis is poor because of frequent macular involvement. Final visual acuity is usually less than 20/200. Disseminated aspergillosis has a high mortality rate.

Spadea L, Giannico MI. Diagnostic and management strategies of *Aspergillus* endophthalmitis: current insights. *Clin Ophthalmol.* 2019;13:2573–2582.

CHAPTER 15

Masquerade Syndromes

This chapter includes a related video. Go to www.aao.org/bcscvideo_section09 or scan the QR code in the text to access this content.

Highlights

- Uveitic masquerade syndromes are neoplastic and nonneoplastic conditions that mimic immune-mediated entities. Because the underlying diseases often have serious consequences, early diagnosis and prompt treatment are vital.
- The most common condition to mimic uveitis is vitreoretinal lymphoma (VRL).
- VRL typically presents with vitritis, subretinal infiltrates, subretinal pigment epithelium infiltrates, and/or intraretinal infiltrates. Definitive diagnosis is made by cytologic analysis of intraocular fluid or tissue.
- More than two-thirds of patients with VRL will develop central nervous system (CNS) lymphoma; thus, all patients with suspected VRL should be evaluated for CNS lymphoma even in the absence of neurologic symptoms.

Introduction

Uveitic masquerade syndromes are a heterogeneous group of conditions noteworthy for mimicking immune-mediated uveitis and therefore are often difficult to diagnose. They can be divided into neoplastic and nonneoplastic conditions. The underlying diseases often have harmful consequences, so early diagnosis and prompt treatment may preserve life and/or vision.

Neoplastic Masquerade Syndromes

Neoplastic masquerade syndromes may account for 2%–3% of all patients evaluated in tertiary uveitis clinics. Vitreoretinal lymphoma is the most common entity.

Grange LK, Kouchouk A, Dalal MD, et al. Neoplastic masquerade syndromes in patients with uveitis. *Am J Ophthalmol.* 2014;157(3):526–531.

Read RW, Zamir E, Rao NA. Neoplastic masquerade syndromes. *Surv Ophthalmol.* 2002;47(2): 81–124.

Vitreoretinal Lymphoma

Vitreoretinal lymphoma (VRL), formerly known as *primary intraocular lymphoma,* is a subset of primary central nervous system lymphoma (PCNSL). It is an uncommon but potentially fatal malignant neoplasm that may occur with or without CNS lesions. The mean age at onset is between 50 and 70 years, and there is no convincing gender predilection. Immunosuppressed patients are at increased risk of VRL. Nearly all (98%) cases of VRL are B-cell, non-Hodgkin lymphomas. Approximately 2% are T-cell lymphomas.

Chan CC, Rubenstein JL, Coupland SE, et al. Primary vitreoretinal lymphoma: a report from an international primary central nervous system lymphoma collaborative group symposium. *Oncologist.* 2011;16(11):1589–1599.

Clinical features and findings

Approximately 25% of patients with intracranial lymphoma will develop intraocular disease. The most common presenting symptoms are decreased vision and floaters. Sites of ocular involvement include the vitreous, retina, and subretinal pigment epithelium (sub-RPE), or any combination thereof.

Examination reveals a variable degree of vitritis and anterior chamber cells. Posterior segment involvement may appear as cream-colored or yellow subretinal or sub-RPE infiltrates (Figs 15-1, 15-2) with overlying RPE detachments and discrete white lesions that may mimic those of acute retinal necrosis, toxoplasmosis, "frosted-branch" angiitis, or retinal arteriolar occlusion with coexisting multifocal chorioretinal scars and retinal vasculitis. Due to the challenge of diagnosing VRL, clinicians often prescribe anti-inflammatory medications that temporarily improve the vitreous cellular infiltration. In cases of presumed autoimmune uveitis that do not respond to appropriate noninfectious uveitis treatment, VRL should be a diagnostic consideration.

More than two-thirds of patients with VRL will develop CNS disease—usually within 29 months of diagnosis. CNS manifestations range from behavioral changes, hemiparesis, and cerebellar signs to epileptic seizures and cranial nerve palsies.

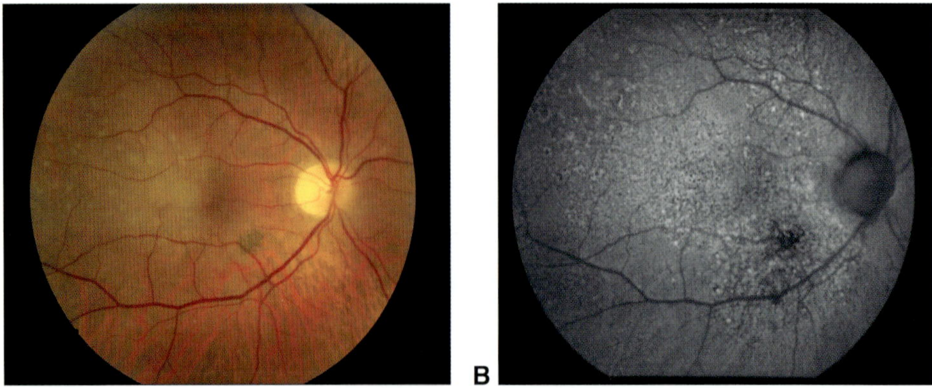

Figure 15-1 Ocular involvement in primary central nervous system (CNS) lymphoma. **A,** Fundus photograph demonstrates multifocal, cream-colored subretinal infiltrates. **B,** On fundus autofluorescence, these infiltrates appear as hyperautofluorescent and hypoautofluorescent granular changes. *(Courtesy of H. Nida Sen, MD/National Eye Institute.)*

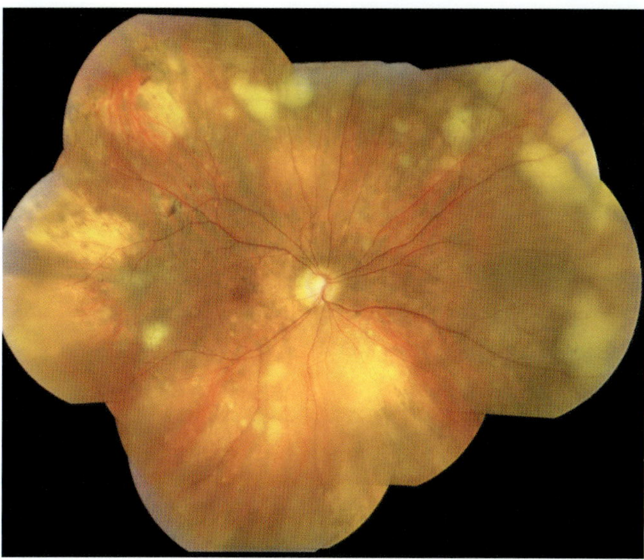

Figure 15-2 Vitreoretinal lymphoma. Fundus photograph montage shows varied multifocal lesions, some of which are cream colored/yellow and elevated while others are more atrophic. There are punctate and granular retinal pigment epithelial changes throughout the fundus. *(Courtesy of H. Nida Sen, MD/National Eye Institute.)*

Diagnostic testing

Ultrasonography may reveal vitreous debris, elevated subretinal lesions, and exudative retinal detachment. Fluorescein angiography (FA) may show hypofluorescent areas due to choroidal fluorescence blockage from a sub-RPE tumor or from RPE clumping. Hyperfluorescent window defects may be caused by RPE atrophy from resolved RPE infiltration. An unusual leopard-spot pattern of alternating hyperfluorescence and hypofluorescence may also be noted on FA. Hyperautofluorescent and hypoautofluorescent granular changes may be present on fundus autofluorescence (Fig 15-3; see also Fig 15-1B), and optical coherence tomography may reveal nodular elevations at the level of the RPE and sub-RPE and/or vertical hyperreflective lesions. Indocyanine green angiography may show ill-defined hypofluorescent lesions in the late phase of the study.

All patients with suspected VRL should be urgently evaluated for CNS lymphoma, preferably with magnetic resonance imaging, even in the absence of neurologic symptoms. Cerebrospinal fluid analysis reveals lymphoma cells in one-third of patients with suspected VRL.

A vitreous biopsy is the most common procedure performed to definitively diagnose VRL. To increase diagnostic yield, systemic corticosteroids should be stopped at least 2 to 4 weeks before the diagnostic vitrectomy. As much vitreous as possible should be obtained. An ideal biopsy consists of at least 1 mL of undiluted vitreous and a cytospin preparation of diluted vitreous. Because the results of as many as one-third of vitreous biopsies may be falsely negative in VRL, a retinal biopsy and/or an aspirate of sub-RPE material may be considered if there is still a strong clinical suspicion for VRL after a negative result (Video 15-1).

VIDEO 15-1 Vitreoretinal lymphoma.
Courtesy of Emilio M. Dodds, MD.

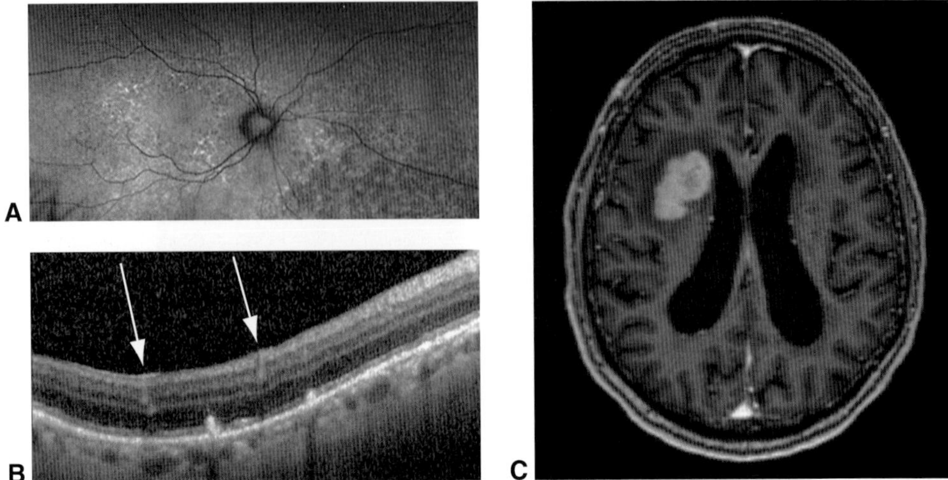

Figure 15-3 Primary CNS lymphoma. **A,** Wide-field fundus autofluorescence shows extensive mixed hyperautofluorescent and hypoautofluorescent granularities. **B,** Optical coherence tomography (OCT) shows vertical hyperreflective lesions *(arrows)* as well as subretinal infiltrates. **C,** The patient was evaluated for CNS lymphoma despite a lack of CNS symptoms, and a frontal lobe lesion was found on magnetic resonance imaging. *(Courtesy of Karen R. Armbrust, MD, PhD.)*

Prior to surgery, it is crucial to communicate with an experienced pathologist to ensure that specimens will be promptly and properly handled. Degeneration of the typically friable lymphoma cells may occur with delays in specimen handling and processing. The diagnosis may be difficult to establish because specimens from eyes with VRL may show sparse cellularity, or they may contain numerous reactive cells that hamper detection of the few lymphoma cells. Aliquots of the vitreous specimen are typically prepared for both cytologic analysis and cell surface marker determination by flow cytometry.

Cytologic specimens obtained from the vitreous typically contain pleomorphic lymphoid cells with scant cytoplasm, hyperchromatic nuclei with multiple irregular nucleoli, and an elevated nuclear-to-cytoplasm ratio (Fig 15-4). Samples that show hypercellularity may reveal numerous small reactive lymphocytes with rare tumor cells. Therefore, additional molecular techniques can be essential to confirm the diagnosis of lymphoma. Because VRL cells can be monoclonal, immunohistochemical immunophenotyping or flow cytometry is used to demonstrate the clonality of B lymphocytes by the presence of (1) abnormal immunoglobulin κ or λ light chain predominance; (2) specific B-lymphocyte markers (CD19, CD20, and CD22); and/or (3) gene or oncogene translocations or gene rearrangements. Abnormal lymphocytes isolated manually or by laser capture can be analyzed in polymerase chain reaction (PCR)–based assays to improve the diagnostic yield of paucicellular samples. A specific mutation (proline for leucine substitution mutation at position 265, L265P) in the gene *MYD88* (myeloid differentiation primary response 88) is present in 62%–88% of VRL cases; thus, detection of this mutation by PCR can be strong

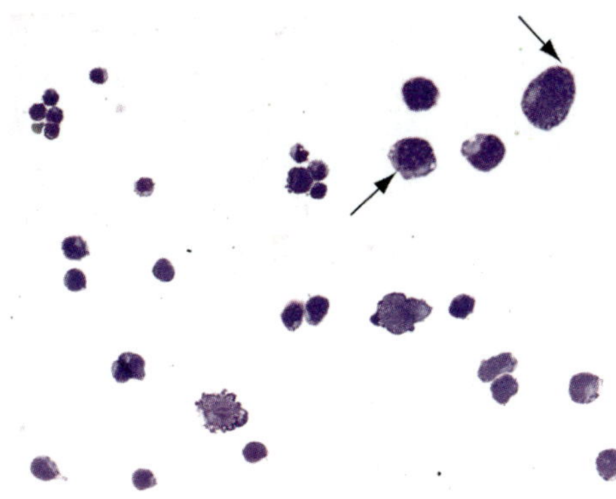

Figure 15-4 Cytologic appearance of vitreoretinal lymphoma in a vitreous specimen. Note the large atypical lymphoid cells *(arrows)*, large irregular nuclei, and scant basophilic cytoplasm consistent with large B-cell lymphoma. *(Courtesy of Chi Chao Chan, MD, and H. Nida Sen, MD/ National Eye Institute.)*

evidence for the diagnosis of VRL. See also BCSC Section 4, *Ophthalmic Pathology and Intraocular Tumors,* for discussion of intraocular lymphoma.

Cytokine analysis of vitreous samples can also provide supportive evidence. Interleukin (IL)-10 levels are elevated in the vitreous of patients with lymphoma, while high levels of IL-6 are found in the vitreous of patients with inflammatory uveitis. An elevated ratio of IL-10 to IL-6 supports the diagnosis of VRL.

Carbonell D, Mahajan S, Chee SP, et al; Study Group for Vitreoretinal Lymphoma Diagnostics. Consensus recommendations for the diagnosis of vitreoretinal lymphoma. *Ocul Immunol Inflamm.* 2021;29(3):507–520.

Deák GG, Goldstein DA, Zhou M, Fawzi AA, Jampol LM. Vertical hyperreflective lesions on optical coherence tomography in vitreoretinal lymphoma. *JAMA Ophthalmol.* 2019;137(2): 194–198.

Gangaputra S, Kodati S, Kim M, Aranow M, Sen HN. Multimodal imaging in masquerade syndromes. *Ocul Immunol Inflamm.* 2017;25(2):160–168.

Treatment

Treatment of VRL may involve intravitreal chemotherapy (methotrexate and/or rituximab), local external beam radiation of the eye, and/or systemic chemotherapy depending on CNS involvement. In cases with concomitant PCNSL, high-dose systemic chemotherapy in conjunction with intrathecal therapy, whole-brain radiotherapy, and/or autologous stem cell transplantation is considered. There are various chemotherapy regimens. Among the most commonly used is high-dose systemic methotrexate with rituximab. Some specialists use prophylactic treatment of the CNS even in patients with seemingly isolated ocular disease.

Pulido JS, Johnston PB, Nowakowski GS, Castellino A, Raja H. The diagnosis and treatment of primary vitreoretinal lymphoma: a review. *Int J Retina Vitreous.* 2018 May 7;4:18. doi:10.1186/s40942-018-0120-4

Prognosis

Vitreoretinal lymphoma responds well to initial treatment; however, it is associated with high rates of relapse and CNS involvement, which usually lead to poor prognosis and limited survival. The prognosis for survival depends on whether there is CNS involvement. Despite the availability of multiple treatment modalities and regimens, the long-term prognosis for patients with PCNSL remains poor. The median survival with supportive care alone is 2–3 months, and with surgery alone, median survival is in the range of 1–5 months. In various reports, the longest median survival approaches 40 months with treatment, and the 5-year overall survival is approximately 60%. Factors that negatively influence outcome include advanced age, worse neurologic functional classification level, multiple CNS lesions, and deep nuclei/periventricular lesions rather than superficial cerebral and cerebellar hemispheric lesions.

Uveal Lymphoma

The uveal tract may be a site for low-grade lymphoma that can mimic chronic posterior uveitis. Presenting symptoms may include vision loss that is gradual, painless, and unilateral or bilateral. Early-stage disease shows multifocal cream-colored or yellow choroidal lesions that may mimic those of sarcoidosis-associated uveitis or birdshot chorioretinopathy (Fig 15-5). Macular edema may be present. Anterior uveitis with acute signs and symptoms of pain, redness, and photophobia may also occur. Angle structures may be infiltrated by lymphocytes, resulting in elevation of intraocular pressure (IOP). The presentation may overlap with that of posterior scleritis and uveal effusion syndrome.

Fleshy salmon-pink episcleral or conjunctival masses may be present. Unlike subconjunctival lymphomas, these masses are not mobile and are attached firmly to the sclera. Histologic examination of biopsy specimens demonstrates mature lymphocytes and plasma cells, quite different from the histologic appearance of VRL specimens. In cases of uveal lymphoma, ancillary testing to evaluate for systemic lymphoma is indicated. This testing typically consists of skull base to mid-thigh computed tomography with or without positron emission tomography.

Therapy consisting of corticosteroids, radiation, or both has been used with variable results. Systemic and periocular corticosteroid therapy can lead to rapid regression of the lesions, as can external beam radiotherapy.

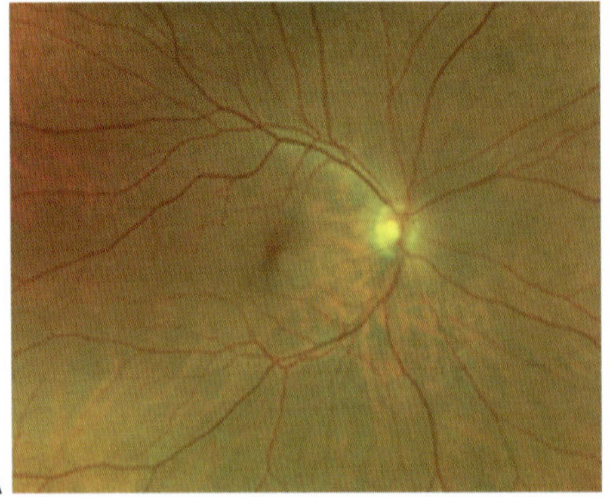

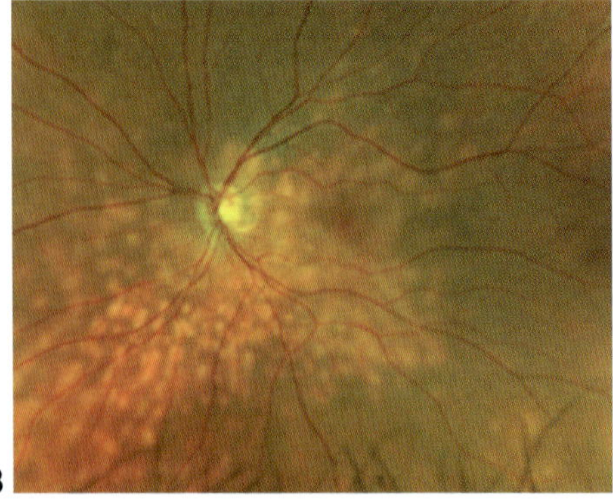

Figure 15-5 Primary uveal lymphoma. **A,** Fundus image of the right eye is unremarkable. **B,** Fundus image of the left eye shows multifocal yellow choroidal lesions. *(Courtesy of Karen R. Armbrust, MD, PhD.)*

Aronow ME, Portell CA, Sweetenham JW, Singh AD. Uveal lymphoma: clinical features, diagnostic studies, treatment selection, and outcomes. *Ophthalmology.* 2014;121(1):334–341.

Ocular Manifestations of Systemic Lymphoma

Systemic lymphomas can spread hematogenously to the choroid, subretinal space, vitreous, and anterior chamber, although this is rare. These entities can manifest with a pseudohypopyon, vitritis, cream-colored subretinal infiltrates, retinal vasculitis, necrotizing retinitis, and diffuse choroiditis or uveal masses.

Ocular Manifestations of Leukemia

Patients with leukemia may have retinal findings, including intraretinal hemorrhages, cotton-wool spots, white-centered hemorrhages, microaneurysms, and peripheral neovascularization. In rare instances, leukemic cells may invade the vitreous cavity. If the choroid is involved, exudative retinal detachment (Fig 15-6) and angiographic findings may be reminiscent of Vogt-Koyanagi-Harada syndrome. Leukemia may also manifest with a hypopyon or hyphema; iris heterochromia; or a pseudohypopyon, which can be gray yellow.

Nonlymphoid Tumors

Uveal melanoma

Approximately 5% of patients with uveal melanoma present with signs of ocular inflammation, including episcleritis, anterior or posterior uveitis, or panuveitis. Most tumors that manifest in this fashion are epithelioid-cell or mixed-cell choroidal melanomas. Ultrasonography

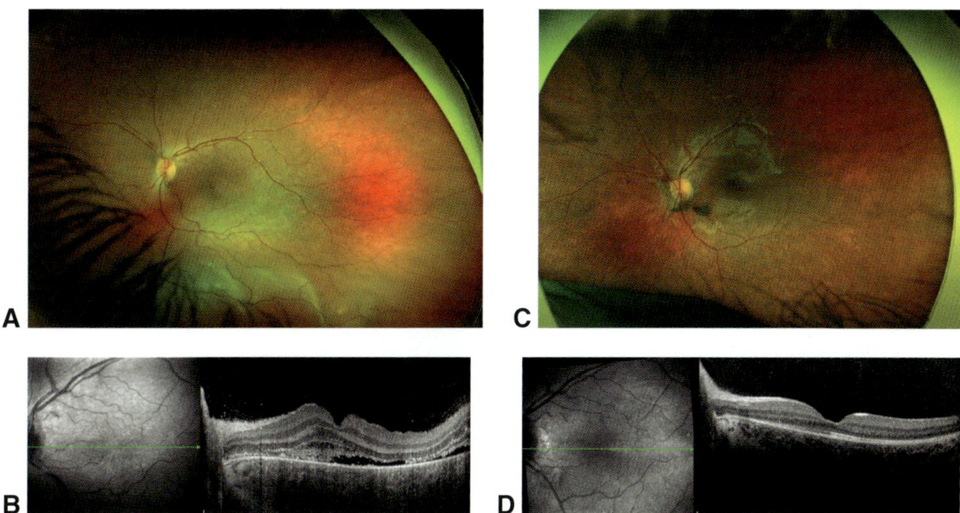

Figure 15-6 Exudative retinal detachment in acute leukemia. **A,** Wide-field fundus image shows inferior exudative retinal detachment. **B,** OCT shows that subretinal fluid and infiltration extend to the fovea. **C, D,** Resolution with systemic treatment of leukemia. *(Courtesy of Polly A. Quiram, MD, PhD, and Karen R. Armbrust, MD, PhD.)*

is useful in diagnosing atypical cases because of the characteristically low internal reflectivity of these lesions. Diagnosis and management of uveal melanomas is discussed in BCSC Section 4, *Ophthalmic Pathology and Intraocular Tumors.*

Retinoblastoma

Approximately 1%–3% of retinoblastomas, primarily the relatively rare form of retinoblastoma termed *diffuse infiltrating retinoblastoma,* may manifest with the appearance of inflammation. Affected patients are usually between age 4 and 6 years at presentation. Diffuse infiltrating retinoblastoma can be diagnostically confusing because of the limited visibility of the fundus and minimal or absent calcification on radiography or ultrasonography. Patients may have conjunctival chemosis, anterior chamber cells, pseudohypopyon, iris nodules (Fig 15-7), and vitritis. The pseudohypopyon typically shifts with changes in head position and is usually white as opposed to the yellowish color of inflammatory hypopyon.

Juvenile xanthogranuloma

Juvenile xanthogranuloma is the result of a histiocytic process affecting mainly the skin and eyes and, in rare instances, viscera. Patients usually present before 1 year of age with characteristic reddish-yellow skin lesions. Histologic examination of the lesions shows large histiocytes with foamy cytoplasm and Touton giant cells. Ocular lesions can involve the iris and result in a spontaneous hyphema (Fig 15-8). Histologically, iris biopsy samples show fewer foamy histiocytes and fewer Touton giant cells than do skin biopsy specimens. In rare cases, other ocular structures may be affected. If the eyelid skin is involved, the globe is usually spared.

Intraocular lesions may respond to topical, periocular, or systemic corticosteroid therapy. Resistant cases may require local resection, radiation, or immunomodulatory therapy. See BCSC Section 4, *Ophthalmic Pathology and Intraocular Tumors,* for additional discussion.

Samara WA, Khoo CT, Say EA, et al. Juvenile xanthogranuloma involving the eye and ocular adnexa: tumor control, visual outcomes, and globe salvage in 30 patients. *Ophthalmology.* 2015;122(10):2130–2138.

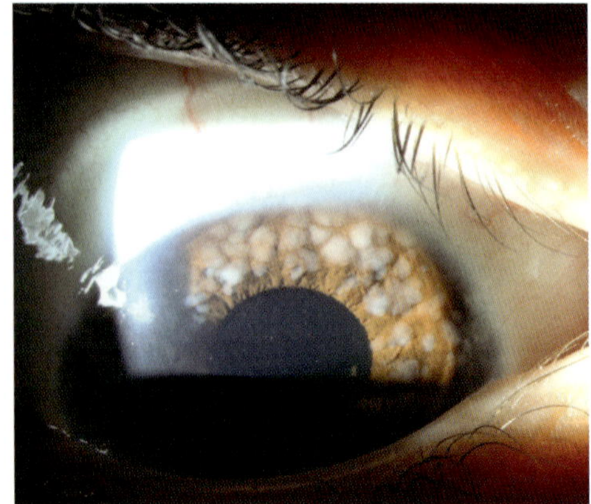

Figure 15-7 Diffuse infiltrating retinoblastoma. Slit-lamp photograph from a child with retinoblastoma shows iris tumor nodules and anterior chamber cells. *(Courtesy of Laura J. Kopplin, MD, PhD.)*

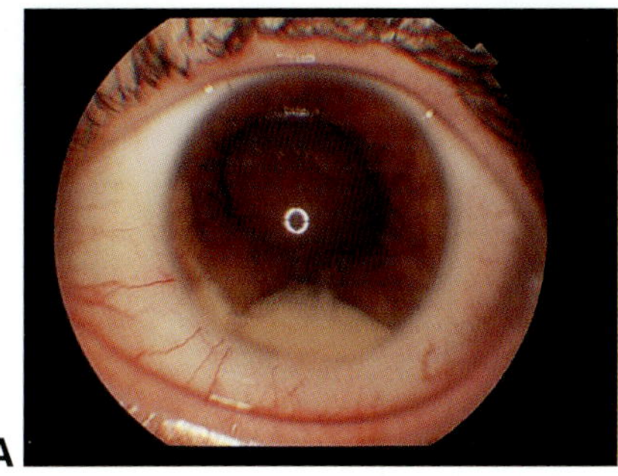

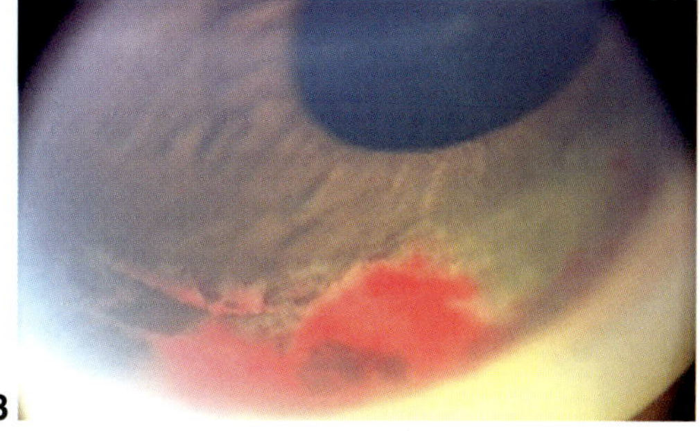

Figure 15-8 Juvenile xanthogranuloma (JXG). **A,** Iris JXG. **B,** JXG presenting as a yellow iris lesion with associated atraumatic hyphema in a child. *(Part A courtesy of Emilio M. Dodds, MD; part B courtesy of Raymond G. Areaux Jr, MD.)*

Metastatic Tumors

Most intraocular malignancies in adults are metastatic tumors. The most common primary cancers metastasizing to the eye include lung and breast carcinoma. Patients with anterior uveal metastasis may present with cells in the aqueous humor, iris nodules, neovascularization of the iris, and elevated IOP. Anterior chamber paracentesis may help confirm the diagnosis. Retinal metastases are extremely rare. Primary cancers metastatic to the retina include cutaneous melanoma (the most common), followed by lung, gastrointestinal, and breast cancer. Metastatic melanoma often produces brown spherules in the retina, whereas other metastatic cancers appear white to yellow and may result in perivascular sheathing, simulating a retinal vasculitis or necrotizing retinitis. Choroidal metastasis may be marked by vitritis, exudative retinal detachment, and occasionally macular edema. These lesions are often bilateral and multifocal. See BCSC Section 4, *Ophthalmic Pathology and Intraocular Tumors,* for additional discussion and images showing metastases to the eye.

Bilateral Diffuse Uveal Melanocytic Proliferation

Bilateral diffuse uveal melanocytic tumors have been associated with systemic malignancy. Such tumors can be accompanied by rapid vision loss, cataracts, multiple pigmented and nonpigmented placoid iris and choroidal nodules, and exudative retinal detachments. This condition can mimic Vogt-Koyanagi-Harada syndrome. Histologic examination shows diffuse infiltration of the uveal tract by benign nevoid or spindle-shaped cells. Necrosis within the tumors may be present, and scleral involvement is common. The cause of this entity is unknown. Treatment should be directed at finding and treating the underlying malignancy. See BCSC Section 12, *Retina and Vitreous,* for additional information about this condition.

Nonneoplastic Masquerade Syndromes

Retinitis Pigmentosa

Patients with retinitis pigmentosa (RP) often have variable numbers of vitreous and anterior chamber cells and can develop macular edema. Features of RP that differentiate it from uveitis include nyctalopia, positive family history of RP, waxy optic disc pallor, attenuation of arterioles, and a bone-spicule pattern of pigmentary changes in the midperiphery. Electroretinographic responses of patients with RP often appear severely depressed or extinguished, even early in the disease. However, these findings can also occur in some types of posterior uveitis, such as late-stage birdshot chorioretinopathy, making differentiation between the entities very difficult in some cases. See BCSC Section 12, *Retina and Vitreous,* for additional information.

Ocular Ischemic Syndrome

Ocular ischemic syndrome (OIS) results from hypoperfusion of the entire eye and sometimes the orbit, usually because of carotid artery obstruction. Patients with OIS are typically men aged 65 years or older. Examination findings may include corneal edema, anterior chamber cells, and moderate anterior chamber flare that is often greater than and out of proportion to the number of cells. Anterior segment neovascularization may also be present.

Dilated fundus examination and FA help distinguish OIS from uveitis. In OIS, fundus examination typically shows dilated retinal venules, narrowed arterioles, and medium to large intraretinal blot hemorrhages scattered in the midperiphery and far periphery. FA shows delayed arteriolar filling, diffuse leakage in the posterior pole as well as from the optic disc, and signs of capillary nonperfusion.

Diagnostic studies for OIS include carotid Doppler ultrasonography; ipsilateral carotid stenosis greater than 90% supports the diagnosis of OIS. See BCSC Section 12, *Retina and Vitreous,* for discussion of OIS treatment.

Mendrinos E, Machinis TG, Pournaras CJ. Ocular ischemic syndrome. *Surv Ophthalmol.* 2010;55(1):2–34.

Chronic Peripheral Rhegmatogenous Retinal Detachment

Chronic peripheral rhegmatogenous retinal detachment can be associated with anterior chamber cell and flare and vitreous inflammatory and pigment cells. Patients often have good vision unless they develop macular edema. Careful dilated fundus examination with scleral depression is crucial to establishing the diagnosis. Findings may include peripheral pigment demarcation lines, subretinal fluid, retinal breaks, subretinal fibrosis, and peripheral retinal cysts.

Photoreceptor outer segments liberated from the subretinal space may be present in the anterior chamber, simulating inflammatory cells. In such situations, the photoreceptor outer segments may obstruct trabecular outflow, resulting in elevated IOP and secondary open-angle glaucoma. This condition is called *Schwartz-Matsuo syndrome.*

Matsuo T. Photoreceptor outer segments in aqueous humor: key to understanding a new syndrome. *Surv Ophthalmol.* 1994;39(3):211–233.

Intraocular Foreign Bodies

Open-globe injury may result in an intraocular foreign body. Retained intraocular foreign bodies may produce chronic intraocular inflammation as the result of mechanical, chemical, toxic, or inflammatory irritation of uveal tissues (particularly the ciliary body). In some cases of retained intraocular foreign bodies, the ocular trauma is unrecognized or perceived as mild by the patient. A high index of suspicion and the following are essential for accurate diagnosis: a careful history; clinical examination; and ancillary testing, including gonioscopy, ultrasonography, and computed tomography of the eye and orbits. If this condition is suspected and recognized quickly, removal of the foreign body is often curative. If the diagnosis is delayed, ocular complications, such as proliferative vitreoretinopathy and endophthalmitis, result in a poorer visual prognosis.

Pigment Dispersion Syndrome

Pigment dispersion syndrome is characterized by pigment granules released into the anterior chamber from the iris and/or ciliary body. These granules may be confused with the cells of anterior uveitis. Careful examination of the corneal endothelium, iris, and iridocorneal angle can help distinguish between uveitis and pigment dispersion syndrome. See BCSC Section 10, *Glaucoma,* for a complete discussion of pigment dispersion syndrome.

Infectious Uveitis

Certain infectious uveitic entities may be mistaken for immune-mediated uveitis and thus are included in nonneoplastic masquerade syndromes. These entities are discussed in Chapters 11 and 12.

CHAPTER 16

Complications of Uveitis

This chapter includes a related video. Go to www.aao.org/bcscvideo_section09 or scan the QR code in the text to access this content.

Highlights

- In uveitis, vision loss can result from multiple complications involving the cornea, lens, vitreous, retina, and optic nerve. Consequently, consultations with multiple ophthalmic subspecialists can help improve the management of challenging cases.
- When surgical intervention is required in patients with uveitis, strict perioperative control of inflammation is paramount.
- Uveitic macular edema, which is a common cause of vision loss, can be diagnosed with optical coherence tomography; treatment is typically focused on controlling inflammation, often with adjunctive local corticosteroids.

Calcific Band Keratopathy

Band keratopathy, or calcium deposition along the epithelial basement membrane and Bowman layer, may develop in patients with chronic uveitis, especially children. Most often seen in juvenile idiopathic arthritis–associated anterior uveitis or undifferentiated chronic anterior uveitis, band keratopathy may arise within months of uveitis onset. The deposition is typically located in the interpalpebral zone and becomes visually significant when it extends into the visual axis. It may also cause foreign body sensation. Because the calcium deposits are located beneath the corneal epithelium, their removal requires epithelial debridement followed by chelation with disodium EDTA. Recurrences may require repeated EDTA treatments. Photorefractive keratotomy may also be considered as an alternative to chelation with EDTA.

Cataracts

Chronic inflammation and/or long-term corticosteroid use can provoke cataract development. Indications for cataract surgery include functional impairment that interferes with activities of daily living, decreased vision, and amblyopia prevention. In uveitic eyes, an additional consideration for surgery is whether the cataract obscures the view of the fundus and interferes with monitoring of posterior segment inflammation. A careful preoperative evaluation will help determine whether the cataract is actually contributing to visual dysfunction.

Other potential causes of vision loss in uveitic eyes include corneal or vitreous opacity, macular edema, macular atrophy or fibrosis, and glaucoma.

Management

Uveitic eyes are at greater risk for complications after cataract surgery than are nonuveitic eyes. Thus, careful planning, such as preoperative medical management that includes control of inflammation and timing of the procedure, is key to a successful visual outcome. To decrease the risk of severe postoperative inflammation, the general guideline is to achieve well-controlled uveitis without flare-ups for at least 3 months before cataract surgery. However, this recommendation is based on retrospective clinical case series and clinical experience; no prospective or controlled trials have provided definitive data on the 3-month guideline. As such, exceptions to this guideline may be warranted, for example, in eyes with mild uveitis lacking sequelae, in patients with uveitic disorders that have a good surgical prognosis (eg, Fuchs uveitis syndrome), or in special circumstances such as lens-induced uveitis or when the posterior segment must be visible (eg, to repair a rhegmatogenous retinal detachment).

Of note, the "best possible control" of uveitis may not be achieved with corticosteroids alone. Before proceeding with surgery, the clinician should use all appropriate means for uveitis control, including systemic immunosuppression and/or referral to a specialist for help with systemic treatment.

Once long-term control of uveitis has been achieved, perioperative management may include oral corticosteroids (0.5–1.0 mg/kg/day, started 3 days before and subsequently tapered in the weeks after surgery) and/or intensive topical corticosteroids. Sub-Tenon or intravitreal corticosteroids may also be used. There are no prospective comparative data on optimal perioperative inflammatory control, so surgeons typically rely on preference and experience.

Patients with certain infectious uveitic entities (eg, those caused by *Toxoplasma gondii* infection and herpetic viral infections) may require perioperative prophylactic antimicrobial therapy to prevent surgically induced recurrence. Preoperative oral corticosteroids are usually not given to these patients.

In general, cataract surgery in uveitic eyes is more complex than in nonuveitic eyes because of possible sequelae of the disorder, including posterior synechiae, pupillary membranes, corneal edema or opacity, and hypotony. Entrance into the eye through a clear corneal approach is typical and may be particularly desirable in patients with scleritis to reduce the risk of postoperative scleral necrosis. Posterior synechiae and pupillary miosis may require mechanical or viscoelastic pupil stretching, sphincterotomies, or the use of flexible iris retractors (Video 16-1).

VIDEO 16-1 Synechiolysis, placement of iris dilator, and capsular staining in a patient with uveitis.
Courtesy of Russell W. Read, MD, PhD.

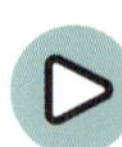

Although a curvilinear capsulorrhexis is preferred for uveitic eyes, a can-opener capsulotomy may be the only way to open a fibrotic anterior capsule. In eyes with zonular insufficiency, options include the use of a capsular tension ring or pars plana lensectomy and vitrectomy with a 3-piece sulcus intraocular lens (IOL) or scleral-fixated IOL. In some situations, the eye may be left aphakic. Relative contraindications for IOL implantation in uveitic eyes include prior development of rubeosis, a history of extensive membrane formation, and hypotony; however, even in these circumstances, an IOL may be used in select cases if inflammation is well controlled before and after surgery. In patients with vision-limiting vitreous opacity or macular pathology, such as epiretinal membranes or macular hole, phacoemulsification with IOL implantation can also be done in conjunction with pars plana vitrectomy. Meticulous cortical cleanup is important to minimize proinflammatory material in the eye. For IOL choice, many surgeons prefer hydrophobic acrylic posterior chamber IOLs placed in the capsular bag. Studies have shown that phacoemulsification with implantation of a posterior chamber (in-the-bag) IOL effectively improves vision and is well tolerated in many eyes with uveitis, even over long periods. Silicone IOLs are rarely used in uveitic cataracts.

At the conclusion of surgery, periocular or intravitreal corticosteroids may be administered. Postoperatively, systemic immunomodulation is continued and supplemented with liberal use of topical corticosteroids, which are slowly tapered. Dosages of topical and/or oral corticosteroids may be tapered over weeks to months after surgery based on the severity of the preexisting uveitis and the postoperative inflammatory response. In patients who had extensive posterior synechiae and/or peripheral anterior synechiae before surgery, cycloplegic drops may be continued for a week or 2 after surgery to prevent re-formation of posterior synechiae to the anterior capsule or IOL.

In children with juvenile idiopathic arthritis–associated uveitic cataracts, the debate regarding IOL placement is ongoing. Recent studies have shown favorable outcomes of IOL placement with or without combined pars plana vitrectomy. Although avoiding aphakia in children is desirable, it may not always be in their best interest because of the potential complications of IOL placement in uveitic eyes. Choosing the proper IOL power, especially in children younger than 10 years, can also be challenging because of normal ocular/orbital growth. (For more information about IOL use in children, see BCSC Section 6, *Pediatric Ophthalmology and Strabismus.*) In-the-bag implantation of acrylic IOLs and primary posterior capsulorrhexis are generally preferred. Some surgeons may also perform a core anterior vitrectomy through the posterior capsulorrhexis before IOL placement. Regardless, the most important step in treating these children is stringent control of preoperative and postoperative intraocular inflammation with corticosteroids and immunomodulatory therapy (IMT). Administration of intraocular corticosteroids at the end of the procedure is extremely useful for controlling postoperative inflammation and uveitic macular edema (UME). When these methods are used, 75% of patients have obtained a visual acuity of better than 20/40.

Bolletta E, Coassin M, Iannetta D, et al. Cataract surgery with intraocular lens implantation in juvenile idiopathic arthritis-associated uveitis: outcomes in the era of biological therapy. *J Clin Med.* 2021;10(11):2437. doi:10.3390/jcm10112437

Lu LM, McGhee CNJ, Sims JL, Niederer RL. High rate of recurrence of herpes zoster–related ocular disease after phacoemulsification cataract surgery. *J Cataract Refract Surg.* 2019; 45(6):810–815.

Schmidt DC, Al-Bakri M, Rasul A, et al. Cataract surgery with or without intraocular lens implantation in pediatric uveitis: a systematic review with meta-analyses. *J Ophthalmol.* 2021 Jun 11;2021:5481609. doi:10.1155/2021/5481609

Complications

After cataract surgery, close monitoring of the patient for inflammation or complications is critical, as strict control reduces the risk of inflammatory debris and membrane accumulation on the surface of the IOL. In addition, aggressive dosing of topical and local corticosteroids as well as IMT are often necessary. In patients with major postoperative anterior segment inflammation, cycloplegic drops should be used to reduce the chance of developing posterior synechiae with iris adherence to either the IOL or the anterior capsule. Inflammatory cocooning of the IOL–lens capsule complex and uncontrolled inflammation necessitate IOL explantation in 5%–10% of patients.

Postoperative UME rates may be reduced by delaying surgery until the uveitis has been controlled for at least 3 months and through the use of perioperative corticosteroids. Postoperative use of topical nonsteroidal anti-inflammatory drugs (NSAIDs) has not been studied in uveitic eyes; however, similar to their use in nonuveitic eyes, topical NSAIDs may be employed to prevent postoperative macular edema. The incidence of posterior capsule opacification is higher in uveitic eyes than in nonuveitic eyes, leading to earlier use of Nd:YAG laser capsulotomy in this population. However, Nd:YAG laser capsulotomy may exacerbate uveitis, so patients should be monitored carefully after the procedure.

Bélair M-L, Kim SJ, Thorne JE, et al. Incidence of cystoid macular edema after cataract surgery in patients with and without uveitis using optical coherence tomography. *Am J Ophthalmol.* 2009;148(1):128–135.e2.

Mehta S, Linton MM, Kempen JH. Outcomes of cataract surgery in patients with uveitis: a systematic review and meta-analysis. *Am J Ophthalmol.* 2014;158(4):676–692.e7.

Moshirfar M, Somani AN, Motlagh MN, Ronquillo YC. Management of cataract in the setting of uveitis: a review of the current literature. *Curr Opin Ophthalmol.* 2020;31(1):3–9.

Sen HN, Abreu FM, Louis TA, et al; Multicenter Uveitis Steroid Treatment (MUST) Trial and Follow-up Study Research Group. Cataract surgery outcomes in uveitis: the Multicenter Uveitis Steroid Treatment trial. *Ophthalmology.* 2016;123(1):183–190.

Glaucoma

In uveitic eyes, elevated intraocular pressure (IOP) may be acute, chronic, or recurrent. Multiple mechanisms may contribute to uveitic glaucoma, including mechanical factors (obstruction of the angle with peripheral anterior synechiae or inflammatory debris) and biochemical changes. Active uveitis alone is not necessarily the cause of elevated IOP, especially in the case of posterior uveitis. Acute anterior uveitis can even be associated with a *decrease* in IOP due to inflammation of the ciliary body. In eyes with long-term ciliary body inflammation, the IOP may fluctuate between abnormally high and low values. When acute anterior uveitis is accompanied by acute ocular hypertension, a herpes virus–associated anterior uveitis should be suspected. Another major contributor to uveitic glaucoma is overuse of topical and/or regional corticosteroids. Uncontrollable or barely controlled corticosteroid-induced glaucoma can be an indication to add systemic IMT.

Assessment of patients with uveitis and elevated IOP should include the same measures used for other cases of ocular hypertension: slit-lamp and dilated fundus examination, pachymetry, gonioscopy, evaluation of the optic nerve head with disc photographs and optical coherence tomography (OCT), and serial automated visual fields.

Kesav N, Palestine AG, Kahook MY, Pantcheva MB. Current management of uveitis-associated ocular hypertension and glaucoma. *Surv Ophthalmol.* 2020;65(4):397–407.

Uveitic Ocular Hypertension

Unilateral uveitis of sudden onset with open angles and increased IOP may have an infectious origin, particularly a viral cause or *Toxoplasma* infection. Thus, when IOP elevation occurs early in the course of uveitis, clinicians should resist the urge to prematurely taper corticosteroids because of a fear of steroid-induced ocular hypertension (which rarely occurs before 3 weeks of corticosteroid therapy). In patients with unilateral uveitis, early IOP elevations with active anterior segment inflammation almost always require aggressive anti-inflammatory treatment in addition to IOP-lowering medication.

Daniel E, Pistilli M, Kothari S, et al; Systemic Immunosuppressive Therapy for Eye Diseases Research Group. Risk of ocular hypertension in adults with noninfectious uveitis. *Ophthalmology.* 2017;124(8):1196–1208.

Uveitic Glaucoma

Uveitic glaucoma is classified by morphologic changes in angle structure as either secondary angle-closure glaucoma or secondary open-angle glaucoma. These disorders can be further subdivided into acute and chronic types. In cases of chronic uveitic glaucoma, corticosteroid-induced ocular hypertension and glaucoma should also be addressed. See also BCSC Section 10, *Glaucoma.*

Secondary angle-closure glaucoma

Acute disease with central shallowing of the anterior chamber Acute secondary angle-closure glaucoma may occur when choroidal inflammation results in forward rotation of the ciliary body and lens–iris diaphragm. It may also be the presenting sign of Vogt-Koyanagi-Harada syndrome or sympathetic ophthalmia. Affected patients present with pain, elevated IOP, and no posterior synechiae. The diagnosis is confirmed by ultrasound biomicroscopy (UBM) or ultrasonography showing choroidal thickening and anterior rotation of the ciliary body. Treatment involves aggressive corticosteroid therapy, aqueous suppressants, and cycloplegia to induce a posterior rotation of the ciliary body. As the inflammation subsides, the anterior chamber deepens and the IOP normalizes. Peripheral laser iridotomy or surgical iridectomy is not useful in acute disease because the underlying cause is not pupillary block.

Acute disease without central shallowing of the anterior chamber Chronic or acute recurrent anterior segment inflammation may lead to the formation of circumferential posterior synechiae with pupillary block. This is typically due to seclusion of the pupil and resultant iris bombé, which produces secondary peripheral angle closure. Although synechiae usually form over time, iris bombé may be an acute event. Peripheral laser iridotomy or surgical iridectomy results in resolution of the bombé and angle closure if the procedure is performed before peripheral anterior synechiae become permanent. If peripheral anterior synechiae have started to develop, the procedure may be supplemented with goniosynechialysis; however, this approach is controversial. Iridotomies should involve multiple holes that are as large as possible. Intensive topical corticosteroid and cycloplegic therapy is administered after laser iridotomy. In patients with brown irides, pretreatment of the iris with an argon laser before Nd:YAG laser use may lessen the chance of bleeding and facilitate a wider opening. Exacerbation of inflammation after the laser procedure may cause closure of the iridotomy and necessitate re-treatment or surgical iridectomy.

Chronic disease Chronic intraocular inflammation may cause posterior and peripheral anterior synechiae as well as chronic secondary angle-closure glaucoma. In these cases, chronic secondary open-angle glaucoma and corticosteroid-induced glaucoma are often superimposed. Topical aqueous suppressants may not prevent progression of optic nerve head damage, requiring goniosynechialysis and trabeculectomy with mitomycin C or placement of a glaucoma drainage device. See BCSC Section 10, *Glaucoma,* for more details on the surgical treatment of glaucoma.

Secondary open-angle glaucoma

Acute disease Inflammatory open-angle glaucoma occurs when the trabecular meshwork is inflamed (ie, trabeculitis). The trabeculitis commonly occurs with infectious causes of uveitis such as *Toxoplasma* retinochoroiditis, necrotizing herpetic retinitis, herpes simplex and varicella-zoster anterior uveitis, cytomegalovirus anterior uveitis (including the Posner-Schlossman type), and sarcoidosis-associated uveitis or when inflammatory debris clogs the angle. This type of glaucoma often responds to treatment targeting the infectious agent, supplemented by topical cycloplegics and corticosteroids.

Chronic disease Chronic outflow obstruction is caused by direct damage to the trabecular meshwork. The management of chronic secondary open-angle glaucoma is similar to that of primary open-angle glaucoma (see BCSC Section 10, *Glaucoma*), with the addition of IMT to strictly control intraocular inflammation.

Combined-mechanism uveitic glaucoma

As noted previously, multiple mechanisms may be responsible for elevated IOP in uveitic eyes. Thus, a multimodal treatment approach that incorporates both medical and surgical therapies aimed at the responsible mechanisms should be used to control inflammation and IOP.

Corticosteroid-Induced Ocular Hypertension and Glaucoma

Elevated IOP in patients with uveitis should prompt consideration of one of the aforementioned angle issues or a corticosteroid-induced disorder. In patients with uveitis, corticosteroids in any formulation—topical, periocular, intraocular (injection and sustained release), or systemic—may also induce an elevation of IOP that may be difficult to distinguish from other causes of ocular hypertension. Fluocinolone intraocular implants are associated with an eventual need for glaucoma surgery in approximately 3% to 40% of eyes depending on the implant corticosteroid dose. Topical difluprednate also appears to be associated with substantial and sometimes very rapid increases in IOP. This IOP rise may be avoided by use of a less-potent topical corticosteroid preparation, a less-frequent administration schedule, or both. Although fluorometholone and loteprednol may be less likely to elevate IOP than other corticosteroids are, they are also less effective in controlling intraocular inflammation.

Management

Medical management of uveitic ocular hypertension and uveitic glaucoma requires aggressive control of both intraocular inflammation and IOP to prevent progressive glaucomatous optic nerve damage and visual field loss (see BCSC Section 10, *Glaucoma*). Aqueous suppressants are generally the first-line treatment. Prostaglandin analogues may also be used to treat uveitic ocular hypertension and glaucoma and generally do not exacerbate intraocular inflammation, especially when used concomitantly with IMT and corticosteroids. However, caution is important when prostaglandin analogues are used in eyes with herpetic uveitis, because the medication may lead to viral reactivation. Pilocarpine should be avoided in uveitis, as pilocarpine breaks down the blood–aqueous barrier, and posterior synechiae may be more likely to form in the immobile small pupil.

When medical management fails, glaucoma filtering surgery is indicated. Although standard trabeculectomy has an increased risk of failure in uveitic eyes, results may be improved by using mitomycin C with intensive topical corticosteroids. After surgery, IOP control with 0 or 1 medication is achieved in up to 90% of patients 1 year after surgery and in approximately 62% of patients 5 years after surgery. Surgical complications include cataract formation, early and late bleb leakage (with increased risk of endophthalmitis), and choroidal effusions.

Several alternatives to classic trabeculectomy have shown short-term success in treating uveitic glaucoma. Nonpenetrating deep sclerectomy with or without a drainage implant controlled IOP in up to 90% of uveitic eyes for 1 year after surgery. Viscocanalostomy has shown even higher success rates in a limited number of studies. Among pediatric patients with uveitis, goniotomy has up to a 75% chance of reducing IOP to 21 mm Hg or less after 2 operations. However, this procedure may be complicated by transient hyphema and worsening of the preexisting cataract. Trabeculodialysis and laser sclerostomy have high rates of failure in treating uveitic glaucoma because of recurrent postoperative inflammation. The role of minimally invasive glaucoma surgery in uveitis remains unclear, with isolated reports of inflammation induced by devices placed in the angle.

Most cases of uveitic glaucoma, especially in pseudophakic or aphakic eyes, require aqueous drainage devices. These devices may be tunneled into the anterior chamber or placed through the pars plana directly into the vitreous cavity after vitrectomy. Use of a unidirectional valve design (ie, valve implant) can prevent postoperative hypotony. Compared with trabeculectomy, these implants are more likely to successfully control IOP in the long term; in studies, they reduced preoperative IOP by up to 75% as well as controlled IOP with 0 or 1 medication in nearly 75% of patients after 4 years. Unlike trabeculectomy, the drainage devices continue to function despite chronic, recurrent inflammation.

Complications of glaucoma drainage device surgery (10% per patient-year) have included shallow anterior chamber; hypotony; suprachoroidal hemorrhage; and occlusion of the drainage device by blood, fibrin, or iris. Long-term complications have included device erosion through the conjunctiva, valve migration, drainage device–cornea touch, corneal decompensation, and retinal detachment.

Cyclodestructive procedures to treat glaucoma may worsen ocular inflammation and lead to macular edema, hypotony, and phthisis bulbi. Although laser trabeculoplasty is generally thought to be ineffective in eyes with uveitis, it is considered a lower-risk first step in management than incisional surgery.

As with all surgical procedures in uveitic eyes, tight and meticulous control of perioperative inflammation not only helps ensure the success of glaucoma surgery but also limits sight-threatening complications such as UME and hypotony. However, when the need for glaucoma surgery is urgent, it should not be delayed because of the attempt to attain at least 3 months of controlled uveitis. Management of perioperative inflammation includes preoperative regimens similar to those applied before cataract surgery as well as use of immunomodulators and corticosteroids. Additional details and information on surgical procedures for uveitic glaucoma are described in BCSC Section 10, *Glaucoma.*

Bello NR, LaMattina KC, Minor JM, Utz VM, Dong K, Levin AV. The risk of uveitis due to prostaglandin analogs in pediatric glaucoma. *J AAPOS.* 2022;26(3):126.e1–126.e5.

Bohnsack BL, Freedman SF. Surgical outcomes in childhood uveitic glaucoma. *Am J Ophthalmol.* 2013;155(1):134–142.

Dupas B, Fardeau C, Cassoux N, Bodaghi B, LeHoang P. Deep sclerectomy and trabeculectomy in uveitic glaucoma. *Eye (Lond).* 2010;24(2):310–314.

Hu J, Vu JT, Hong B, Gottlieb C. Uveitis and cystoid macular oedema secondary to topical prostaglandin analogue use in ocular hypertension and open angle glaucoma. *Br J Ophthalmol.* 2020;104(8):1040–1044.

Kanaya R, Kijima R, Shinmei Y, et al. Surgical Outcomes of Trabeculectomy in Uveitic Glaucoma: a long-term, single-center, retrospective case-control study. *J Ophthalmol.* 2021 May 21;2021:5550776. doi:10.1155/2021/5550776

Markomichelakis NN, Kostakou A, Halkiadakis I, Chalkidou S, Papakonstantinou D, Georgopoulos G. Efficacy and safety of latanoprost in eyes with uveitic glaucoma. *Graefes Arch Clin Exp Ophthalmol.* 2009;247(6):775–780.

Sungur G, Yakin M, Eksioglu U, Satana B, Ornek F. Assessment of conditions affecting surgical success of Ahmed glaucoma valve implants in glaucoma secondary to different uveitis etiologies in adults. *Eye (Lond).* 2017;31(10):1435–1442.

van Meerwijk CLLI, Jansonius NM, Los LI. Uveitic glaucoma in children: a systematic review on surgical outcomes. *J Ophthalmic Inflamm Infect.* 2022;12(1):35. doi:10.1186/s12348-022-00313-2

William A, Spitzer MS, Doycheva D, Dimopoulos S, Leitritz MA, Voykov B. Comparison of ab externo trabeculotomy in primary open-angle glaucoma and uveitic glaucoma: long-term outcomes. *Clin Ophthalmol.* 2016;10:929–934.

Hypotony

Acute inflammation of the ciliary body may cause aqueous hyposecretion and low IOP. This reduction in IOP is reversible by control of intraocular inflammation. In contrast, chronic inflammation may lead to ciliary body damage and atrophy of the ciliary processes, resulting in permanent hypotony. Low IOP may result in hypotony maculopathy, vision loss, and/or phthisis bulbi. The hypotony is often accompanied by serous choroidal detachment, which complicates management. Prolonged choroidal effusions may require surgical drainage. In some cases, chronic hypotony can be treated with long-term local corticosteroid administration. If ciliary processes are atrophic (as demonstrated on UBM), vitrectomy with intraocular silicone oil or viscoelastic may help maintain ocular anatomy and increase IOP. If the ciliary body processes are preserved and there is ciliary body traction from a cyclitic membrane, surgical removal of the membrane may be considered. In some cases, vision may improve after surgery, but these gains can be transient. In general, chronic hypotony often responds poorly to treatment, so prevention (through strict control of uveitis) is the best strategy.

Kapur R, Birnbaum AD, Goldstein DA, et al. Treating uveitis-associated hypotony with pars plana vitrectomy and silicone oil injection. *Retina.* 2010;30(1):140–145.

Moradi A, Stroh IG, Reddy AK, et al. Risk of hypotony in juvenile idiopathic arthritis-associated uveitis. *Am J Ophthalmol.* 2016;169:113–124.

Sen HN, Drye LT, Goldstein DA, et al; Multicenter Uveitis Steroid Treatment (MUST) Trial Research Group. Hypotony in patients with uveitis: the Multicenter Uveitis Steroid Treatment (MUST) trial. *Ocul Immunol Inflamm.* 2012;20(2):104–112.

Uveitic Macular Edema

Uveitic macular edema (UME) is a common cause of vision loss in eyes with uveitis. The edema is usually due to active intraocular inflammation that causes retinal vascular leakage and retinal pigment epithelium dysfunction, although UME severity may not correspond to the level of inflammatory disease activity. UME appears to be mediated by the proinflammatory cytokines vascular endothelial growth factor (VEGF), tumor necrosis factor-α (TNF-α), interleukin 6, and interleukin 1. Patterns of UME on OCT include diffuse intraretinal edema, cystoid macular edema, and serous retinal detachment. Macular thickening due to mechanical vitreomacular traction is not considered UME. Fluorescein angiography should also be used to evaluate UME, as retinal vascular leakage may be more extensive than appreciated on examination and macular OCT. UME is often slow to respond to treatment and may persist even after other signs of active inflammation have resolved. Cigarette smoking appears to be associated with a greater prevalence of UME, especially in intermediate uveitis and panuveitis.

Lin P, Loh AR, Margolis TP, Acharya NR. Cigarette smoking as a risk factor for uveitis. *Ophthalmology.* 2010;117(3):585–590.

Rothova A. Inflammatory cystoid macular edema. *Curr Opin Ophthalmol.* 2007;18(6): 487–492.

Treatment

The initial approach to treatment of UME is to control intraocular inflammation. If UME persists after inflammation has been controlled, additional regional or systemic treatment is required. Ruling out infectious uveitis is crucial before administering local corticosteroids, especially intravitreal formulations. See Chapter 6 for additional information on the use of corticosteroids and systemic IMT to treat uveitis and UME.

Once infectious uveitis has been sufficiently investigated, periocular corticosteroid injections may be delivered into the orbital floor or the sub-Tenon space. Ultrasonography studies comparing periocular injection locations suggest that a superotemporal posterior sub-Tenon injection delivers juxtascleral corticosteroid closest to the macula. Periocular triamcinolone acetonide injections of 20–40 mg may be repeated monthly, but they are only rarely appropriate as monotherapy.

Intravitreal preservative-free triamcinolone acetonide (2–4 mg) can also be effective for reducing UME, particularly in nonvitrectomized eyes. (In vitrectomized eyes, the corticosteroid is eliminated more quickly from the vitreous cavity.) In the PeriOcular vs. INTravitreal Corticosteroids for Uveitic Macular Edema (POINT) Trial, intravitreal corticosteroids were superior to periocular sub-Tenon triamcinolone acetonide for treating UME. After intravitreal injection, visual improvement and UME reduction typically occur within 4 weeks. Risk factors for poor prognosis with intravitreal corticosteroids are chronic UME and worse visual acuity at the time of diagnosis. Intravitreal corticosteroid–induced IOP elevation may occur in up to 40% of patients, especially those younger than 40 years.

The use of implants for sustained delivery of intravitreal corticosteroid is also effective for UME, but they should be avoided in aphakic eyes. In the United States, implants include Retisert (Bausch + Lomb; fluocinolone 0.59 mg), Ozurdex (AbbVie; dexamethasone 0.7 mg), and Yutiq (EyePoint Pharmaceuticals Inc; fluocinolone 0.18 mg). In Europe, the Iluvien implant (Alimera Sciences Inc; fluocinolone 0.19 mg) is available. The risk of ocular hypertension is lower for the dexamethasone delivery system than for the fluocinolone 0.59 mg implant; in the other fluocinolone implants mentioned, lower concentrations of the corticosteroid may be associated with lower risk of IOP elevation as well.

Topical corticosteroids are usually insufficient for treating UME; however, topical difluprednate 0.05% emulsion reaches the retina and choroid at a higher concentration than topical prednisolone acetate. Small studies suggest that topical difluprednate can reduce UME; however, IOP should be monitored closely because of the risk of rapid and severe elevation.

Intravitreal anti-VEGF agents such as bevacizumab (1.25 mg in 0.05 mL) and ranibizumab (0.5 mg in 0.05 mL) are used primarily for neovascular complications of uveitis. They may be considered as second-line treatment for UME when periocular or intravitreal corticosteroids are contraindicated or ineffective; however, they have demonstrated only moderate short-term reductions in edema. When UME is reduced by anti-VEGF agents, it often recurs 1–3 months later, so ongoing injections may be needed. Intravitreal methotrexate (400 µg/0.1 mL) may also reduce UME; clinical trial data are pending.

Systemic IMT can be increased or added to treat UME. Agents that target specific cytokines or other proinflammatory molecules may be particularly effective. Options include TNF-α inhibitors (eg, adalimumab, infliximab), anti–interleukin-6 antibody (tocilizumab), and interferon alfa-2a/2b. See Chapter 6 for further discussion of systemic IMT.

Topical NSAIDs can be beneficial in treating pseudophakic macular edema, but their efficacy in UME has not been established. Oral acetazolamide, 500 mg once or twice daily, may also reduce UME, particularly when inflammation is otherwise well controlled.

Surgical therapy for UME is still controversial. When there is hyaloidal traction on the macula (best seen on OCT), pars plana vitrectomy may improve anatomy and vision. In the absence of vitreomacular traction, pars plana vitrectomy may be beneficial in managing recalcitrant UME; however, this application requires further investigation.

Radosavljevic A, Agarwal M, Bodaghi B, Smith JR, Zierhut M. Medical therapy of uveitic macular edema: biologic agents. *Ocul Immunol Inflamm.* 2020;28(8):1239–1250.
Schallhorn JM, Niemeyer KM, Browne EN, Chhetri P, Acharya NR. Difluprednate for the treatment of uveitic cystoid macular edema. *Am J Ophthalmol.* 2018;191:14–22.
Schilling H, Heiligenhaus A, Laube T, Bornfeld N, Jurklies B. Long-term effect of acetazolamide treatment of patients with uveitic chronic cystoid macular edema is limited by persisting inflammation. *Retina.* 2005;25(2):182–188.
Taylor SRJ, Habot-Wilner Z, Pacheco P, Lightman SL. Intraocular methotrexate in the treatment of uveitis and uveitic cystoid macular edema. *Ophthalmology.* 2009;116(4):797–801.
Thorne JE, Sugar EA, Holbrook JT, et al; Multicenter Uveitis Steroid Treatment Trial Research Group. Periocular Triamcinolone vs. Intravitreal Triamcinolone vs. Intravitreal Dexamethasone Implant for the Treatment of Uveitic Macular Edema: The PeriOcular vs. INTravitreal Corticosteroids for Uveitic Macular Edema (POINT) Trial. *Ophthalmology.* 2019;126(2):283–295.
Tran THC, de Smet MD, Bodaghi B, Fardeau C, Cassoux N, Lehoang P. Uveitic macular oedema: correlation between optical coherence tomography patterns with visual acuity and fluorescein angiography. *Br J Ophthalmol.* 2008;92(7):922–927.
Tsui E, Rathinam SR, Gonzales JA, et al; FAST Research Group. Outcomes of uveitic macular edema in the First-line Antimetabolites as Steroid-Sparing Treatment Uveitis Trial. *Ophthalmology.* 2022;129(6):661–667.

Epiretinal Membrane and Macular Hole

Epiretinal membranes and macular holes can occur in patients with active or inactive uveitis and are often associated with substantial vision loss. In some cases, epiretinal membranes and macular holes have improved with medical management alone. Although pars plana vitrectomy and membrane peel may also benefit these patients, consensus is lacking on the optimal techniques, timing, and case selection for surgical therapy. In general, the posterior hyaloid and epiretinal membranes are more adherent and resistant to removal in uveitic eyes than in nonuveitic eyes. Standard vitreoretinal techniques are described in BCSC Section 12, *Retina and Vitreous.* Similar to the approach to uveitic cataract surgery, well-controlled preoperative and postoperative inflammation improves the chances of successful anatomical and visual outcomes with epiretinal membranes and macular holes.

Branson SV, McClafferty BR, Kurup SK. Vitrectomy for epiretinal membranes and macular holes in uveitis patients. *J Ocul Pharmacol Ther.* 2017;33(4):298–303.
Callaway NF, Gonzalez MA, Yonekawa Y, et al. Outcomes of pars plana vitrectomy for macular hole in patients with uveitis. *Retina.* 2018;38(suppl 1):S41–S48.

Vitreous Opacification and Vitritis

Even when uveitis activity is reduced or controlled with treatment, visually significant vitreous membranes may persist. In a small study of eyes with controlled inflammation, vitrectomy improved visual acuity in 69%. A standard small (23- to 27-gauge) 3-port pars plana vitrectomy is the preferred technique, with a few minor variations (see BCSC Section 12, *Retina and Vitreous*).

Bansal R, Dogra M, Chawla R, Kumar A. Pars plana vitrectomy in uveitis in the era of microincision vitreous surgery. *Indian J Ophthalmol.* 2020;68(9):1844–1851.

Henry CR, Becker MD, Yang Y, Davis JL. Pars plana vitrectomy for the treatment of uveitis. *Am J Ophthalmol.* 2018;190:142–149.

Rhegmatogenous Retinal Detachment

Rhegmatogenous retinal detachment (RRD) occurs in 3% of patients with uveitis. Panuveitis and infectious uveitis are most frequently associated with RRD, although pars planitis and posterior uveitis have also been associated with rhegmatogenous and tractional retinal detachments. Patients with RRD often still have active uveitis. Up to 30% may also have proliferative vitreoretinopathy on presentation, a rate that is significantly higher than in patients with primary RRD without uveitis. Repair is challenging and often complicated by preexisting proliferative vitreoretinopathy, vitreous membranes, and poor visualization. Aggressive control of inflammation is essential in the perioperative period.

Retinal detachments due to acute retinal necrosis and cytomegalovirus retinitis are also difficult to repair because of multiple, often occult, posterior retinal breaks. However, the benefits of prophylactic laser treatment in acute retinal necrosis and cytomegalovirus retinitis are unclear. Pars plana vitrectomy and endolaser treatment with internal silicone oil tamponade are most often required to repair these detachments.

De Hoog J, Ten Berge JC, Groen F, Rothova A. Rhegmatogenous retinal detachment in uveitis. *J Ophthalmic Inflamm Infect.* 2017;7(1):22. doi:10.1186/s12348-017-0140-5

Choroidal and Retinal Neovascularization

Choroidal neovascularization (CNV) complicates some uveitic entities (eg, multifocal choroiditis, punctate inner choroiditis, or serpiginous choroiditis), whereas retinal neovascularization is more likely to occur in other entities (eg, retinal vasculitis, including Eales disease). The prevalence of uveitic CNV varies; for example, it can occur in up to 10% of patients with Vogt-Koyanagi-Harada syndrome versus 69% in those with punctate inner choroiditis. Risk factors for CNV in uveitis include disruptions in the Bruch membrane from chorioretinal inflammation and the presence of inflammatory cytokines that promote angiogenesis. Symptoms include metamorphopsia and scotoma, and diagnosis is based on clinical, angiographic, and OCT findings. Treatment includes medication to reduce uveitis activity in combination with intravitreal anti-VEGF. Improved control of inflammation with local corticosteroids and/or systemic IMT may also reduce the risk of CNV recurrence and the need for repeated anti-VEGF injections.

Uveitis-associated retinal neovascularization results from chronic inflammation and/or capillary nonperfusion. Unless there is vision-obscuring vitreous hemorrhage or extensive angiographic ischemia, first-line treatment is usually focused on reducing inflammation. Treatment with panretinal photocoagulation is not necessary in all cases, especially when inflammation is controlled. For example, sarcoidosis-associated panuveitis may manifest as neovascularization of the optic disc that resolves completely with IMT and corticosteroids alone. Intravitreal anti-VEGF injections may be used as a short-term adjunct to systemic or local treatment of inflammation and/or laser photocoagulation. Dramatic regression of neovascularization typically occurs after 1 or 2 intravitreal anti-VEGF injections. Uveitic retinal neovascularization may also resolve after posterior vitreous detachment, particularly in young patients.

Baxter SL, Pistilli M, Pujari SS, et al. Risk of choroidal neovascularization among the uveitides. *Am J Ophthalmol.* 2013;156(3):468–477.e2.

Patel AK, Newcomb CW, Liesegang TL, et al; Systemic Immunosuppressive Therapy for Eye Diseases Research Group. Risk of retinal neovascularization in cases of uveitis. *Ophthalmology.* 2016;123(3):646–654.

Woronkowicz M, Niederer R, Lightman S, Tomkins-Netzer O. Intravitreal antivascular endothelial growth factor treatment for inflammatory choroidal neovascularization in noninfectious uveitis. *Am J Ophthalmol.* 2022;236:281–287.

Vision Rehabilitation

Despite optimal treatment, inflammatory disorders of the eye may lead to vision loss. Worldwide, inflammatory disease is a major cause of blindness and low vision. In the United States, 10% of all blindness is attributed to uveitis. Clinicians can assist their patients by asking whether vision loss is affecting day-to-day functions, such as reading, or mobility. Referral to vision rehabilitation is recommended for patients with visual acuity less than 20/40 in the better eye, reduced contrast sensitivity, disabling glare, or central or peripheral visual field loss (see BCSC Section 3, *Clinical Optics and Vision Rehabilitation*). The low vision section of the American Academy of Ophthalmology website (www.aao.org/low-vision-and-vision-rehab) defines *low vision* and discusses associated symptoms, diagnosis, treatment, rehabilitation, vision aids, and how patients can identify vision rehabilitation resources in their community.

For parents of children with uveitis, clinicians are encouraged to provide information about rehabilitation to optimize functions at school and in other activities. A useful guide for teachers and parents can be found at www.uveitis.org/patients/education/patient-guides.

Fontenot JL, Bona MD, Kaleem MA, et al; American Academy of Ophthalmology Preferred Practice Pattern Vision Rehabilitation Committee. Vision Rehabilitation Preferred Practice Pattern. *Ophthalmology.* 2018;125(1):P228–P278. doi:10.1016/j.ophtha.2017.09.030

APPENDIX A

Diagnostic Survey for Uveitis

FAMILY HISTORY

These questions refer to your grandparents, parents, aunts, uncles, brothers and sisters, children, or grandchildren.

To your knowledge, has anyone in your family ever had any of the following?

Arthritis or rheumatism	Yes	No
Multiple sclerosis or other autoimmune disease	Yes	No
Sickle cell disease or trait	Yes	No
Uveitis, or inflammation in the eye	Yes	No

SOCIAL HISTORY

Your age (years):		
Your current job:		
Have you ever traveled outside the United States?	Yes	No
If yes, where and when?		
Have you ever owned a dog or cat?	Yes	No
Have you ever eaten raw meat or uncooked sausage?	Yes	No
Have you ever had unpasteurized milk or cheese?	Yes	No
Have you ever been exposed to sick animals?	Yes	No
Do you drink untreated stream, well, or lake water?	Yes	No
Have you gone hunting or camping?	Yes	No
Do you smoke cigarettes?	Yes	No
Have you ever used recreational intravenous drugs?	Yes	No
Have you ever had sexual relations with a person of the same sex or with a person who engages in same-sex relations?	Yes	No

PERSONAL MEDICAL HISTORY

Are you allergic to any medications?	Yes	No
If yes, which medications?		
Have you been vaccinated recently?	Yes	No
If yes, which vaccines?		

Please list the medications that you are currently taking, including nonprescription or over-the-counter drugs, nutritional supplements, and herbal or other alternative remedies:

Please list all the eye operations you have had (including laser surgery) and the dates of the procedures:

Please list all the operations you have had (excluding those on the eye) and the dates of the operations:

Have you ever been told by a medical doctor that you have the following conditions?

Anemia (low blood count)	Yes	No
Cancer	Yes	No
Diabetes	Yes	No
Hepatitis	Yes	No
High blood pressure	Yes	No
Pleurisy	Yes	No
Pneumonia	Yes	No
Ulcers	Yes	No
Herpes (sores in or on the mouth or genitals)	Yes	No
Chickenpox	Yes	No
Shingles (zoster)	Yes	No
German measles (rubella)	Yes	No
Measles (rubeola)	Yes	No
Mumps	Yes	No
Chlamydia or trachoma	Yes	No
Syphilis	Yes	No
Gonorrhea	Yes	No
Any other sexually transmitted disease	Yes	No
Tuberculosis	Yes	No
Leprosy	Yes	No
Leptospirosis	Yes	No
Lyme disease	Yes	No
Histoplasmosis	Yes	No
Candida infection or moniliasis	Yes	No
Coccidioidomycosis	Yes	No
Sporotrichosis	Yes	No
Toxoplasmosis	Yes	No
Toxocariasis	Yes	No
Cysticercosis	Yes	No
Trichinosis	Yes	No
Whipple disease	Yes	No
HIV infection or AIDS	Yes	No
Hay fever	Yes	No
Allergies	Yes	No
Vasculitis	Yes	No
Arthritis	Yes	No
Rheumatoid arthritis	Yes	No
Lupus (systemic lupus erythematosus)	Yes	No
Scleroderma	Yes	No
Reactive arthritis	Yes	No
Colitis (Crohn disease, ulcerative colitis)	Yes	No
Behçet disease	Yes	No
Sarcoidosis	Yes	No
Ankylosing spondylitis	Yes	No
Erythema nodosa	Yes	No
Temporal arteritis	Yes	No
Multiple sclerosis	Yes	No

Have you had any of the following symptoms or conditions in the past 3 months?

GENERAL HEALTH

Chills	Yes	No
Fever (persistent or recurrent)	Yes	No
Painful or swollen glands	Yes	No
Night sweats	Yes	No
Fatigue (tire easily)	Yes	No
Poor appetite	Yes	No
Unexplained weight loss	Yes	No
Do you feel sick?	Yes	No

HEAD

Headaches	Yes	No
Fainting	Yes	No
Numbness or tingling in your body	Yes	No
Paralysis in parts of your body	Yes	No
Seizures or convulsions	Yes	No

EARS

Hard of hearing or deafness	Yes	No
Ringing or noise in your ears	Yes	No
Frequent or severe ear infections	Yes	No
Painful or swollen ear lobes	Yes	No

NOSE AND THROAT

Sores in your nose or mouth	Yes	No
Severe or recurrent nosebleeds	Yes	No
Frequent sneezing	Yes	No
Sinus trouble	Yes	No
Persistent hoarseness	Yes	No
Tooth or gum infections	Yes	No

SKIN

Rashes	Yes	No
Skin sores	Yes	No
Sunburn easily (photosensitivity)	Yes	No
White patches of skin or hair	Yes	No
Loss of hair	Yes	No
Tick or insect bites	Yes	No
Painfully cold fingers	Yes	No
Severe itching	Yes	No

RESPIRATORY

Severe or frequent colds	Yes	No
Constant coughing	Yes	No
Coughing up blood	Yes	No
Recent flu or viral infection	Yes	No
Wheezing or asthma attacks	Yes	No
Difficulty breathing	Yes	No

CARDIOVASCULAR		
Chest pain	Yes	No
Shortness of breath	Yes	No
Swelling of your legs	Yes	No
BLOOD		
Frequent or easy bruising	Yes	No
Frequent or easy bleeding	Yes	No
Have you received blood transfusions?	Yes	No
GASTROINTESTINAL		
Trouble swallowing	Yes	No
Diarrhea	Yes	No
Bloody stools	Yes	No
Stomach ulcers	Yes	No
Jaundice or yellow skin	Yes	No
BONES AND JOINTS		
Stiff joints	Yes	No
Stiff lower back	Yes	No
Back pain while sleeping or awakening	Yes	No
Muscle aches	Yes	No
GENITOURINARY		
Kidney problems	Yes	No
Bladder trouble	Yes	No
Blood in your urine	Yes	No
Urinary discharge	Yes	No
Genital sores or ulcers	Yes	No
Prostatitis	Yes	No
Testicular pain	Yes	No
Are you pregnant?	Yes	No
Do you plan to become pregnant in the future?	Yes	No

Adapted from Foster CS, Vitale AT. *Diagnosis and Treatment of Uveitis*. 2nd ed. Jaypee Brothers Medical Publishers; 2012:123–128.

APPENDIX B

Antimicrobial Agents for Intraocular Injection

Table B-1 Intravitreal Antimicrobial Agents

Agent	Standard Dose	Susceptible Microorganisms	Frequency of Repeated Injections
Antibacterial			
Amikacin	400 μg/0.1 mL	Aerobic GNB (eg, *Pseudomonas aeruginosa*)	24–48 h
Ceftazidime	2.25 mg/0.1 mL	Aerobic GNB (eg, *P aeruginosa*); GPB	48–72 h
Clindamycin	1 mg/0.1 mL	GPC (staphylococci, pneumococci); GPB (*Bacillus* spp); GNB (*Bacteroides* spp, *Fusobacterium* spp); *Toxoplasma gondii*	72 h
Vancomycin	1 mg/0.1 mL	GPC (MRSA and MDR *Staphylococcus epidermidis*)	72 h
Antifungal			
Amphotericin B	5–10 μg/0.1 mL	Yeasts, filamentous fungi (resistance reported for various species of *Aspergillus*)	NA
Voriconazole	100 μg/0.1 mL	Broad-spectrum activity against yeasts and molds	NA
Antiviral			
Foscarnet	2.4 mg/0.1 mL	HSV-1, HSV-2, and VZV > CMV	Adjunct to systemic antiviral: 2–3×/wk until retinitis is stable; then weekly if necessary
Ganciclovir	2 mg/0.5 mL or 0.1 mL	CMV > HSV-1, HSV-2, and VZV	Adjunct to systemic antiviral: 2–3×/wk until retinitis is stable; then weekly if necessary

CMV = cytomegalovirus; GNB = gram-negative bacilli; GPB = gram-positive bacilli; GPC = gram-positive cocci; HSV-1 = herpes simplex virus type 1; HSV-2 = herpes simplex virus type 2; MDR = multidrug resistant; MRSA = methicillin-resistant *Staphylococcus aureus;* NA = not applicable; VZV = varicella-zoster virus.

Information from Radhika M, Mithal K, Bawdekar A, et al. Pharmacokinetics of intravitreal antibiotics in endophthalmitis. *J Ophthalmic Inflamm Infect.* 2014 Sep 10;4:22. Also from Sallam AB, Kirkland KA, Barry R, Soliman MK, Ali TK, Lightman S. A review of antimicrobial therapy for infectious uveitis of the posterior segment. *Med Hypothesis Discov Innov Ophthalmol.* 2018;7(4):140–155.

Additional Materials and Resources

Related Academy Materials

The American Academy of Ophthalmology is dedicated to providing a wealth of high-quality clinical education resources for ophthalmologists.

Print Publications and Electronic Products

For a complete listing of Academy clinical education products, including the BCSC Self-Assessment Program, visit our online store at https://store.aao.org/clinical-education.html. Or call Customer Service at 866.561.8558 (toll free, US only) or +1 415.561.8540, Monday through Friday, between 8:00 AM and 5:00 PM (PST).

Online Resources

Visit the **Ophthalmic News and Education (ONE®) Network** at aao.org/uveitis to find relevant videos, podcasts, webinars, online courses, journal articles, practice guidelines, self-assessment quizzes, images, and more. The ONE Network is a free Academy-member benefit.

The **Residents page** on the ONE Network (aao.org/residents) offers resident-specific content, including courses, videos, flashcards, and OKAP and Board Exam study tools. A learning plan, Uveitis Rotation, offers resources designed to support residents in their uveitis rotation.

Find comprehensive **resources for diversity, equity, and inclusion** in ophthalmology on the ONE Network at aao.org/diversity-equity-and-inclusion.

Access free, trusted articles and content with the Academy's collaborative online encyclopedia, **EyeWiki,** at aao.org/eyewiki.

Get mobile access to the *Wills Eye Manual* and *EyeWiki,* watch the latest 1-minute videos, challenge yourself with weekly Diagnose This activities, and set up alerts for clinical updates relevant to you with the free **AAO Ophthalmic Education App.** Download today: search for "AAO Ophthalmic Education" in the Apple app store or in Google Play.

Basic Texts and Additional Resources

Albert DM, Miller JW, Azar DT, Young LH, eds. *Albert and Jakobiec's Principles and Practice of Ophthalmology.* 4th ed. Springer; 2022.

Delves PJ, Martin SJ, Burton DR, Roitt IM. *Roitt's Essential Immunology.* 13th ed. Wiley-Blackwell; 2017.

Foster CS, Gonzalez-Gonzalez LA, Anesi SD, Palafox SKV. *Childhood Uveitis.* OIUF; 2019.

Foster CS, Vitale AT, eds. *Diagnosis & Treatment of Uveitis.* 2nd ed. Jaypee Brothers Medical Publishers; 2013.

Garg, SJ. ed. *Uveitis.* 2nd ed. Lippincott Williams & Wilkins; 2018. *Color Atlas & Synopsis of Clinical Ophthalmology.*

Gupta V, Nguyen QD, LeHoang P, Agarwal A. *The Uveitis Atlas.* Springer New Delhi; 2020.

Papaliodis GN, ed. *Uveitis: A Practical Guide to the Diagnosis and Treatment of Intraocular Inflammation.* Springer International Publishing AG; 2017.

Rao NA, section ed. Part 7: Uveitis and other intraocular inflammations. In: Yanoff M, Duker JS, eds. *Ophthalmology.* 6th ed. Elsevier; 2023.

Salmon JF. *Kanski's Clinical Ophthalmology: A Systematic Approach.* 9th ed. Elsevier; 2019.

Watson PG, Hazleman BL, McCluskey P, Pavésio CE. *The Sclera and Systemic Disorders.* 3rd ed. Jaypee Medical Ltd; 2012.

Whitcup SM, Sen HN. *Whitcup and Nussenblatt's Uveitis: Fundamentals and Clinical Practice.* 5th ed. Elsevier; 2021.

Zierhut M, Pavésio C, Ohno S, Oréfice F, Rao NA. *Intraocular Inflammation.* Springer-Verlag Berlin Heidelberg; 2016.

Requesting Continuing Medical Education Credit

The American Academy of Ophthalmology is accredited by the Accreditation Council for Continuing Medical Education (ACCME) to provide continuing medical education for physicians.

The American Academy of Ophthalmology designates this enduring material for a maximum of 10 *AMA PRA Category 1 Credits*™. Physicians should claim only the credit commensurate with the extent of their participation in the activity.

To claim *AMA PRA Category 1 Credits*™ upon completion of this activity, learners must demonstrate appropriate knowledge and participation in the activity by taking the posttest for Section 9 and achieving a score of 80% or higher.

There is no formal American Board of Ophthalmology (ABO) approval process for self-assessment activities. Any CME activity that qualifies for ABO Continuing Certification credit may also be counted as "self-assessment" as long as it provides a mechanism for individual learners to review their own performance, knowledge base, or skill set in a defined area of practice. For instance, grand rounds, medical conferences, or journal activities for CME credit that involve a form of individualized self-assessment may count as a self-assessment activity.

To take the posttest and request CME credit online:

1. Go to www.aao.org/cme-central and log in.
2. Click on "Claim CME Credit and View My CME Transcript" and then "Report AAO Credits."
3. Select the appropriate media type and then the Academy activity. You will be directed to the posttest.
4. Once you have passed the test with a score of 80% or higher, you will be directed to your transcript. *If you are not an Academy member, you will be able to print out a certificate of participation once you have passed the test.*

CME expiration date: June 1, 2026. *AMA PRA Category 1 Credits*™ may be claimed only once between June 1, 2023 (original release date), and the expiration date.

For assistance, contact the Academy's Customer Service department at 866.561.8558 (US only) or +1 415.561.8540 between 8:00 AM and 5:00 PM (PST), Monday through Friday, or send an e-mail to customer_service@aao.org.

Study Questions

Please note that these questions are not part of your CME reporting process. They are provided here for your own educational use and for identification of any professional practice gaps. The required CME posttest is available online (see "Requesting Continuing Medical Education Credit"). Following the questions are answers with discussions. Although a concerted effort has been made to avoid ambiguity and redundancy in these questions, the authors recognize that differences of opinion may occur regarding the "best" answer. The discussions are provided to demonstrate the rationale used to derive the answer. They may also be helpful in confirming that your approach to the problem was correct or, if necessary, in fixing the principle in your memory. The Section 9 faculty thanks the Resident Self-Assessment Committee for developing these self-assessment questions and the discussions that follow.

1. What are the main effector cells of the innate immune system?
   a. $CD4^+$ T cells and $CD8^+$ T cells
   b. macrophages and neutrophils
   c. mast cells and dendritic cells
   d. plasma cells and B lymphocytes

2. What type of macrophage produces the full spectrum of inflammatory and cytotoxic cytokines?
   a. resting macrophage
   b. primed macrophage
   c. activated macrophage
   d. stimulated macrophage

3. Which type of white blood cell can become an antigen-presenting cell?
   a. basophil
   b. eosinophil
   c. monocyte
   d. neutrophil

4. What is the term for antigenic sites on antibodies?
   a. allotopes
   b. epitopes
   c. idiotopes
   d. isotopes

5. What agent used in therapy for uveitis may induce anti-idiotypic antibodies?
   a. infliximab
   b. interferon alfa-2a/2b
   c. methotrexate
   d. tacrolimus

6. What feature allows the ocular surface to mount an antibody-mediated effector response to influenza viral antigens after a patient is administered an intranasal influenza vaccine?
   a. abundance of antigen-presenting cells in the conjunctiva
   b. predominance of immunoglobulin (Ig) A within the tear film
   c. presence of conjunctiva-associated lymphoid tissue
   d. high density of mast cells within the conjunctiva

7. What is a major component that affords immune privilege to the cornea?
   a. complement
   b. conjunctival-associated lymphoid tissue
   c. cytokines (eg, interleukin 1)
   d. limbal physiology

8. What immune cells are present in the choroid under normal physiologic conditions?
   a. B lymphocytes
   b. eosinophils
   c. macrophages
   d. neutrophils

9. What ocular inflammatory disease has the strongest human leukocyte antigen (HLA) association?
   a. birdshot chorioretinopathy and HLA-A29
   b. acute anterior uveitis and HLA-B27
   c. Behçet disease and HLA-B51
   d. intermediate uveitis and HLA-DR15

10. HLA-DR4 is weakly associated with what ophthalmic disease?
   a. acute anterior uveitis
   b. Behçet disease
   c. birdshot chorioretinopathy
   d. sympathetic ophthalmia

11. A patient is treated with topical corticosteroids for anterior uveitis in the right eye. At the 1-month visit, the eye is quiet without medication. Four months later, the patient returns

and is again found to have anterior uveitis in the right eye. According to the Standardization of Uveitis Nomenclature (SUN) Working Group classification, what is the best description of this patient's uveitis?

a. acute

b. chronic

c. limited

d. recurrent

12. What medication used to treat uveitis may exacerbate multiple sclerosis?

a. adalimumab

b. interferon alfa-2a/2b

c. methylprednisolone

d. rituximab

13. A patient is being treated for first-time presentation of undifferentiated granulomatous iridocyclitis. She responds very well to hourly topical corticosteroid, but in the past 3 months, the intraocular inflammation recurred every time the ophthalmologist tried to taper the corticosteroid frequency to less than 4 times per day. A posterior subcapsular cataract is beginning to develop, and the intraocular pressure is now 23 mm Hg despite the patient's use of 3 types of antiglaucoma eyedrops. What is the most appropriate next step in management of this case?

a. Continue topical corticosteroids and schedule the patient for glaucoma drainage implant surgery.

b. Continue topical corticosteroids and initiate therapy with methotrexate.

c. Increase topical corticosteroids and initiate therapy with oral acetazolamide.

d. Increase topical corticosteroids and initiate therapy with an oral nonsteroidal anti-inflammatory drug (NSAID).

14. What type of scleritis is most likely to be associated with life-threatening systemic disease?

a. nodular scleritis

b. posterior scleritis

c. diffuse scleritis

d. necrotizing scleritis

15. What finding is associated with an increased risk of uveitis in patients with juvenile idiopathic arthritis (JIA)?

a. antinuclear antibody positivity

b. polyarticular involvement

c. rheumatoid factor positivity

d. systemic involvement

16. Abnormal urinalysis findings, with increased β_2-microglobulin level, in a patient with uveitis should prompt initiation of what systemic treatment?
    a. antibiotics
    b. anticoagulants
    c. corticosteroids
    d. xanthine oxidase inhibitor

17. A 23-year-old man purchases a genetic testing kit and learns that he is positive for HLA-B27. He becomes worried about developing acute anterior uveitis after reading stories on the Internet and presents for an eye examination. What is the most likely finding on this patient's slit-lamp examination?
    a. hypopyon
    b. posterior synechiae
    c. posterior subcapsular cataract
    d. quiet anterior chamber

18. How often should a 6-year-old girl with a 2-year history of antinuclear antibody–positive oligoarticular JIA be screened for uveitis?
    a. every 3 months
    b. every 6 months
    c. every 9 months
    d. every 12 months

19. A patient is referred for evaluation of anterior uveitis in the right eye. On examination, there is conjunctival injection, 1+ cell, and granulomatous keratic precipitates (KPs). The patient is on topical therapy (dorzolamide, timolol, and brimonidine) for glaucoma and is also undergoing treatment for latent tuberculosis with oral rifampin. What medication is most likely to be responsible for this patient's presentation?
    a. brimonidine
    b. dorzolamide
    c. rifampin
    d. timolol

20. What is the typical onset and disease course for birdshot chorioretinopathy?
    a. acute onset with progressive course
    b. acute onset with self-limiting course
    c. insidious onset with progressive course
    d. insidious onset with self-limiting course

21. Peripheral necrotizing retinochoroiditis resembling acute retinal necrosis can be seen in patients infected with what pathogen?
    a. *Mycobacterium tuberculosis*
    b. *Nocardia asteroides*

c. *Pneumocystis jirovecii*
d. *Treponema pallidum*

22. When stellate KPs are present in intraocular infections caused by herpes simplex virus type 1 (HSV-1), what description best characterizes their appearance on the corneal endothelium?
    a. They are distributed diffusely, often extending above the corneal equator.
    b. They are distributed inferiorly, specifically only in the Arlt triangle.
    c. They manifest as ring-shaped clusters.
    d. KPs are not found in HSV-1 intraocular infections.

23. What is an appropriate induction treatment option for a patient with varicella-zoster virus–associated acute retinal necrosis?
    a. oral acyclovir 800 mg 5 times/day
    b. oral valacyclovir 1 g 3 times/day
    c. oral valacyclovir 2 g 3 times/day
    d. oral valganciclovir 900 mg twice/day

24. A patient is referred with a history of disseminated coccidioidomycosis. Which form of inflammation is the most common ocular manifestation of the disease?
    a. phlyctenular and granulomatous conjunctivitis
    b. hypertensive anterior uveitis
    c. intermediate uveitis
    d. multifocal choroidal granulomas

25. What pathogen is associated with the development of Kaposi sarcoma?
    a. cytomegalovirus
    b. Epstein-Barr virus
    c. HSV-1
    d. human herpesvirus 8

26. A patient with a history of AIDS (last $CD4^+$ T-lymphocyte count 89 cells/μL) presents for evaluation of decreased vision and is diagnosed with ocular toxoplasmosis. What test should be ordered promptly for this patient?
    a. serologic tests for syphilis (rapid plasma reagin/fluorescent treponemal antibody absorption test)
    b. serologic tests for *Toxoplasma gondii* (IgG and IgM)
    c. computed tomography of the chest
    d. magnetic resonance imaging of the brain

27. A patient with AIDS presents with bilateral pale-yellow, placoid retinal lesions. What testing and treatment should be ordered?
    a. Check $CD4^+$ helper T-lymphocyte count and start antiretroviral therapy.
    b. Check $CD4^+$ helper T-lymphocyte count and start systemic corticosteroids.
    c. Check syphilis antibodies and rapid plasmin reagin and start intramuscular benzathine penicillin G, 2.4 million units.
    d. Check syphilis antibodies and rapid plasmin reagin and start intravenous penicillin G, 18–24 million units.

28. An immunosuppressed patient presents with features consistent with unilateral endophthalmitis. A pars plana vitrectomy is performed, and analysis of vitreous fluid specimens reveals septate hyphae with dichotomous branching on silver stain. What is the most likely organism?
    a. *Aspergillus fumigatus*
    b. *Candida albicans*
    c. *Coccidioides immitis*
    d. *Cryptococcus neoformans*

29. A patient with candidemia is found to have yellow-white chorioretinal lesions without vitritis. What is the most appropriate initial treatment option?
    a. intravitreal vancomycin
    b. oral voriconazole
    c. pars plana vitrectomy
    d. posterior sub-Tenon injection of triamcinolone

30. Four months after cataract surgery in the right eye, a patient had recurrent 1–2+ anterior chamber cell and flare each time topical corticosteroids were tapered. Now, a hypopyon, an iris mass, necrotizing scleritis, and vitreous snowballs have developed. Infection with what organism most likely caused this condition?
    a. *Candida* species
    b. *Histoplasma* species
    c. *Pseudomonas* species
    d. *Streptococcus* species

31. A 78-year-old man presents for a routine eye examination. His ocular history is notable only for uncomplicated bilateral cataract surgery 5 years earlier. On examination, intraocular pressure is 6 mm Hg in the right eye and 13 mm Hg in the left eye. The right-eye examination is notable for 1+ cell and 2+ flare in the anterior chamber. Findings from the left-eye examination are unremarkable. The fundus examination shows clear vitreous in both eyes and dilated retinal venules and narrowed arterioles, worse in the right eye. What is the most appropriate next step in the care of this patient?
    a. Start topical corticosteroid drops.
    b. Perform a vitreous biopsy to obtain a specimen for flow cytometry.

c. Order carotid Doppler ultrasonography.

d. Reassure the patient that these are normal findings after cataract surgery.

32. A 65-year-old woman with vitritis and negative results on the treponemal antibody test and interferon-gamma release assay responds well initially to systemic corticosteroids; however, as the corticosteroids are tapered, the vitritis recurs. A vitreous biopsy is performed, and cytologic analysis shows pleomorphic lymphoid cells with a high nuclear-to-cytoplasm ratio. Approximately what proportion of patients with this condition will develop intracranial lesions characterized by the same cells?

    a. less than 1 in 10

    b. 1 in 3

    c. 1 in 2

    d. more than 2 in 3

33. A child with a history of reddish-yellow skin lesions presents with unilateral recurrent hyphema and anterior chamber cells. A few iris lesions are noted. What is the best test to identify the etiology of this patient's intraocular inflammation and hyphema?

    a. anterior chamber paracentesis with directed polymerase chain reaction (PCR) for cytomegalovirus

    b. skin or iris biopsy to evaluate for foamy macrophages

    c. anterior chamber paracentesis with directed PCR for rubella virus

    d. skin or iris biopsy to evaluate for caseating granulomas

34. A patient who is being treated with mycophenolate mofetil for bilateral pars planitis has persistent macular edema in the right eye. Examination of the anterior chamber and vitreous shows no evidence of active inflammation. What is the most appropriate next step to manage the macular edema in this patient?

    a. Switch to cyclophosphamide.

    b. Administer intravenous methylprednisolone 1 g daily for 3 days.

    c. Administer periocular or intravitreal triamcinolone acetonide injection.

    d. Perform pars plana vitrectomy with membrane peeling.

35. A 12-year-old patient with a 7-year history of JIA-associated chronic anterior uveitis (CAU) presents for her regular follow-up appointment. She uses prednisolone drops once daily and is asymptomatic. What finding can be observed on examination?

    a. band keratopathy

    b. fibrinous anterior chamber reaction

    c. hypopyon

    d. vitritis

36. A child with JIA-associated chronic bilateral nongranulomatous uveitis has developed band keratopathy. What pathologic finding can be observed in this patient's cornea?
    a. subepithelial urate deposition
    b. subepithelial calcium deposition
    c. pre-Descemet urate deposition
    d. pre-Descemet calcium deposition

Answers

1. **b.** The innate immune system is a relatively broad-acting rapid reaction force that recognizes "nonself" (foreign) substances, proteins, or lipopolysaccharides. The innate response can be thought of as a preprogrammed reaction that is immediate, requires no prior exposure to the foreign substance, and is similar for all encountered triggers. The result is the generation of biochemical mediators and cytokines that recruit innate effector cells, especially macrophages and neutrophils, to remove the offending stimulus through phagocytosis or enzymatic degradation.
2. **c.** Activated macrophages are classically defined as macrophages that produce the full spectrum of inflammatory and cytotoxic cytokines; thus, they mediate and amplify acute inflammation, tumor killing, and major antibacterial activity. Epithelioid cells and giant cells represent different terminal differentiations of the activated macrophage.

   Resting macrophages are the classic scavenging cell, capable of phagocytosis and uptake of dead cell membranes, chemically modified extracellular protein (ie, acetylated or oxidized lipoproteins), sugar ligands, naked nucleic acids, and bacterial pathogens. Resting monocytes express at least 3 types of scavenging receptors but synthesize very low levels of proinflammatory cytokines. Scavenging can occur in the absence of inflammation. Primed macrophages are derived from resting macrophages that become primed by exposure to certain cytokines. Upon priming, these cells become positive for human leukocyte antigen (HLA) class II molecules and capable of functioning as antigen-presenting cells (APCs) to T lymphocytes. Primed macrophages thus resemble dendritic cells. They can exit tissue sites by afferent lymphatic vessels to reenter the lymph node. Stimulated (or reparative) macrophages are partially activated and produce some inflammatory cytokines that contribute to fibrosis and wound healing.
3. **c.** Monocytes can be primed and induced to become APCs. Basophils, eosinophils, and neutrophils generally do not have the ability to act as APCs.
4. **c.** Because they are proteins, antibodies themselves can be antigenic. Their antigenic sites are called *idiotopes,* as distinguished from *epitopes*, which are the antigenic sites on foreign molecules. An allotope is a site on the constant or nonvarying part of an antibody molecule that is recognizable by a combining site of other antibodies. Isotopes are 2 or more atoms whose nuclei have the same number of protons but different numbers of neutrons.
5. **a.** Infliximab is a mouse/human-chimeric monoclonal antibody directed against tumor necrosis factor α (TNF-α). One study showed that as many as 75% of patients receiving more than 3 infusions develop antinuclear antibodies, causing drug-induced lupus syndrome and the formation of human anti-idiotypic (anti-chimeric) antibodies, which can lead to reduced efficacy of infliximab.

   Methotrexate, interferon alfa-2a/2b, and tacrolimus are not associated with formation of anti-idiotypic antibodies. Methotrexate is an antimetabolite drug that is often coadministered with biologics for synergistic effect and to *reduce* the risk of developing antidrug antibodies. Interferon alfa-2a/2b, administered subcutaneously, has been beneficial in some patients with uveitis. Interferon alfa-2a has antiviral, immunomodulatory, and antiangiogenic effects. Tacrolimus, a product of *Streptomyces tsukubaensis,* is a calcineurin inhibitor that eliminates T-cell receptor signal transduction and downregulates interleukin-2 gene transcription and receptor expression of $CD4^+$ T lymphocytes.

6. **c.** Conjunctiva-associated lymphoid tissue (CALT) is part of the mucosal immune system, which utilizes innate and adaptive immune responses to maintain the homeostasis of mucosal surfaces. Although there is an abundance of APCs (macrophages, dendritic cells) in CALT, their role is to convey antigen to local lymph nodes for processing. They do not create a population of memory B cells. While immunoglobulin A (IgA) is present abundantly in tears, IgA does not provide for a secondary adaptive immune response. One defining feature of the mucosal immune system is that it is an interconnected system of lymphatic function, such that prior exposure at any mucosal immune system site will allow for a secondary adaptive immune response (eg, via a population of memory B cells) at every mucosal immune system site. Prior exposure at a non-mucosal location in the body (eg, abrasion of the skin or vaccination within a muscle) does not sensitize and prime the mucosal immune system for future exposure. Although there is a high density of mast cells within the conjunctiva, these cells do not explain the ability of an intranasal vaccine to facilitate an antibody-mediated effector response on the ocular surface.
7. **d.** Normal limbal physiology is a major component of corneal immune privilege, especially the maintenance of avascularity and the scarcity of APCs in the paracentral and central cornea. The lack of APCs and lymphatic channels partially inhibits the afferent response in the central cornea. The absence of postcapillary venules centrally can limit the efficiency of effector recruitment, although effector cells and molecules can infiltrate even avascular cornea.

   Cytokines and complement help recruit immune mediators to the central cornea, which is otherwise relatively devoid of immune effectors. CALT is responsible for antigen processing, but the effector limb of this system can extend to the corneal surface, resulting in recruitment of immune effectors to the cornea.
8. **c.** Both the choroid and the retina have abundant potential APCs, including macrophages and dendritic cells in the choroid and choriocapillaris and microglia in the retina. Effector cells such as B lymphocytes typically are very rare in normal retina and choroid. Eosinophils and neutrophils are also absent but may be induced to infiltrate the retina and choroid by various stimuli.
9. **a.** The ocular inflammatory disease with the strongest HLA association is birdshot chorioretinopathy (BCR); nearly all patients with BCR are HLA-A29 positive (relative risk up to 224 for North American and European populations). HLA-B27, HLA-B51, and HLA-DR15 are associated with low relative risks (between 2 and 10) for acute anterior uveitis, Behçet disease, and intermediate uveitis, respectively. It is important to remember that the HLA association identifies individuals at risk, but it is not a diagnostic marker. The associated haplotype is not necessarily present in all people with the disease, nor does its presence ensure the associated diagnosis.
10. **d.** HLA-DR4 has been weakly associated with both Vogt-Koyanagi-Harada syndrome and sympathetic ophthalmia.
11. **d.** This patient has *recurrent uveitis,* a term used to describe repeated episodes of uveitis separated by periods of quiescence lasting 3 months or more without therapy. *Acute uveitis* refers to episodes characterized by sudden onset and limited (eg, <3 months') duration. *Chronic uveitis* refers to episodes of uveitis that recur less than 3 months after treatment has been discontinued. *Limited* refers to episodes lasting 3 months or less.
12. **a.** TNF-α is believed to play a major role in the pathogenesis of juvenile idiopathic arthritis, ankylosing spondylitis, and other spondyloarthropathies. Adalimumab, infliximab, certolizumab, golimumab, and etanercept are TNF-α inhibitors. TNF inhibitors have been associ-

ated with central nervous system demyelination (promoting or unmasking multiple sclerosis [MS]), hepatitis B reactivation, and deep fungal and other serious atypical infections. This class of medication is not recommended in patients with demyelinating disease. Screening for tuberculosis and viral hepatitis is performed before starting these medications.

A number of immunomodulatory agents, including interferon β preparations, alemtuzumab, dimethyl fumarate, ocrelizumab, rituximab, and teriflunomide, have important beneficial effects for patients with MS. Acute attacks of MS are typically treated with glucocorticoids. Systemic corticosteroids such as methylprednisolone can safely be used in uveitis associated with MS.

13. **b.** The increasing intraocular pressure (IOP) is a concern; however, if additional anti-inflammatory treatment is not added, it is very likely that the cataract will become visually significant and the uveitis will not be sufficiently controlled to safely perform cataract extraction. A systemic immunomodulatory medication should be added to attain control of inflammation and allow the eventual taper of topical corticosteroids. Glaucoma surgery is likely to worsen the uveitis, which already requires topical corticosteroids at least 4 times per day. While oral acetazolamide may improve IOP control, the increase in topical corticosteroids will likely result in cataract progression, and cataract surgery will be contraindicated as long as very frequent topical treatment is necessary to control the uveitis. Although an oral nonsteroidal anti-inflammatory drug (NSAID) may decrease the amount of topical corticosteroids necessary to control chronic anterior uveitis, it is unlikely that this class of medication will adequately control the patient's uveitis and allow the discontinuation of topical corticosteroids.

14. **d.** Necrotizing scleritis is the most severe and destructive type of scleritis. Approximately 50%–60% of cases are associated with systemic disease, including life-threatening systemic vasculitides. Necrotizing scleritis is more likely than the other forms of anterior scleritis to lead to vision loss. In the past, mortality rates of patients with necrotizing scleritis associated with systemic inflammatory diseases were as high as 30%; prompt diagnosis as well as the use of biologic therapies can improve prognosis.

15. **a.** Juvenile idiopathic arthritis (JIA; formerly referred to as *juvenile chronic arthritis* and *juvenile rheumatoid arthritis*) is the most common systemic disorder associated with anterior uveitis in the pediatric age group. It is characterized by arthritis beginning before age 16 years and lasting for at least 6 weeks. Girls younger than 5 years who are positive for antinuclear antibody (ANA) have an increased risk of developing chronic anterior uveitis. Ocular involvement is rare in children with systemic arthritis (Still disease) or polyarticular involvement and in those with positive rheumatoid factor. In JIA-associated uveitis, affected eyes are frequently white and asymptomatic. Children with JIA, especially those who are ANA positive or who have oligoarticular disease, should undergo regular slit-lamp examinations to screen for uveitis.

16. **c.** Tubulointerstitial nephritis and uveitis (TINU) syndrome occurs predominantly in adolescent girls and women. The median age at onset is 15 years. The uveitis is typically a bilateral nongranulomatous anterior uveitis. Posterior segment involvement may include vitritis, multifocal chorioretinal lesions or scars, and retinal vascular leakage, as well as optic disc and macular edema. Patients may present with systemic symptoms before the development of uveitis. Abnormal laboratory findings include elevated serum creatinine level or decreased creatinine clearance, increased *urinary* β_2-microglobulin level, proteinuria, presence of urine eosinophils, pyuria or hematuria, urinary white cell casts, and normoglycemic

glycosuria. TINU syndrome is responsive to high-dose oral corticosteroids, but patients with a prolonged inflammatory course may require systemic immunomodulatory therapy.

17. **d.** The prevalence of HLA-B27 varies by population. Although approximately 8% of the US population is positive for HLA-B27, only 0.012% of them (or 1 in 667) will develop acute anterior uveitis (AAU). Therefore, the most likely finding on this patient's slit-lamp examination is a quiet anterior chamber; eye examination results would be normal. Hypopyon, posterior synechiae, and posterior subcapsular cataract can occur in patients with AAU; however, these findings are unlikely in this patient, who is asymptomatic and who has a very low risk of developing AAU.
18. **a.** This patient demonstrates all the high-risk characteristics for developing uveitis and should be screened for uveitis every 3 months. High-risk children are those with antinuclear antibodies and oligoarticular arthritis, polyarticular arthritis (rheumatoid factor negative), psoriatic arthritis, or undifferentiated arthritis; those who were younger than 7 years at the time of JIA onset; and those with JIA duration of 4 years or less. All other children with JIA should be screened every 6–12 months.
19. **a.** A common presentation of brimonidine-associated uveitis is a red and irritated eye with extensive (often granulomatous) keratic precipitates (KPs) and low-grade anterior uveitis in a patient receiving long-term brimonidine therapy. Corneal edema and vitreous inflammation may also be present. Dorzolamide and timolol are not associated with drug-induced uveitis. While rifabutin is associated with drug-induced uveitis, rifampin is not.
20. **c.** Birdshot chorioretinopathy typically has an insidious onset. While a small subset of patients may have self-limited disease, the clinical course of BCR is characteristically chronic and progressive.
21. **d.** Syphilis should be considered in the differential diagnosis of any intraocular inflammatory disease. It is caused by the spirochete *Treponema pallidum* and is associated with numerous ocular manifestations. Posterior segment findings of acquired syphilis include vitritis, chorioretinitis, focal or multifocal retinitis, necrotizing retinochoroiditis, retinal vasculitis, exudative retinal detachment, isolated papillitis, and neuroretinitis. Syphilis may present as a focal retinitis or as a peripheral necrotizing retinochoroiditis that may resemble acute retinal necrosis or progressive outer retinal necrosis.
22. **a.** Stellate KPs are very suggestive of a viral intraocular infection and are a frequent finding in these cases. However, larger nongranulomatous or granulomatous KPs can also occur in herpetic intraocular infections, including herpes simplex virus (HSV) types 1 and 2 and varicella-zoster virus (VZV). When stellate KPs are present, they are often distributed diffusely. The KPs localizing only to the Arlt triangle may be granulomatous or nongranulomatous and classically occur in noninfectious intraocular inflammation. Ring-shaped clusters of corneal endothelial lesions or small, white-domed KPs have been observed in cytomegalovirus (CMV) anterior uveitis.
23. **c.** Induction therapy for VZV-associated acute retinal necrosis may consist of intravenous (IV) acyclovir 10 mg/kg every 8 hours for 10–14 days or oral valacyclovir 2 g 3 times/day. Valacyclovir 1 g 3 times/day is the dosage used for HSV-associated acute retinal necrosis or active herpetic keratitis. Oral valganciclovir is appropriate for CMV-associated intraocular infections.
24. **a.** Ocular manifestations of coccidioidomycosis (caused by *Coccidioides immitis*) such as phlyctenular and granulomatous conjunctivitis are more common than uveal involvement.

Uveal manifestations can include granulomatous KPs and iris nodules, which are granulomas on histologic examination. Hypertensive anterior uveitis does not occur, however. Choroidal involvement manifests as multifocal choroidal granulomas most frequently located in the postequatorial fundus.

25. **d.** The pathogen associated with the development of Kaposi sarcoma is human herpesvirus (HHV)-8. Epstein-Barr virus (HHV-4) is associated with the development of primary central nervous system lymphomas and vitreoretinal lymphomas in HIV-infected individuals. HSV-1 (HHV-1) and CMV (HHV-5) are not associated with any specific neoplasias in persons with HIV infection.

26. **d.** Ocular toxoplasmosis in immunocompromised patients may be associated with cerebral or disseminated toxoplasmosis. For patients with AIDS who have active ocular toxoplasmosis, neuroimaging (preferably magnetic resonance imaging) should be performed to evaluate for central nervous system involvement. Although syphilis is reemerging globally, particularly in association with HIV coinfection, there is no indication for urgent syphilis testing in this patient. Since the patient has already been diagnosed with ocular toxoplasmosis, serologic testing is not immediately useful. Computed tomography of the chest might be indicated if there is concern for pulmonary infection or inflammation, but in this case, expeditious investigation for toxoplasmic encephalitis is necessary.

27. **d.** Suspicion for syphilis should be high in this patient. Syphilis is a common coinfection in HIV-infected individuals. A classic manifestation of syphilis in patients with AIDS is unilateral or bilateral pale-yellow, placoid retinal lesions that preferentially involve the macula. Checking syphilis antibodies (treponemal test) and the rapid plasmin reagin (RPR, nontreponemal test) will help confirm the diagnosis and assess response to treatment. Ocular cases of syphilis should be treated in the same manner as neurosyphilis, and 18–24 million units of IV penicillin G administered daily for 10–14 days is indicated. Syphilis without neurologic or ocular involvement may be treated intramuscularly as a single dose.

    Checking $CD4^+$ helper T-lymphocyte count and starting antiretroviral therapy (ART) would be appropriate if the patient exhibited features of HIV retinopathy (cotton-wool spots, microaneurysms, and retinal hemorrhages) only. Systemic corticosteroids may be used in treating immune recovery uveitis, an inflammatory process that affects patients with a history of CMV retinitis and AIDS whose immune status improves with ART. Systemic corticosteroids may also be used if there is a prominent inflammatory reaction in syphilis, but this medication should not be started until after treatment with IV penicillin has commenced.

28. **a.** Histologically, *Aspergillus* species is characterized by septate hyphae with dichotomous branching. *Candida* species are recognized as budding yeast with a characteristic pseudohyphate appearance. Histologically, *C immitis* appears as spherules with multiple endospores. *Cryptococcus neoformans* does not appear as hyphae but rather as round capsules with a halo on India ink; periodic acid–Schiff (PAS) and Gomori methenamine silver (GMS) stain the organism and leave the capsule unstained.

29. **b.** In this case, the hematogenous dissemination of *Candida* organisms involves only the choroid, so appropriate initial treatment includes systemic antifungal medication and close monitoring. Oral voriconazole has excellent intraocular penetration. If there is vitreal involvement, pars plana vitrectomy in conjunction with systemic and intravitreal antifungals may be necessary. Monotherapy with periocular or intraocular depot corticosteroids will worsen the infectious endophthalmitis. Intravitreal injection of the antibiotic vancomycin will not treat the *Candida* infection.

30. **a.** Recurrent inflammation in an eye that has previously undergone surgery is concerning for chronic postoperative endophthalmitis. While the presentation of chronic postoperative fungal endophthalmitis may be similar to that of a bacterial infection, certain clinical signs make a fungal etiology more likely, including a corneal infiltrate or edema, a mass in the iris or ciliary body, necrotizing scleritis, vitreous snowballs, or a "string-of-pearls" appearance in the vitreous. Chronic postoperative bacterial endophthalmitis is most commonly caused by *Cutibacterium acnes* (formerly *Propionibacterium acnes*), a gram-positive anaerobe. Other gram-positive bacteria, gram-negative bacteria, *Mycobacterium* species, and fungi (such as *Candida parapsilosis, Aspergillus flavus,* and *Torulopsis candida*) can also cause chronic postoperative endophthalmitis.

31. **c.** The most likely diagnosis is ocular ischemic syndrome, which can masquerade as uveitis. Carotid Doppler ultrasonography should be ordered to assess for ipsilateral stenosis of the carotid artery. Given the lack of symptoms and lack of previous uveitic episodes, this presentation in an older man is unlikely to be caused by uveitis; therefore, empiric topical corticosteroid therapy is not indicated. Given this patient's age, it is appropriate to consider lymphoma in the differential diagnosis. however, the patient's vitreous cavity is clear, and the diagnosis of vitreoretinal lymphoma (formerly called *primary intraocular lymphoma*) is unlikely. While extensive intraocular surgery can result in breakdown of the blood–aqueous barrier, this breakdown does not typically result from uncomplicated cataract surgery (nor would it explain the hypotony and absence of cells in the left eye).

32. **d.** The case described clinically is consistent with vitreoretinal lymphoma (VRL), and the cytopathologic findings confirm the diagnosis. In more than two-thirds of cases of VRL, patients will have or will go on to develop intracranial disease. In fact, VRL is a subset of primary central nervous system lymphoma (PCNSL). Approximately 25% of patients with PCNSL (who do not yet have intraocular involvement) will go on to develop VRL.

33. **b.** The case described is consistent with juvenile xanthogranuloma, which may feature reddish-yellow skin lesions. Intraocular features may include recurrent hyphema. Histologically, skin or iris biopsy specimens would be expected to show large histiocytes with foamy cytoplasm and Touton giant cells. Caseating granulomas are a feature of tuberculous granulomas, but tuberculosis-associated uveitis does not feature recurrent hyphemas. CMV and rubella virus have been associated with forms of hypertensive anterior uveitis, but they are not associated with the skin lesions described in this case.

34. **c.** Uveitic macular edema is a frequent complication of uveitis and may occur or persist even when inflammation seems otherwise controlled. The use of periocular or intravitreal corticosteroids is the most appropriate next step to resolve this patient's uveitic macular edema. The PeriOcular vs. INTravitreal Corticosteroids for Uveitic Macular Edema (POINT) trial demonstrated superior visual outcomes with intravitreal triamcinolone and intravitreal dexamethasone implant compared with sub-Tenon triamcinolone injection.

    Macular optical coherence tomography can help identify factors contributing to the macular edema, such as vitreomacular traction. Since there is no evidence of prominent vitreomacular traction in this case, a pars plana vitrectomy with membrane peeling is not indicated. Although macular edema can result in irreversible vision loss, an alkylating agent such as cyclophosphamide would be reserved for more aggressive, sight-threatening ocular inflammation. Similarly, pulses of IV methylprednisolone are more typically used to rapidly control acute, high-grade inflammation.

35. **a.** Chronic anterior uveitis (CAU) associated with JIA is an indolent, relatively asymptomatic anterior uveitis in children. After years of low-grade inflammation, these eyes may develop signs of chronic inflammation, which include band keratopathy, cataracts, and/or synechiae. Fibrinous anterior chamber reaction and hypopyon are characteristic of acute anterior uveitis, which is usually symptomatic. Although patients with JIA-associated CAU may have anterior vitreous cells, the vitreous is not the predominant site of inflammation and therefore vitritis is usually not present.
36. **b.** Band keratopathy results from the deposition of calcium hydroxyapatite at the level of the Bowman membrane. Aside from chronic inflammation associated with uveitis, other etiologies of calcific band keratopathy include systemic disorders that cause hypercalcemia or elevated serum phosphorus levels, as well as silicone oil (particularly in an aphakic eye), exposure to mercurial vapors or preservative, and primary hereditary band keratopathy.

Index

(*f*=figure; *t*=table)